SPACE, TIME AND NUMBER IN THE BRAIN

SEARCHING FOR THE FOUNDATIONS OF MATHEMATICAL THOUGHT

T0324184

SPACE, TIME AND NUMBER IN THE BRAIN

SEARCHING FOR THE FOUNDATIONS OF MATHEMATICAL THOUGHT

AN ATTENTION AND PERFORMANCE SERIES VOLUME

Edited by

STANISLAS DEHAENE AND ELIZABETH M. BRANNON

AMSTERDAM • BOSTON • HEIDELBERG • LONDON
NEW YORK • OXFORD • PARIS • SAN DIEGO
SAN FRANCISCO • SINGAPORE • SYDNEY • TOKYO
Academic Press is an imprint of Elsevier

Academic Press is an imprint of Elsevier
32 Jamestown Road, London NW1 7BY, UK
30 Corporate Drive, Suite 400, Burlington, MA 01803, USA
525 B Street, Suite 1800, San Diego, CA 92101-4495, USA

First edition 2011

Copyright © 2011 Elsevier Inc. All rights reserved

Except chapters 4, 6, 12, 13, 16 & 17 which are reprinted from Trends in Cognitive
Sciences with permission from Elsevier

No part of this publication may be reproduced, stored in a retrieval system or transmitted in
any form or by any means electronic, mechanical, photocopying, recording or otherwise without
the prior written permission of the publisher. Permissions may be sought directly from Elsevier's
Science & Technology Rights Department in Oxford, UK: phone (+44) (0) 1865 843830;
fax (+44) (0) 1865 853333; email: permissions@elsevier.com. Alternatively, visit the Science
and Technology Books website at www.elsevierdirect.com/rights for further information

Notice
No responsibility is assumed by the publisher for any injury and/or damage to persons
or property as a matter of products liability, negligence or otherwise, or from any use or
operation of any methods, products, instructions or ideas contained in the material herein.
Because of rapid advances in the medical sciences, in particular, independent verification of
diagnoses and drug dosages should be made

British Library Cataloguing-in-Publication Data
A catalogue record for this book is available from the British Library

Library of Congress Cataloging-in-Publication Data
A catalog record for this book is available from the Library of Congress

ISBN : 978-0-12-385948-8

For information on all Academic Press publications
visit our website at elsevierdirect.com

Typeset by MPS Limited, a Macmillan Company, Chennai, India
www.macmillansolutions.com

Printed in the United States of America
Transferred to Digital Printing, 2012

Working together to grow
libraries in developing countries

www.elsevier.com | www.bookaid.org | www.sabre.org

ELSEVIER   BOOK AID International   Sabre Foundation

Contents

Contributors

Marilena Aiello Dipartimento di Psicologia, Università degli Studi "La Sapienza", Roma, Italy & Fondazione Santa Lucia IRCCS, Roma, Italy

Paola Binda Istituto di Neuroscienze del CNR, Pisa, Italy & Italian Institute of Technology, Genova, Italy

Lera Boroditsky Psychology Department, Stanford University, Stanford, CA

Elizabeth M. Brannon Center for Cognitive Neuroscience, Duke University, Durham, NC

Claudio Brozzoli ImpAct, Centre des Neurosciences de Lyon, Institut National de la Santé et de la Recherche Médicale, Université Claude Bernard Lyon, Bron, France

Dean V. Buonomano Departments of Neurobiology and Psychology, UCLA, Los Angeles, CA

Christopher Burgess UCL Institute of Cognitive Neuroscience and UCL Institute of Neurology, University College London, UK

Neil Burgess UCL Institute of Cognitive Neuroscience and UCL Institute of Neurology, University College London, UK

David Burr Istituto di Neuroscienze del CNR, Pisa, Italy & Department of Psychology, Universitá Degli Studi di Firenze, Firenze, Italy

Brian Butterworth Institute of Cognitive Neuroscience & Department of Psychology, University College London, UK

Patrick Cavanagh Laboratoire Psychologie de la Perception, Université Paris Descartes, France

Nicky Clayton Department of Experimental Psychology, University of Cambridge, UK

Roi Cohen Kadosh Department of Experimental Psychology and Oxford Centre for Functional Magnetic Resonance Imaging of the Brain, University of Oxford, UK

Jennifer T. Coull Laboratoire de Neurobiologie de la Cognition, CNRS—Université de Provence, Marseille, France

Stanislas Dehaene Collège de France, Paris, France & INSERM, Cognitive Neuroimaging Unit, NeuroSpin center, Saclay, France

Dori Derdikman Department of Physiology, Faculty of Medicine, Technion, Haifa, Israel

Jean-Philippe van Dijck Department of Experimental Psychology, Ghent University, Belgium

Fabrizio Doricchi Dipartimento di Psicologia, Università degli Studi "La Sapienza", Roma, Italy & Fondazione Santa Lucia IRCCS, Roma, Italy

Lisa Feigenson Department of Psychological and Brain Sciences, Johns Hopkins University, Baltimore, MD

Wim Fias Department of Experimental Psychology, Ghent University, Belgium

C. R. Gallistel Department of Psychology and Rutgers Center for Cognitive Science, Rutgers University, New Brunswick, NJ

Limor Gertner Department of Psychology, and Zlotowski Center for Neuroscience, Ben-Gurion University of the Negev, Beer-Sheva, Israel

Wim Gevers Unité de Recherches en Neurosciences Cognitives, Université Libre de Bruxelles, Belgium

Daniel Haun Max Planck Institute for Evolutionary Anthropology, Leipzig, Germany, & Max Planck Institute for Psycholinguistics, Nijmegen, The Netherlands, & University of Portsmouth, UK

Sheng He Department of Psychology, University of Minnesota, Minneapolis, MN

Danielle Hinchey Department of Psychology, Harvard University, Cambridge, MA

Masami Ishihara Department of Health Promotion Sciences, Tokyo Metropolitan University, Japan

Véronique Izard Laboratoire Psychologie de la Perception, Université Paris Descartes, Paris, France & CNRS UMR 8158, Paris France & Department of Psychology, Harvard University, Cambridge, MA

Sophie Jacquin-Courtois ImpAct, Centre des Neurosciences de Lyon, Institut National de la Santé et de la Recherche Médicale, Université Claude Bernard Lyon, Bron, France, & Mouvement et Handicap, Hôpital Henry Gabrielle, Hospices Civils de Lyon, St Genis Laval, France

Fiona Jordan Max Planck Institute for Psycholinguistics, Nijmegen, The Netherlands

R. Laje Departments of Neurobiology and Psychology, UCLA, Los Angeles, CA, & Department of Science and Technology, University of Quilmes, Argentina

Matthew R. Longo Department of Psychological Sciences, Birbeck, University of London, UK

Stella F. Lourenco Department of Psychology, Emory University, Atlanta, GA

Dustin J. Merritt Center for Cognitive Neuroscience, Duke University, Duke University, Durham, NC

Concetta Morrone Department of Physiological Sciences, University of Pisa & Scientific Institute Stella Maris, Pisa, Italy

Edvard I. Moser Kavli Institute for Systems Neuroscience and the Centre for the Biology of Memory, Norwegian University of Science and Technology, Trondheim, Norway

Andreas Nieder Animal Physiology Institute of Neurobiology, University of Tübingen, Germany

Manuela Piazza INSERM, U562, Cognitive Neuroimaging Unit, CEA/SAC/DSV/DRM/Neurospin center, Gif-sur-Yvette, France, & Center for Mind/Brain Sciences and Dipartimento di Scienze della Cognizione e della Formazione University of Trento, Italy

Pierre Pica "Formal Structure of Language", CNRS and Université Paris 8, Paris, France

Geetha B. Ramani Department of Human Development, University of Maryland, College Park, MD

John Ross Department of Psychology University of Western Australia, Nedlands, Perth, Western Australia

Yves Rossetti ImpAct, Centre des Neurosciences de Lyon, Institut National de la Santé et de la Recherche Médicale, Université Claude Bernard Lyon, Bron, France, & Mouvement et Handicap, Hôpital Henry Gabrielle, Hospices Civils de Lyon, St Genis Laval, France

Nicolas W. Schuck Department of Psychology, Humboldt Universität zu Berlin, Germany

Robert S. Siegler Department of Psychology, Carnegie Mellon University, Pittsburgh, PA

Elizabeth S. Spelke Department of Psychology, Harvard University, Cambridge, MA

Giorgio Vallortigara Centre for Mind/Brain Sciences, University of Trento, Rovereto, Italy

Foreword

by Stanislas Dehaene and Elizabeth M. Brannon

The knowledge of first principles, as space, time, motion, number, is as sure as any of those which we get from reasoning. And reason must trust these intuitions of the heart, and must base on them every argument.

Blaise Pascal, Pensées
(translated by W. F. Trotter)

What do the representations of space, time and number have in common that justifies our dedicating an entire book to them? In his *Critique of Pure Reason*, Immanuel Kant famously argued that they provide *"a priori* intuitions" that precede and structure how we experience our environment. Indeed, these concepts are so basic to our understanding of the external world that we find it hard to imagine how any animal species could survive without possessing mechanisms for spatial navigation, temporal orienting (e.g., time-stamped memories), and elementary numerical computations (e.g., choosing the food patch with the largest expected return) [1]. In the course of their evolution, humans and many other animal species have internalized basic codes and operations isomorphic to the physical and arithmetic laws that govern the interaction of objects in the external world [2]. Indeed, there is now considerable evidence that space, time and number are part of the essential toolkit that adult humans share with infants and with many other nonhuman animals. One of the main purposes of the present book is therefore to review this work in detail. From grid cells to number neurons, the richness and variety of the mechanisms used by animals and humans, including infants, to represent the dimensions of space, time and number is bewildering and suggests evolutionary processes and neural mechanisms which may universally give rise to Kantian intuitions.

But a second issue motivates our present focus on the representations of space, time and number: they all raise deep computational issues for cognitive neuroscience. In all three domains, the nervous system must encode and compute with quantities. Behavioral evidence suggests that these computations can be remarkably accurate, even in miniature organisms such as desert ants or in immature systems such as the infant brain. Animal spatial navigation implies the mental storage of spatial coordinates and their updating through path integration [1]. Temporal decisions imply that memorized representations of time are subjected to operations analogous to addition, subtraction and comparison [3]. In the number domain, human infants as well as other animal species readily anticipate the outcome of analogs of arithmetic operations performed with concrete sets of objects [4]. Does this mean that a common set of coding and computation mechanisms underlies quantity manipulations in all three domains? Do these systems share similar brain circuitry? An exciting research program consists of mapping the range of the possible implementations of quantitative operations in the nervous system, and testing whether evolution has arrived at the same computational solutions in distinct organisms or for distinct domains.

The 24th Attention & Performance meeting on "Space, Time, and Number: Cerebral Foundations of Mathematical Intuitions", held from July 6 to 10, 2010, in Vaux de Cernay near Paris, was organized with this goal in mind: to clarify the fundamental points of convergence and divergence between the representations of number, space, and time. The present book is the outcome of this enterprise (six of its chapters also appeared in a special issue of *Trends in Cognitive Neuroscience* entitled "Space, Time and Number").

As the meeting unfolded, it became clear that, although remarkable progress had been made in mapping out the behavioral competence, brain areas and occasionally the single-cell mechanisms underlying specific spatial, temporal or numerical tasks, the domain as a whole remains unsystematically explored. A general research program lies ahead, which may aptly be termed a Kantian research project, since it aims to understand how basic intuitions arise, how they can be related to their neural mechanisms, which aspects of these mechanisms arise independent of experience, and which can be enriched by training and education. Rather than attempt to summarize the diversity of insights and discoveries that have been made in this field, and which can be found in the chapters of this book, our aim in this introduction is to highlight the range of questions that we believe should be part of this Kantian research program and which can indeed, be productively formulated in the light of present-day cognitive neuroscience methods.

QUANTITY CODES

How are quantities such as spatial coordinates, distances, times, durations or numbers encoded in the nervous system? Electrophysiology in animal models has uncovered mechanisms that include neurons tuned to specific values; neurons with monotonically increasing or decreasing firing as a function of quantity; neurons with periodical firing patterns, such as grid cells; and neurons with a rich diversity of dynamics capable of generating a unique, partially random collective code for any quantity. Do these mechanisms exhaust the range of possibilities? How do these mechanisms account for the many orders of magnitudes that can be simultaneously represented in the brain, for instance in the time domain? And can we extrapolate from animal models to the human neural code for space, time and number?

DEVELOPMENTAL ORIGINS

Are neural codes for space, time and number available early enough in development to play a determining role in structuring subsequent experience, as postulated by Kant? Or are they, on the contrary, extracted from exposure to a richly structured physical world through learning mechanisms? The hypothesis that "innate" mechanisms underlie spatial orientation mechanisms has received a major boost recently with the finding, by two independent groups, that several (but by no means all) aspects of the underlying neural machinery of head direction cells, grid cells and place cells are already in place in newly born rats prior to any significant navigation experience [5,6]. This research is stimulating innovative research focusing on the search for representations of space, time and number inherited from evolution. We must, however, acknowledge that the word "innate", meaning "independent of experience", is an idealization which will ultimately have to be replaced by detailed research into the underlying genetic and developmental mechanisms.

CROSS-DIMENSIONAL INTERACTIONS AND METAPHORS

Do the representations of space, time and number share neural resources? Or do they interact through systematic cross-dimensional mappings? Does a generalized sense of "magnitude" underlie them all, as recently suggested by the discovery that human infants spontaneously link the dimensions of size, numerosity and duration [7–9]? Or is a single dimension, for instance space, used as a reference for all the others, as is perhaps suggested by the observation that, in human languages, spatial terms are frequently used metaphorically to refer to time and number?

QUANTITATIVE COMPUTATIONS

What are the brain mechanisms by which basic arithmetic operations are implemented? At the very least, behavioral research indicates that operations of larger-smaller comparison, addition and subtraction must be available in all three domains of space, time and number. Multiplication and division are also frequently needed, for instance to compute speed (space divided by time) or rate of return (number divided by time). Are these operations always implemented by *ad hoc* evolved devices (e.g., neurons in the middle temporal area MT acting as motion filters; or in the lateral intraparietal are LIP performing "addition" of retinal position and eye gaze vectors)? Or is there a more general and shared brain machinery by which all quantities, regardless of their domain of origin, can be operated upon?

THOUGHT WITH OR WITHOUT SYMBOLS

Are quantity computations implemented by analog devices? Or do digital or symbolic coding devices exist even in nonhuman species? How do we move from approximate computations in animals to exact truth values in human mathematics? How is the neural code for number specifically changed in humans by the acquisition of cultural symbols such as Arabic numerals? Do symbolic computations "recycle" evolutionarily older mechanisms for non-symbolic quantity processing [10]?

HUMAN TURING MACHINE

In humans at least, quantities enter into sophisticated multi-step calculation and decision algorithms which can be likened to computer programs. Do these computations imply specifically human brain mechanisms that grant us the computational power of a Turing machine? Does the human brain contain dedicated mechanisms for the necessary operations of "routing" [11] (selecting one out of many input-output mappings), "chaining" [12] (re-using the output of a process as the input to another), "if-then" branching, or "for" and "while" loops? Can multi-step operations unfold automatically or are they necessarily under conscious control?

IMPACT OF CULTURE AND EDUCATION

Education to formal mathematical concepts can considerably enhance the human ability to reason about number, time and space. This is clearest in the case of number, where many concepts are traceable to a recent cultural invention (e.g. decimal numbers, zero, fractions, negative numbers). Is this the case for space and time too? Exactly what changes? Can the concept of "mathematical intuition", as put forward by many mathematicians such as Henri Poincaré and Jacques Hadamard, be traced back to pre-experiential Kantian representations already present in other animals, or can even our intuitions change as we acquire advanced mathematical knowledge?

None of the papers in this book solve these difficult problems. However, they all shed light on how they can be addressed empirically, with a combination of behavioral, neuro-imaging and neurophysiological methods in animals, preverbal infants, children and adults. The development of mathematical and simulation models of quantity processing in the nervous system is also progressing rapidly. We are therefore optimistic that the research program we have outlined will progress significantly in the next decade, and lead to important advances, not only at the conceptual level, but also in practical terms, illuminating the issue of how human education impacts on the brain and how brain sciences can inform educational practices. If Immanuel Kant or Blaise Pascal were born today, they would probably be cognitive neuroscientists!

ACKNOWLEDGMENTS

The 24th Attention & Performance meeting on "Space, Time, and Number: Cerebral Foundations of Mathematical Intuitions" was sponsored by Commissariat à l'Energie Atomique et aux Energies Alternatives (CEA), Ecole des Neurosciences de Paris (ENP), European Society for Cognitive Psychology (ESCOP), the Bettencourt-Schueller Foundation, the Fondation de France, the Hugot Foundation of the Collège de France, the IPSEN Foundation, Institut National de la Santé et de la Recherche Médicale (INSERM), the James D. McDonnell Foundation, National Institute of Child Health & Human Development (NICHD R13HD065378), the National Science Foundation (NSF award #0950686), and Ministère de l'Enseignement Supérieur et de la Recherche. We are extremely grateful to Laurence Labruna and Giovanna Santoro for their help in organizing the meeting. Our special thanks go to Susana Franck, for her indefatigable help in supervising all aspects of the meeting and of this book; and to Stavroula Kousta, whose informed and pertinent suggestions contributed dramatically towards the shape of the meeting and its publication both as a special issue of *Trends in Cognitive Science* and in this book.

References

[1] C.R. Gallistel, The Organization of Learning, MIT Press (1990).

[2] R.N. Shepard, Perceptual-cognitive universals as reflections of the world, Behav. Brain. Sci. 24 (2001) 581–601 (discussion 652–571).

[3] J. Gibbon, Scalar expectancy theory and Weber's law in animal timing, Psych. Rev. 84 (1977) 279–325.

[4] S. Dehaene, The Number Sense, second ed., Oxford University Press (2011).

[5] T.J. Wills, Development of the hippocampal cognitive map in preweanling rats, Science 328 (2010) 1573–1576.

[6] R.F. Langston, Development of the spatial representation system in the rat, Science 328 (2010) 1576–1580.

[7] S.F. Lourenco, M.R. Longo, General magnitude representation in human infants, Psychol. Sci. 21 (2010) 873–881.

[8] M. Srinivasan, S. Carey, The long and the short of it: on the nature and origin of functional overlap between representations of space and time, Cognition 116 (2010) 217–241.

[9] M.D. de Hevia, E. Spelke, Number-space mapping in human infants, Psychol. Sci. 21 (2010) 653–660.

[10] S. Dehaene, L. Cohen, Cultural Recycling of Cortical Maps, Neuron 56 (2007) 384–398.

[11] A. Zylberberg, The brain's router: a cortical network model of serial processing in the primate brain, PLoS Comput. Biol. 6 (2010) e1000765.

[12] J. Sackur, S. Dehaene, The cognitive architecture for chaining of two mental operations, Cognition 111 (2009) 187–211.

MENTAL MAGNITUDES AND THEIR TRANSFORMATIONS

Introduction, by Elizabeth M. Brannon

In *The descent of* man, Charles Darwin made an insightful and, at the time, highly provocative statement: "As man possesses the same senses as the lower animals, his fundamental intuitions must be the same." Since the cognitive revolution, students of the mind have been driven by the darwinian canon. Human cognitive mechanisms must have been shaped by evolution, and therefore they must follow universal principles of mental architecture. One of the principles that emerged is that at least some of our mental life reflects analog coding. For example, Roger Shepard's work has elegantly demonstrated that when we rotate objects in our mind we perform an operation that is a mental analog of an external rotation of the object in space. Moyer and Landauer's classic work on the distance and size effect in symbolic number comparison provides another example of analog coding: when we compare two numbers, even if they are displayed in symbolic form, for instance as Arabic numerals, the underlying comparison operation is performed on analog quantities, as attested by the fact that a subject's response time is dependent on the distance between the two values being compared. Indeed further research demonstrated that humans, like many other animals, possess sophisticated mechanisms for manipulating magnitudes, whether numerical, temporal or spatial.

Charles R. Gallistel's research career has pioneered the study of space, time and number and their corresponding mental magnitudes. It was therefore fitting that he deliver the keynote association address at the 24th Attention and Performance meeting on space, time, and number and that his chapter is the first in this book. Gallistel champions the notion that the ability to represent numbers as mental magnitudes that can be manipulated in arithmetic operations evolved throughout the animal kingdom and emerges early in human development. Like Shepard, Gallistel argues that these analog representations evolved because they capture important properties of the world. Gallistel emphasizes that discrete quantity (i.e. number) and continuous quantity (e.g., space and time) must be represented by a common mental currency to enable us to perform arithmetic operations across domains. Consider the calculation of the rate of return in a food patch, clearly an essential survival tool. We can make such calculations, Gallistel argues, because we represent time and number in a single currency. He proposes that the need for arithmetic likely shaped how we represent quantity and should constrain our search for the neurobiological underpinnings of quantity representation.

Lisa Feigenson explores the interface between working memory and quantification. She highlights the paradox that although quantification relies on working memory for keeping track of counted *vs* uncounted items, or for holding operands in memory during calculation, we are nonetheless able to estimate, enumerate, compare, and calculate with more than three items at a time. Feigenson outlines an elegant and plausible solution to this puzzle: our short-term store is hierarchically organized, so that not only objects, but also entire sets of objects and even ensembles can function as items in working memory.

Patrick Cavanaugh and **Sheng He** focus on one mechanism by which mental magnitudes are derived: counting. They explore the relationship between attention and counting and debunk the idea that eye movements are essential for counting. A set of elegantly simple experiments show that the counting process does not require eye movements but instead requires the ability to individuate and locate targets with covert attention. Their results suggest that prior studies which claimed that eye movements were essential for counting suffered from element crowding which prevented individuation. Cavanaugh and He demonstrate that when elements are sparsely spaced in a circle around fixation, eye movements become unnecessary for counting. Thus while Feigenson's work illustrates some of the flexibility of our calculating minds, Cavanaugh's work is a counterpoint illustrating that the counting process requires just the right environment to support its work.

The papers presented in this section give us a sense of the computational feats that the brain must accomplish when it constructs mental magnitudes and transforms them. As the works of both Roger Shepard and Charles R. Gallistel have emphasized, the mind is fundamentally constrained by the structure of the world in which it evolved in. While it took mathematicians thousands of years to define irrational numbers as an infinite series of rational numbers Gallistel argues that they were only discovering what the human and animal mind was already universally doing: representing all quantities with continuous internal magnitudes.

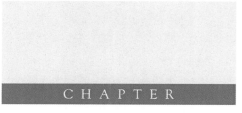

CHAPTER 1

Mental Magnitudes

C.R. Gallistel

Department of Psychology and Rutgers Center for Cognitive Science, Rutgers
University, New Brunswick, USA

Summary

Mental magnitudes are physically realized symbols in the brain. They refer to continuous
and discrete quantities an animal has experienced, and they enter into arithmetic processing. Arithmetic is special because of its extraordinary representational power. The processing
machinery is strongly constrained by both referential and computational considerations.

As is evident from the other chapters in this volume, the experimental study of the
mind's foundational abstractions has become an important part of cognitive science.
Prominent among those abstractions are space, time, number, rate and probability, which
have now been shown to play a fundamental role in the mentation of nonverbal animals
and preverbal humans [1–5]. The results have moved cognitive science in a rationalist direction. In an empiricist theory of mind, these concepts are somehow induced from primitive
sensory experience. Because language has often been thought to mediate the induction,
these abstractions were often supposed to be absent in the mentation of nonverbal or preverbal beings. In a rationalist epistemology, by contrast, these abstractions are foundational.
They make sensory experience possible. I suggest that the brain's ability to represent these
foundational abstractions depends on a still-more basic ability, the ability to store, retrieve
and arithmetically manipulate signed magnitudes [6]. If this is true, then the discovery of
the physical basis of this ability is a *sine qua non* for a well-founded cognitive neuroscience.

By magnitude I mean computable number, a magnitude that can be subjected to arithmetic manipulation in a physically realized system (see Box 1.1). I use 'magnitude' to avoid
confusions that arise from 'number'. 'Number' may denote the numerosity of a set, or it
may denote the symbols in a system of arithmetic, which may or may not refer to numerosities. The symbol '1' may denote the numerosity of a set, or the height in meters of a large
dog, or the multiplicative identity element in the system of arithmetic.

© 2011 Elsevier Inc. All rights reserved.

BOX 1.1

WHY ARITHMETIC IS SPECIAL

Eugene Wigner [20] called attention to "The unreasonable efficacy of mathematics in the natural sciences." Mathematics rests on arithmetic. Representations constructed on this simple foundation have proved surprisingly successful in representing the natural world. Based on ethnographic and psychological evidence, Fiske has argued that humans, at least, also use mental magnitudes to represent the social world [21]. Box 1.1 Fig. 1 reminds the reader of the ways in which magnitudes may be used to represent space, time, number,

probability, and rate. It uses the lengths of lines in place of number symbols, because length instantiates magnitude.

The representations shown are conventional and elementary. The brain's representations are likely more sophisticated, hence less transparent. See, for example, Chapter 5 in this volume. Nonetheless, they, like those portrayed here, must enable arithmetic processing to be brought to bear in behaviorally useful ways. What makes arithmetic special is its representational power.

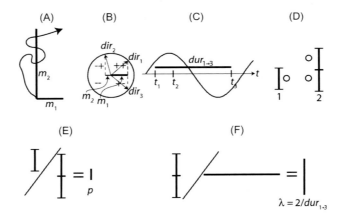

BOX 1.1 FIGURE 1   (A) The representation or location in two or three dimensions, as in dead reckoning while foraging (trace ending in location arrow), may be mediated by a vector composed of two or three magnitudes (m_1 & m_2). (B) The representation of direction, which is critical in dead reckoning, may be reduced to a magnitude proportional to the cosine of the direction angle and two signs. The signs code the quadrant. The magnitude codes direction within it: dir_1 is encoded by $\langle m_1,+,+ \rangle$, dir_2 by $\langle m_2,-,+ \rangle$ and dir_3 by $\langle m_1,+,- \rangle$. (C) Durations are represented by single magnitudes ($dur_{1\rightarrow3}$), which may be computed from differences in temporal locations (t_1,t_2,t_3): $dur_{1\rightarrow3} = t_3 - t_1$. Temporal locations may be represented by the phases of endogenous clocks, like the circadian clock [22], and phase may be represented in the same way as directions: $\langle m_1,+,+ \rangle$, $\langle m_2,-,+ \rangle$ and $\langle m_1,+,- \rangle$ could represent t_1,t_2,t_3 as readily as dir_1, dir_2, and dir_3. (D) Numerosity is also represented by analog-like magnitudes [23]. (E) Dividing magnitudes representing numerosity (discrete quantity) generates magnitudes representing probability and proportion (continuous quantities). (F) Dividing magnitudes representing numerosity by magnitudes representing duration yields magnitudes representing rates.

I begin with a short review of some of the behaviorally implied representations that would seem to be constructed from mental magnitudes, emphasizing the basic computational operations that appear to be performed on them. This leads me to consider the constraints this usage would impose on the system of mental magnitudes. One constraint is that mental magnitudes must cover a huge range. Logarithmic mappings from real-world magnitudes to mental magnitudes would be one way of accomplishing this, but such a mapping leads to computational problems. I suggest an alternative: autoscaling. I then argue that one constraint links a computational role to a referential role: the mental magnitude that functions as the multiplicative identity in the brain's computations must refer to numerosity one in the mapping from discrete quantity (numerosity) to mental magnitudes. I conclude that the properties of mental magnitudes are strongly constrained, not just by their reference, but also by the computational considerations. Awareness of these constraints can focus neurobiological inquiry.

COMPUTATIONAL IMPLICATIONS OF BEHAVIORAL RESULTS

The representation of space arises in its most basic form in the process of dead reckoning (aka path integration), which is the foundation of an animal's ability to find its way back whence it came and to construct a representation of the locations of landscapes and locations relative to a home base [2]. It requires summing successive displacements in a framework in which the coordinates of locations other than that of the animal do not change as the animal moves. By summing successive small displacements (small changes in its location), the animal maintains a representation of its location. This representation makes it possible to record locations of places and objects of interest as it encounters them, thereby constructing a cognitive map of the experienced environment. Computational considerations make it likely that this representation is Cartesian and allocentric. Polar and egocentric representations rapidly become inaccurate, because they integrate the step-by-step errors in the signals for the direction and distance of displacements in such a way that the inaccuracy of each step in the integration is increased by inaccuracies incorporated at earlier steps [2].

The representations of locations are vectors, ordered sets of magnitudes. A fundamental operation in navigation is computing courses—the range and bearing of a destination from the current location. If the vectors are Cartesian, the range and bearing are the modulus and angle of the difference between the destination vector and the current–location vector. This difference is the element-by-element differences between the two vectors. Thus, putting a representation of spatial location to use in navigational computations depends on the arithmetic processing of the magnitudes that constitute the vector.

The representation of time takes two forms: the representation of phase (location within one or more cycles) and the representation of temporal intervals. Nonverbal animals represent both [2], and they compute signed temporal differences: how long it will be, and how long it has been. A behavioral manifestation of the first computation (how long it will be) is the anticipation of time of feeding seen when animals are fed at regular times of day (for review, see [2]). A behavioral manifestation of the latter is the cache-revisiting behavior of scrub jays: their choice of which caches to visit first depends on their knowledge of how long it has been since they buried what where and on their acquired knowledge of the (experimenter-determined) rotting-times for the different foods they have cached [7].

It has been widely supposed that the representation of temporal intervals is generated by an interval-timing mechanism [8]. There is a conceptual problem with this hypothesis: the ability to record the first occurrence of an interesting temporal interval would seem to require the starting of an infinite number of timers for each of the very large number of experienced events that might turn out to be the start of something interesting. There is no knowing what may follow, so one would need to start a timer in anticipation of any eventuality, but the eventualities are infinite. Moreover, if one does not record the first occurrence of an interval, then every recurrence is effectively the first. Resolving this paradox seems to require the assumption that temporal intervals are derived from the representation of temporal locations, just as displacements (directed spatial intervals) are derived from differences in spatial locations. This, in turn, leads to arithmetic operations on temporal vectors (see [2] for details).

Rats represent rates (numbers of events divided by the durations of the intervals) and combine them multiplicatively with reward magnitudes [9]. Both mice and adult human subjects represent the uncertainty in their estimates of elapsing durations (a probability distribution defined over a continuous variable). They also represent the probabilities of short- and long-duration trials (the proportions between the numbers of trials of each kind and the total number of trials). They combine their representations of these two distributions, one continuous, one discrete, multiplicatively to estimate an optimal time for switching from the short option to the long option [1]. Human adult subjects generalize spontaneously from the proportion between two durations to the proportion between two integers [10]. These are but a few of the many experimental results that imply two important conclusions: (1) the analog magnitude system of mental magnitudes represents both discrete and continuous quantity; and (2) mental magnitudes enter into arithmetic processing that is closed under order, addition, multiplication, subtraction and division.

CONSTRAINTS ON MENTAL MAGNITUDES

Closure

Closure is an important constraint on the mechanisms that implement arithmetic processing in the brain. Closure means that there are no inputs that crash the machine. Closure under subtraction requires that magnitudes have sign (direction); otherwise, entering a subtrahend greater than the minuend would crash the subtraction machine; it would not be able to produce an output. Rats learn directed (signed) temporal differences; they distinguish between whether the reward comes before or after a signal, and they can sum one directed temporal difference with another of opposite sign [11]—see Box 1.2. When humans are asked to tap out the estimated sums or differences between two sequences of rapid arhythmic flashes, one on the right side of a screen and one on the left, their mean numbers of taps are proportional to the true sums and differences; and, the variability in their estimates increases in proportion to the magnitude of the operands [12]. Both the mean taps and the variability are smooth as the true differences approach and pass through 0, reversing their sign (hence, the key on which the subject taps). Thus, the mechanism that subtracts analog magnitudes does not appear to engage any special processing mechanism as differences pass through 0 and reverse their sign.

Closure under division requires that there be magnitudes that represent non-integer proportions, including proportions less than one. The magnitudes that represent probability

BOX 1.2

MENTAL MAGNITUDES HAVE SIGN

Experiment shows that nonverbal animals (pigeons and rats) subtract mental magnitudes representing both continuous and discrete time. In the time-left experiment [16], the subject is free to switch between two possible outcomes at any time up to some unpredictable moment of irrevocable commitment. Commitment to one outcome will necessitate waiting a fixed delay to food, say 20 s. Commitment to the other outcome necessitates waiting a delay that grows shorter in proportion as the pre-commitment time grows longer. The delay for this option starts out much longer, say 40 s, so it is a poor choice at first. However, as the trial goes on, it becomes a better choice at the point where the time-left is shorter than the standard delay associated with the other option. Pigeons and rats choose appropriately, switching from the standard option to the time-left option when the time-left becomes less than the standard delay. In the number-left experiment [24], the pigeon's pecks on a center key occasionally produce key flashes. After an unpredictable number of these flashes, the center key goes dark and two side keys light up. Pecking either one will again occasionally cause it to flash, and after some number of flashes, yield food. However, the number of flashes that must be produced on one key is fixed (at, say, four), while the number that must be produced on the other is a fixed large initial number, say eight, minus however many flashes were generated on the center key. Thus, on a trial where the center key had generated only two flashes, the fixed option would be preferable, but on a trial where it had generated six flashes, the number-left key would be preferable. Again, pigeons choose appropriately, and they do so on the basis of number not duration. If a rat is taught that noise onset follows light onset after 1 min and, separately, that shock precedes noise onset by 1 s, it is afraid of the light, but not of the noise, even though it has never experienced shock following light and it has experienced shock preceding noise [11]. The sequence in which the rat learns the positively signed (forward) interval and the negatively signed (backward) interval does not matter. In either case, the rat adds the two oppositely signed intervals to get the anticipated interval from light onset to shock onset.

These results and others like them imply that mental magnitudes have sign (binary direction, forward and back, left and right). That in turn implies an additive identity, the mental magnitude for 0, where the sign reverses.

(a continuous variable) may be generated by the division of magnitudes representing discrete numerosities.

Large Dynamic Range

Weber's law was experimentally established at the dawn of empirical psychology. It has traditionally been seen as a fact about sensory discrimination: the discriminability of two sensed magnitudes (e.g., two weights) is a function of their ratio. However, it turns out to apply just as much to the abstract magnitudes of number and duration [8,13]. This suggests that it is a fundamental aspect of the brain's machinery for representing magnitudes. What that implies about that machinery is, however, still not understood. Is it a feature or a bug?

One constraint on the encoding and arithmetic processing of magnitude is that the system functions over a very large range, because the distances and durations that must be encoded are like light and sound intensities in that they range over many orders of magnitude.

One widely advocated explanation of Weber's law is that the mapping from an objective magnitude to its subjective counterpart is logarithmic [14,15]. This could be seen as making Weber's law a feature rather than a bug, because a logarithmic mapping would enable a brain mechanism with a limited dynamic range to represent a much larger objective range. However, the logarithmic representation of objective magnitude makes valid computation problematic: Unless recourse is had to look-up tables, there is no way to implement addition and subtraction, because the addition and subtraction of logarithmic magnitudes corresponds to the multiplication and division of the quantities they refer to (see [16] for an experimental exploitation of this). Also, special processing at 0 is required because the logarithm goes to infinity as magnitude goes to 0. Finally, sign (direction) is a problem, because there is no (real-valued) logarithm of a negative magnitude. Logarithms have sign, but the negative logarithms represent the proportions between 0 and 1, so they cannot be used to represent negative magnitudes.

An alternative explanation is scalar variability: the noise or variability in the representation of magnitude is proportionate to the magnitude [8]. This would make Weber's law a bug, not a feature: mental variability (noise) is simply proportional to magnitude, as it often is for physical quantities. The problem with this suggestion is that it requires a dynamic range in the physical realization of the encoding for which it is hard to imagine a plausible mechanism.

There is a third explanation: autoscaling. Measuring instruments generally have limited dynamic range in their output. It seems likely that the brain's mechanism for representing magnitude is similarly limited. Measuring instruments nonetheless convey information about quantities over a large dynamic range by adjusting their sensitivity to the magnitude of the input signal: the stronger the signal becomes, the more they lower their sensitivity. Automatic scale adjustment makes the minimally representable difference proportional to signal strength, but it does not implement a logarithmic mapping from input to the output. At any scale factor, the mapping from input to output is scalar, which means that the full range of arithmetic operations may be validly carried out on this representation of the input.

The autoscaling explanation puts Weber's law in the feature category. The system is so designed that the amount of information in the representation of a magnitude is independent of the magnitude—a highly desirable design feature.

The autoscaling of sensitivity to stimulus strength has been shown to operate at the single neuron level, with an efficiency close to that imposed by physical considerations [17]. The spike train in a single axon of the fly's visual system conveys a linearly decodable encoding of the yaw waveform (the back and forth swings of the visual scene), while at the same time signaling the scale factor. The scale factor changes quickly as the fly passes from turbulent conditions, which produce large yaws, to calm conditions, which produce only small yaws.

The autoscaling hypothesis is that every mental magnitude is bipartite, like the representation of quantity in scientific notation: one part specifies where the magnitude falls within some range; the other specifies the range (scale). This will, of course, have implications for the machinery that performs arithmetic processing.

Combined Referential and Computational Constraints

The autoscaling explanation suggests that the mechanism(s) for encoding and processing experienced magnitudes have been shaped over evolutionary time by the role that the encoding plays in conveying information about quantities in the world. This imposes a two-fold constraint that enables us to say with unusual precision and explicitness how to recognize this encoding when one has found it in the machinery of the brain: (1) the physical realization of mental magnitudes in the brain must allow them to enter efficiently into the basic arithmetic operations [18]; (2) the mapping from quantities in the world to the mental magnitudes that represent them must be such as to make the results of arithmetic processing validly applicable to the represented world.

Attempts to identify the neural mechanisms mediating the brain's representation of the experienced world must address both aspects of an effective representation. Most neurobiological

---

BOX 1.3

THE SIGNAL PROCESSING SIGNATURE OF THE MULTIPLICATIVE IDENTITY ELEMENT

Identifying the physical mechanism of the mental magnitudes will go hand in hand with identifying the neurobiological machinery for the arithmetic processing of those magnitudes. That machinery must implement the basic arithmetic operations: addition, subtraction, multiplication, division, ordination and negation. In all but the last of these operations, the machinery must combine two inputs (two mental magnitudes) to produce an output that is itself a mental magnitude.

One mental magnitude, the multiplicative identity element, must have distinctive properties that make it easy to recognize, both by its behavior when input to the arithmetic processing machinery and by the mapping from numerosities to mental magnitudes. Its behavior is illustrated in Box 1.3 Fig. 1. The reasons why it must be the representative of numerosity one are explained in the text.

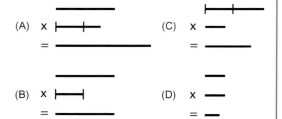

BOX 1.3 FIGURE 1 The behavior of the multiplicative identify element in the multiplication operation, the element whose magnitude is delimited by the two short vertical strokes. (A) Any two magnitudes greater than this produce a magnitude greater than both of them. (B) The product of the identity element and any other magnitude is the other magnitude. (C) The product of an element less than the identity element and an element greater than the identity element is intermediate between the two. (D) The product of two elements less than the identity is smaller than both.

BOX 1.4

UNANSWERED QUESTIONS

A pressing question, the answer to which is likely to have profound consequences for neuroscience, is the coding question: what is the enduring physical change that encodes experienced magnitudes (experienced numerosities, experienced durations, experienced distances, experienced relative frequencies, etc.), carrying this information forward in time in a computationally accessible form. It is very widely assumed that information is encoded in the nervous system in the form of altered synaptic conductances. However, there is almost no discussion of how altered synaptic conductances could code some particular piece of information, and there are reasons to be skeptical that "associative" changes in synaptic conductances are suitable for this purpose [25]. Focusing on how magnitudes may be enduringly encoded is likely to be fruitful for two reasons: first, it poses the question very sharply, to wit, "what is the physical change by which individual neurons or perhaps neuronal circuits encode a computable number?"; second, a mechanism that is capable of encoding a number is capable of encoding any kind of information whatsoever. Thus, answering this question may answer the question of how acquired information is stored in the nervous system, which is arguably the single most important question in behavioral neuroscience.

---

work focuses only on reference, but there is no point in establishing reference if the referring symbols cannot be processed so as to make valid inferences about that to which they refer.

The arithmetically necessary signal-combining properties of the multiplicative identity element (the neural symbol for 1) should make it easy to recognize (Box 1.3). Moreover, it must also be the mental representative of numerosity one, a foundational element in the system of discrete quantity [19]. The scale factors relating mental magnitudes to the quantities they represent cannot generally be specified *a priori*. However, the mapping from numerosity to mental magnitudes is constrained by analytic considerations: numerosity one must map to the multiplicative identity element or the mental books will not balance; the system will be inconsistent.

Suppose, for example, that numerosity one mapped to a magnitude that was not the multiplicative identity, e.g., a magnitude twice the multiplicative identity. This would establish the scale factor for the mapping from numerosity to mental magnitudes: numerosity two would map to a magnitude four times the multiplicative identity, numerosity three to magnitude six times as great, and so on. Consider the effect of two operations on the mental magnitude for numerosity one that ought to have equivalent consequences: adding one or doubling it. Adding one (2 + 2) will give the magnitude that represents numerosity two, but doubling it—multiplying the magnitude that represents numerosity one by the magnitude that represents numerosity two (2 × 4)—gives the magnitude that represents numerosity four. Therefore, for analytic reasons, the scale factor relating numerosity to mental magnitude must itself be one.

CONCLUSIONS

It seems likely that mental magnitudes, by which I mean the neural realization of computable numbers, are used to represent the foundational abstractions of space, time, number, rate, and probability. The growing evidence for the arithmetic processing of the magnitudes in these different domains, together with the 'unreasonable' efficacy of representations founded on arithmetic (see Box 1.1), suggests that there must be neural mechanisms that implement the arithmetic operations. Because the magnitudes in the different domains are interrelated—in, for example, the representation of rate (numerosity divided by duration) or spatial density (numerosity divided by area)—it seems plausible to assume that the same mechanism is used to process the magnitudes underlying the representation of space, time, and number. It should be possible to identify these neural mechanisms by their distinctive combinatorial signal processing, in combination with the analytic constraint that numerosity one be represented by the multiplicative identity symbol in the system of symbols for representing magnitude.

References

[1] F. Balci, D. Freestone, C.R. Gallistel, Risk assessment in man and mouse, Proc. Natl. Acad Sci. USA 106 (7) (2009) 2459–2463.

[2] C.R. Gallistel, The Organization of Learning, Bradford Books/MIT Press, Cambridge, MA, 1990. pp. 648.

[3] S.F. Lourenco, M.R. Longo, General magnitude representation in human infants, Psychol. Sci. 21 (6) (2010) 871–881.

[4] G. Vallortigara, L. Regolin, et al. Rudiments of mind: insights through the chick model on number and space cognition in animals, Comp. Cogn. Behav. Rev. (5) (2010) 78–79.

[5] F. Xu, V. Garcia, Intuitive statistics by 8-month-old infants, Proc. Natl. Acad Sci. USA 105 (13) (2008) 5012–5015.

[6] V. Walsh, A theory of magnitude: Common cortical metrics of time, space and quantity, Trends Cogn. Sci. 7 (11) (2003) 483–488.

[7] N. Clayton, N. Emery, A. Dickinson, The rationality of animal memory: complex caching strategies of western scrub jays, in: M. Nuuds, S. Hurley, (Eds.), Rational Animals? Oxford University Press, Oxford, 2006, pp. 197–216.

[8] J. Gibbon, Scalar expectancy theory and Weber's Law in animal timing, Psychol. Rev. 84 (1977) 279–335.

[9] M.I. Leon, Gallistel, Self-stimulating rats combine subjective reward magnitude and subjective reward rate multiplicatively, J. Exp. Psychol. Anim. Behav. Process. 24 (3) (1998) 265–277.

[10] F. Balci, C.R. Gallistel, Cross-domain transfer of quantitative discriminations: is it all a matter of proportion? Psychon. Bull. Rev. 13 (2006) 636–642.

[11] R.C. Barnet, R.P. Cole, R.R. Miller, Temporal integration in second-order conditioning and sensory preconditioning, Anim. Learn. Behav. 25 (2) (1997) 221–233.

[12] S. Cordes, et al. Nonverbal arithmetic in humans: light from noise, Percept. Psychophys. 69 (2007) 1185–1203.

[13] R.S. Moyer, T.K. Landauer, Time required for judgments of numerical inequality, Nature 215 (1967) 1519–1520.

[14] S. Dehaene, Verbal and nonverbal representations of numbers in the human brain, in: A.M. Galaburda, S.M. Kosslyn, et al. (Eds.), The Languages of the Brain, Harvard University Press, Cambridge, MA, 2002, pp. 179–190.

[15] G. Fechner, Elemente der Psychophysik, Breitkipf & Härtel, Leipzig, 1860.

[16] J. Gibbon, R.M. Church, Time left: linear versus logarithmic subjective time, J. Exp. Psychol. Anim. Behav. Process. 7 (2) (1981) 87–107.

[17] A.L. Fairhall, Efficiency and ambiguity in an adaptive neural code, Nature 412 (2001) 787–792.

[18] S. Dehaene, Arithmetic and the brain, Curr. Opin. Neurobiol. 14 (2) (2004) 218–224.

[19] A.M. Leslie, R. Gelman, C.R. Gallistel, The generative basis of natural number concepts, Trends Cogn. Sci. 12 (6) (2008) 213–218.

[20] E. Wigner, The unreasonable effectiveness of mathematics in the natural sciences, Commun. Pur. Appl. Math. 13 (1) (1960).

[21] A.P. Fiske, Four modes of constituting relationships: consubstantial assimilation; space, magnitude, time and force; concrete procedures; abstract symbolism, in: N. Haslam, (Ed.), Relational Models Theory: A Contemporary Overview, Earlbaum, Mahway, NJ, 2004, pp. 61–146.

[22] J.D. Crystal, Nonlinearities in sensitivity to time: implications for oscillator-based representations of interval circadian clocks, in: W.H. Meck, (Ed.), Functional and Neural Mechanisms of Interval Timing, CRC Press, New York, 2003, pp. 61–76.

[23] C.R. Gallistel, R. Gelman, Mathematical cognition, in: K. Holyoak, R. Morrison, (Eds.), Cambridge Handbook of Thinking and Reasoning, Cambridge University Press, New York, 2005, pp. 559–588.

[24] E.M. Brannon, Numerical subtraction in the pigeon: Evidence for a linear subjective number scale, Psychol. Sci. 12 (3) (2001) 238–243.

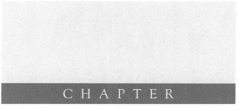

Objects, Sets, and Ensembles

Lisa Feigenson

**Department of Psychological and Brain Sciences,
Johns Hopkins University, Baltimore, USA**

Summary

Observers represent only a tiny fraction of the total amount of information available at any given moment. This small amount of information has been quantified: throughout the lifespan we typically maintain only three or four visual items in working memory at a time. Yet we are also capable of impressive quantificational feats: we can count the objects in arrays containing hundreds, or estimate that a scene contains "about 100" people. Given the strict limits on working memory, how do observers accomplish this? Here I propose that although working memory is limited in the number of items it can store, it is also flexible in what counts as an item. At least three types of representations can serve as an item in working memory: an individual object, a set, and an ensemble. Shifting between these types of representations allows us to bypass some of the strict constraints imposed by WM, thereby empowering quantification.

In order to perform everyday numerical computations like determining the more numerous of two quantities or dividing one number by another, we must make use of memory. For example, exact addition requires holding two numbers in memory, operating only on the immediately relevant digits (e.g., those in the ones column), then maintaining these representations while operating on the next digits (e.g., those in the tens column). Even simple counting requires memory: to achieve an exact count we must accurately remember which items we have already counted. The kind of memory required to support these quantitative computations, whether based on visual information (like seeing an array of objects) or verbal information (like reading a series of Arabic digits) (Box 2.1) must allow for rapid storage and immediate access to memoranda: exactly the functions provided by working memory (WM). Yet, a key signature of WM is the severe constraint on the amount of information it can maintain at any given time. Strikingly, observers of all ages appear able to concurrently represent three or four visual items in WM, but

© 2011 Elsevier Inc. All rights reserved.

BOX 2.1

A DISTINCTION BETWEEN VISUAL AND VERBAL WORKING MEMORY?

Scholars debate whether WM operates separately for visual *vs* verbal material. One view is that, regardless of whether information is presented in the form of a visual object or as a spoken, written, or signed word, these occupy a single shared store within memory [1]. The observation of similar capacity limits across varying kinds of stimuli [2], and the observation that maintenance of verbal material and visual material sometimes mutually interfere have been taken as evidence to support this view of a unitary WM.

Another view is that visual and verbal information occupy entirely independent stores within memory. The observation that memory span for visuo-spatially presented items predicts subjects' performance on standardized visuo-spatial tests but not their performance on the verbal Scholastic Aptitude Test (SAT), and that memory span for written items predicts subjects' SAT performance but not performance on standardized visuo-spatial tests, has been taken as evidence to support this dual-system view of WM [3].

A third proposal is that there are domain-specific visual and verbal stores in memory, but that the process of actively operating on these stored representations is constrained by a domain general resource. One way to conceive of this is that short-term memory (i.e. simply maintaining passive representations) is separable for visual *vs* verbal information, but that working memory (attending to and operating on stored representations) is unified. The locus of this shared domain general working memory resource has been suggested to be the sub-portion of memory that can be maintained in a highly activated state such that it is available for further processing [2], or as the central executive processes needed to coordinate attention to and processing of information stored in short-term memory [4,5].

---

no more [6–8]. Thus it seems that quantitative reasoning is constrained—and numerical actions like adding and counting are governed—by limits on the number of items that can be maintained in WM at any given time. This presents a puzzle for understanding how we think about quantities. How is it possible to estimate, enumerate, compare, or calculate using quantities that contain more than three items, if no more than three items can be held in WM at once?

Here I sketch one possible answer to this problem. I suggest that the hallmark capacity limitation of WM is accompanied by impressive representational flexibility. Only three or four items can be maintained in WM at once; but critically, different types of entities can function as items. These include *individual objects*, *sets* of objects, and *ensembles* (Fig. 2.1). All of these types of representations can be relevant to thinking about quantities, and each supports different kinds of quantity-relevant computations. By shifting between these types of representations [9], WM can offer the representational flexibility required for quantification. This framework for thinking about the role of WM in cognition applies throughout the lifespan, from infancy onward.

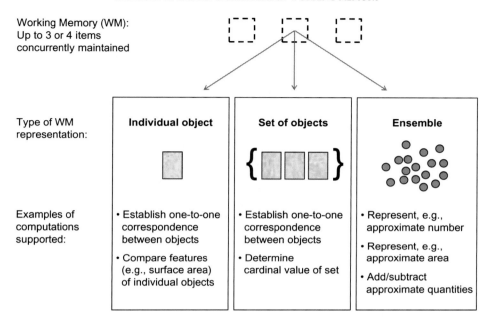

FIGURE 2.1   Schematic of object, set, and ensemble representations being maintained in WM. Up to three or four items can be concurrently maintained. At least three different types of representations can serve as an item. Each of these may enter into a variety of computations, including many that are relevant to numerical processing.

REPRESENTING INDIVIDUAL ITEMS IN WORKING MEMORY

"Individual object" is an important representational unit for attention and memory—we tend to reason about discrete objects, rather than parts of objects or clusters of features [7,10]. Studies suggest a strict limit on the number of individual object representations WM can maintain at any given time. For example, adults shown four or fewer objects easily detect a change to any one of the objects' features, but are much less likely to notice a change when shown more than four [7,11]. The same limit appears to constrain WM from early in development: infants between 10 and 20 months old can remember one, two, or three individual objects at a time, but no more than this [8,12,13]. In one task, infants watched a particular number of identical objects being hidden inside a box, then retrieved just a subset of them. Continued searching of the box indicated that infants remembered the total number of objects originally hidden. In this task, 12- to 20-month old infants searched correctly when three or fewer objects were hidden, but failed when more than four objects were hidden.

These studies and others show that adults and infants can maintain representations of up to three or four individual objects in WM. Although this limit has sometimes been taken to indicate the existence of a "small number system" [14–16], performance in the above tasks is not explicitly numerical in nature. Change detection tasks show that adults use WM representations of objects to notice when an object changes one of its features. The box task with infants shows that WM representations of objects allow infants to detect when an object is missing from an array. However, neither of these tasks requires representing an array's cardinality (i.e. neither task requires an explicit representation of number) [17]. Instead, adults and infants need only represent the individual objects initially seen, and then compare these to the subsequent array, for example, by establishing one-to-one correspondence between the arrays (in change detection: "I saw Object A, Object B; Object C, but now I see Object A, Object B; Object D;" in the box task: "I saw Object A, Object B; Object C, but now I see only Object A and Object B").

These abilities appear to rely on a WM system in which representations of up to three or four individual objects can be maintained. These WM representations of individual objects, while themselves not numerical in nature, are available to play a role in many numerical activities, including the establishment of one-to-one correspondence and the serial counting of small arrays.

REPRESENTING SETS OF ITEMS IN WORKING MEMORY

The strict limit on the number of individual items that can be concurrently maintained in WM might seem to preclude ever representing more than three items at once. What to do, then, when faced with a scene containing more than three or four objects? One way to overcome the three- to four-item limit of WM is to bind together representations of individual objects into representations of sets of objects. Binding multiple individuals into a single higher-order group can increase the number of individual items that can be remembered, as in the well-known demonstrations of chunking by adults. Such chunking can involve either recoding of the group into a new representation that can be stored in Long Term Memory (e.g., recoding the separate letters C–A–T into the word "cat," or recoding a series of digits into a single phone number) or binding without obvious recoding (e.g., representing Bob, Sue, and Mary as a unified set). Critically, in both of these cases, representing sets requires maintaining access to the individual components of the set. Remembering phone numbers would be of little use if one recalled only the number of sets (e.g., remembering that there was an area code, an exchange, and a final string of digits, without remembering the numbers comprising these) or a statistical description of the array (e.g., remembering only the mean of all of the digits comprising the phone number). Yet set-binding manages to evade the three-item limit of WM while still preserving access to individual representations of the sets' contents. This appears to rely on the hierarchical reorganization of items within memory.

Multiple types of information can serve as the basis for this memory reorganization [18,19]. Adults can use spatiotemporal information to bind together items in WM, as in the case of chunking phone numbers into three sets of digits (e.g., 410-516-7364). Adults also can use semantic knowledge to bind items. For example, the subject S.F. used his knowledge of race times to more efficiently remember randomly presented digits (e.g., S.F. chunked 3-4-9-2 as "three forty-nine point two, a near world-record mile time") [20].

Untrained infants have similar abilities. Infants who typically can remember only up to three hidden objects can remember more if given spatial or perceptual grouping cues [21,22]. For example, 14-month-old infants can remember four hidden objects if they are presented as two spatially separated sets of two, but not if they are presented as a single spatially unified set of four. And like adults, infants also can use semantic knowledge to group individual objects into sets. By 14 months infants simultaneously can remember two sets of two cats and two sets of two cars, but not a single set of four different cats or four different cars. Furthermore, besides representing two levels of information in memory (the individual object and the set of chunked objects), both adults and infants appear to construct more complex mental hierarchies. The adult subject S.F. remembered very large numbers of digits by creating elaborate tree structures; for example, he could parse a long digit string into multiple 1-mile running times, ¾-mile running times, or 10,000-meter running times. Within each of those superchunks, S.F. could then store multiple chunks, each of which contained several individual digits [23]. The ability to form superchunks based on spatial and conceptual cues also has been demonstrated in infants [24]. These results demonstrate how chunking empowers the representation of many more items in WM than could be represented individually.

Set representations play a critical role in many numerical processes, including representing the nested relationships between quantities (e.g., that a set of five contains a set of four, which contains a set of three,…), as well as representing the cardinality of an array (that "five" refers to a feature of a set, and not to any particular item within the set). Importantly, WM constrains set representations just as it constrains representations of individual objects [25]. For example, the number of individual items that can be bound into a set never seems to exceed the three- to four-item WM limit [22–25], and the number of chunks that can be bound into a superchunk appears to obey the same principle [23]. This suggests that each set, or chunk, functions much like a single individual object for WM.

REPRESENTING ENSEMBLES IN WORKING MEMORY

Many real-world scenes contain stimuli that do not lend themselves to representation *qua* individual objects or sets of objects. Imagine enumerating a flock containing dozens of individual birds. The number of birds vastly exceeds the number of individual objects that can be represented in WM, and it would be inefficient and perhaps impossible to attempt to serially enumerate the birds in hierarchically organized sets of three. Instead, observers are able to represent quantity information about the flock as a whole, though this information is only approximate. For example, adults can report that there are "about a hundred birds" in the scene. These approximate number representations have been observed in adults, infants, and nonhuman species [14]. In all of these populations, the noisiness of the number representation grows in direct proportion to the size of the stimulus, such that observers show more error when enumerating a flock of 100 birds than a flock of 50.

Approximate number representations are not generated by iteratively representing the individual items in the scene. With large enough arrays, adults and infants do not even detect the disappearance of an individual item [26,27], and adults are often at chance at reporting the features of an individual item from a large array [28–29]. However, observers can report various statistical features that are defined over the array as a whole, including but not limited to its approximate numerosity (Box 2.2). For this reason, representations of arrays in which the individual items are not represented are often called *ensemble representations.* The non-retention of the individual items in the array makes ensemble representations importantly different from object or set representations.

Ensemble representations can support many number-relevant computations, including ordinal judgments (deciding which ensemble contains more items) and approximate arithmetic (adding or subtracting the numerosities of two ensembles) [38–40]. Recent evidence shows that, like representations of individual objects and sets of objects, ensemble representations of approximate numerosity are also constrained by WM. Adults [32,41] and infants [42] can represent the approximate numerosity of up to three arrays at once. For example, when shown spatially intermixed arrays of red and yellow dots, both adults and infants can

---

BOX 2.2

FEATURES BOUND TO ENSEMBLE REPRESENTATIONS

Owing to limits on attention and memory, at any given moment most of the items occupying a visual scene are not individually represented. However, these items can be represented in a coarser way: by contributing to representations of ensembles. Ensemble representations do not offer information about their individual components [29], but instead can provide a statistical summary of portions of a scene. For example, take the simple visual scenes in Box 2.2 Fig. 1. Without storing information about the individual dots that comprise the arrays, observers can easily report that Array A has more dots than Array B [30–32].

Besides representing the approximate numerosity of an ensemble, observers also can represent other features. For example, adults can represent the average size of the items (e.g., recognizing that Array A has dots that are smaller on average than Array B) [29,33,34], the density of the ensemble (e.g., recognizing that Array A has higher density than Array B) [30], and the average spatial location of the ensemble (e.g., recognizing that the center of mass of Array A is shifted rightward relative to that of Array B) [28]. For more complex stimuli, observers also can represent socially relevant features like the average emotion or average

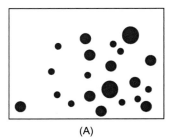 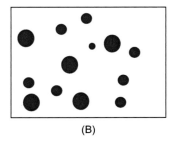

(A)   (B)

BOX 2.2 FIGURE 1   Two simple visual scenes.

BOX 2.2 *(cont'd)*

gender of an ensemble of faces [35]. And ensemble processing need not occur in a single glance: observers are able to represent statistical averages of the size or emotion of stimuli changing over time [34,36]. Finally, ensemble features also are represented by infants. By six months of age, infants respond to changes in both the approximate numerosity [27] and the cumulative surface area of an ensemble [37].

BOX 2.3

OUTSTANDING QUESTIONS

1. Can observers concurrently represent up to three non-numerical features of an ensemble (such as its spatial location, or duration of presentation), much as they can represent up to 3 approximate numerosities?

2. Do individual differences in Working Memory capacity predict individual differences in subjects' reasoning about number, space, and time?

3. Can an item simultaneously be construed at multiple different levels of representation (i.e. as an individual object, as a member of a set, and as a component of an ensemble)? Can WM simultaneously maintain representations of items across different levels (for example, allowing an observer concurrently to represent one individual object, one chunk, and one ensemble)?

4. To what extent is the type of representation that is stored in WM (individual object, set of objects, or ensemble) controlled by top-down *vs* bottom-up processes?

5. Does increasing the number of individual objects, sets of objects, or ensembles held in WM decrease the resolution of those representations?

6. The present framework for thinking about objects, sets, and ensembles draws on slot-based models of WM [2,7,43]. Can resource models of WM, in which capacity is constrained by the total amount of continuous information being stored rather than by the number of items being stored [44] also account for the parallel limits on memory for individual objects, sets, and ensembles?

---

represent the approximate number of red dots, the approximate number of yellow dots, and the approximate number of all of the dots in the array: three ensembles in total. However, neither adults nor infants simultaneously can enumerate more than three ensembles. The same limit is observed for ensembles that are presented sequentially as for ensembles that are presented simultaneously, suggesting that the limit originates in memory rather than in the number of ensembles that can be parsed from a single array using visual attention [41]. These results support the conclusion that, throughout the lifespan, an ensemble functions as an individual item within WM, and therefore that numerical approximation, which is based on ensemble representations, is constrained by limits on WM.

CONCLUSIONS

Thinking about number is one way in which humans use a finite representational system to reason about the infinite. We recognize that there is literally no end to the count list, and that there are infinitely many quantities that lie between any two integers. Yet the methods we use for performing everyday mathematical calculations reveal that the mental processes that underlie numerical thought are themselves far from infinite—they are surprisingly constrained. We often must resort to laborious methods or use external devices such as paper and pencil, abacus, or calculators in order to perform even simple numerical computations. One reason for this is that the number of items that can enter into numerical processing is limited by the strict capacity of WM. At the same time, reasoning about number is aided by WM's representational flexibility. Throughout the lifespan we are able to store in memory representations of at least three types of entities: *individual objects*, *sets* of objects, and *ensembles*. Each of these plays a critical role in numerical thought.

Beyond the domain of number, the constraints imposed by WM also may shape our thinking about non-numerical dimensions. Thinking about space and time also requires immediate access to items being maintained in memory. Furthermore, manipulating representations with spatial and temporal content (e.g., determining the shortest possible route in space or in time) is subject to memory constraints similar to those that limit thinking about quantities. We often jot down a sequence of directions for reaching a new location, or better remember the timing of appointments by marking them on a calendar. An open question is whether the framework offered here for thinking about how representational flexibility expands memory not only captures thinking about number, but also extends to thinking in other domains. Future research may ask whether capacity limits similar to those observed for numerical processing also shape the ways we think about space and time. For example, are we limited to representing up to three or four spatial locations or distances, or three or four temporal durations at once? Future work may also help to determine whether *object-*, *set-*, and *ensemble-* representations support reasoning about space and time, as they do for number. We can remember the spatial location of a single object, or the duration of a single event. Can we also represent the spatial locations or spatial extents of ensembles of many items? Can we hierarchically represent the duration of a series of nested events? Discovering the extent to which objects, sets, and ensembles are employed across varied content domains will help to determine whether these three types of representation instantiate a very general solution to the problem of storing information in a highly limited memory system.

References

[1] R.C. Atkinson, R.M. Shiffrin, Human memory: a proposed system and its control processes, in: K.W. Spence J.T. Spence (Eds.), The Psychology of Learning and Motivation, vol. 2, Academic Press, San Diego, CA, 1968, pp. 89–195.

[2] N. Cowan, The magical number 4 in short-term memory: a reconsideration of mental storage capacity, Behav. Brain Sci. 24 (2000) 87–185.

[3] P. Shah, A. Miyake, The separability of working memory resources for spatial thinking and language processing: an individual differences approach, J. Exp. Psychol. General 125 (1) (1996) 4–27.

[4] A. Baddeley, The episodic buffer: a new component of working memory? Trends Cogn. Sci. 4 (11) (2000) 417–423.

[5] M.J. Kane, D.Z. Hambrick, S.W. Tuholski, O. Wilhelm, T.W. Payne, R.W. Engle, The generality of working memory capacity: a latent-variable approach to verbal and visuospatial memory span and reasoning, J. Exp. Psychol. General 133 (2) (2004) 189–217.

[6] G.A. Alvarez, P. Cavanagh, The capacity of visual short-term memory is set both by visual information load and by number of objects, Psychol. Sci. 15 (2) (2004) 106–111.

[7] S.J. Luck, E.K. Vogel, The capacity of visual working memory for features and conjunctions, Nature 390 (1997) 279–281.

[8] L. Feigenson, S. Carey, Tracking individuals via object-files: evidence from infants' manual search, Dev. Sci. 6 (2003) 568–584.

[9] A. Treisman, How the deployment of attention determines what we see, Vis. Cogn. 14 (4) (2006) 411–443.

[10] B.J. Scholl, Objects and attention: the state of the art, Cognition 80 (2001) 1–46.

[11] G. Sperling, The information available in brief visual presentations, Psychol. Monogr. 74 (11) (1960) 1–29.

[12] D. Barner, D. Thalwitz, J. Wood, S. Carey On the relation between the acquisition of singular–plural morhposyntax and the conceptual distinction between one and more than one, Dev. Sci. 10 (3) (2007) 365–373.

[13] S. Ross-Sheehy, L.M. Oakes, S.J. Luck, The development of visual short-term memory capacity in infants, Child Dev. 74 (6) (2003) 1807–1822.

[14] L. Feigenson, et al. Core systems of number, Trends Cogn. Sci. 8 (7) (2004) 307–314.

[15] F. Xu, Numerosity discrimination in infants: evidence for two systems of representations, Cognition 89 (2003) B15–B25.

[16] S. Dehaene, Origins of mathematical intuitions: the case of arithmetic, Ann. NY Acad. Sci. 1156 (2009) 232–259.

[17] A.M. Leslie, et al. The generative basis of natural number concepts, Trends Cogn. Sci. 12 (6) (2008) 213–218.

[18] G.H. Bower, Perceptual groups as coding units in immediate memory, Psychon. Sci. 27 (1972) 217–219.

[19] G. Orban, et al. Bayesian learning of visual chunks by human observers, P. Natl. Acad. Sci. USA 105 (7) (2008) 2745–2750.

[20] K.A. Ericsson, W.G. Chase, S. Faloon, Acquisition of a memory skill, Science 208 (1980) 1181–1182.

[21] L. Feigenson, J. Halberda, Infants chunk object arrays into sets of individuals, Cognition 91 (2) (2004) 173–190.

[22] L Feigenson, J. Halberda, Conceptual knowledge increases infants' memory capacity, P. Natl. Acad. Sci. USA 105 (29) (2008) 9926–9930.

[23] W.G. Chase, K.A. Ericsson, Skilled memory, in: J.R. Anderson (Ed.), Cognitive Skills and their Acquisition, Erlbaum, Hillsdale, NJ, 1981.

[24] R. Rosenberg, L. Feigenson, Formation of memory superchunks by 14-month old infants, (in preparation).

[25] N. Cowan, Z. Chen, J.N. Rouder, Constant capacity in an immediate serial-recall task, Psychol. Sci. 15 (9) (2004) 634–640.

[26] H. Barth, N. Kanwisher, E. Spelke, The construction of large number representations in adults, Cognition 86 (2003) 201–221.

[27] F. Xu, E.S. Spelke, Large number discrimination in 6-month-old infants, Cognition 74 (1) (2000) B1–B11.

[28] G.A. Alvarez, A. Oliva, The representation of simple ensemble visual features outside the focus of attention, Psychol. Sci. 19 (4) (2008) 392–398.

[29] D. Ariely, Seeing sets: Representation by statistical properties, Psychol. Sci. 19 (4) (2001) 392–398.

[30] J. Ross, D.C. Burr, Vision senses number directly, J Vis. 10 (2) (2010) 1–8.

[31] D. Burr, J. Ross, A visual sense of number, Curr. Biol. 18 (2008) 425–428.

[32] J. Halberda, S.F. Sires, L. Feigenson, Multiple spatially overlapping sets can be enumerated in parallel, Psychol. Sci. 17 (7) (2006) 572–576.

[33] S.C. Chong, A. Treisman, Statistical processing: computing the average size in perceptual groups, Vision Res. 45 (7) (2005) 891–900.

[34] A.R. Albrecht, B.J. Scholl, Perceptually averaging in a continuous visual world: extracting statistical summary representations over time, Psychol. Sci. 21 (4) (2010) 560–567.

[35] J. Haberman, D. Whitney, Rapid extraction of mean emotion and gender from sets of faces, Curr. Biol. 17 (2007) R751–R753.

[36] J. Haberman, T. Harp, D. Whitney, Averaging facial expression over time, J. Vis. 9 (11) (2009) 1–13.

[37] S. Cordes, E.M. Brannon, The difficulties of representing continuous extent in infancy: using number is just easier, Child Dev. 79 (2) (2008) 476–489.

[38] H. Barth, et al. Abstract number and arithmetic in preschool children, P. Natl. Acad. Sci. USA 102 (2005) 14116–14121.

[39] P. Pica, C. Premer, V. Izard, S. Dehaene, Exact and approximate arithmetic in an Amazonian indigene group, Science 306 (2004) 499–503.

[40] K. McCrink, K. Wynn, Large number addition and subtraction by 9-month old infants, Psychol. Sci. 15 (2004) 776–781.

[41] L. Feigenson, Parallel non-verbal enumeration is constrained by a set-based limit, Cognition 107 (2008) 1–18.

[42] J.M. Zosh, L. Feigenson, A capacity–resolution tradeoff in infant working memory, J. Exp. Psychol. General (in press).

[43] J.N. Rouder, R.D. Morey, N. Cowan, C.E. Zwilling, C.C. Morey, M.S. Pratte, An assessment of fixed-capacity models of visual working memory, Proc. Natl. Acad. Sci 105 (16) (2008) 5975–5979.

[44] P.M. Bays, M. Husan, Dynamic shifts of limited working memory resources in human vision, Science 321 (5890) (2008) 851–854.

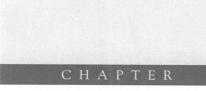

3

Attention Mechanisms for Counting in Stabilized and in Dynamic Displays

Patrick Cavanagh* Sheng He‡

*Laboratoire Psychologie de la Perception, Université Paris Descartes,
Paris, France
‡Department of Psychology, University of Minnesota, Minneapolis, USA

Summary

Numerous studies have claimed that eye movements are a critical or even obligatory part of explicit counting whereas here we will show that counting relies on a set of attention pointers that individuate targets of interest and specify their locations independently of eye movements. We demonstrate that explicit counting can proceed to very high numbers without error in afterimages where eye movements are not possible. Previous studies with afterimages had used displays too dense to allow individuation of items by attention: the displays suffered from crowding. We also show that explicit counting is defeated for displays of more than about six items in motion because there is no mechanism available to mark already-counted items and keep that marking linked to the items as they move. In this case, only the approximate number system can operate and, interestingly, this system shows fairly accurate estimates, rather than the underestimation typically seen for denser displays.

EXPLICIT COUNTING

How do we count the number of caps in Fig. 3.1? We could quickly make a rough estimate without much effort [1] or, if there were only a few, we could "apprehend" the number in a glance (subitizing [2]). However, if there are more than, say, four of them and we want to know the exact number, we have to count explicitly [3–6]. This explicit task has a number

© 2011 Elsevier Inc. All rights reserved.

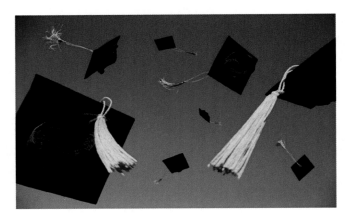

FIGURE 3.1   **Counting graduation caps.**

of components: 1. select an uncounted item; 2. increment the count; 3. mark the just counted item; and, 4. stop when there are no more uncounted items [7,8]. This task offers insights into how we represent the locations of the items, select them one at a time, and discriminate the uncounted from counted items. We study this task because we are interested in how a system of attention pointers [9] might underlie these selection and marking steps.

However, before we can address the attentional processes required by explicit counting, we must deal with an extensive literature that claims that attention cannot count—at least cannot count to more than four. This literature argues that, for more than four items, accurate visual counting relies on eye movements [3,10–12]. In addition to direct recording of eye movements during counting [11,13], experimental evidence supporting this counterintuitive notion comes from studies of counting in afterimages. Because afterimages move with the eyes, it is impossible to bring individual items or subsets of items to the fovea one after the other, eliminating any role for eye movements. The first such study showed that observers could accurately count no more than four items in an afterimage despite durations of up to 60 seconds [3]. This ought to have been enough time to scrutinize many more than four items individually by moving attention from one to the next. Similar results led Simon and Vaishnavi [10] to claim that counting of more than four items "requires the use of eye movements as an individuation mechanism if perfect accuracy is to be achieved" (p. 923).

It seems unlikely that a high-level task like counting would depend on the motor responses of eye movements as an obligatory operation. It is similar to claiming that we can only count using our fingers. But that has been the claim and the data have supported it. However, in our first experiment here we show that this claim does not hold up: accurate counting of sparsely arranged items can be achieved without eye movements up to quite high numbers. The original data was an artifact, as we will show, of the stimulus display.

If eye movements are not obligatory, the alternative is simply that attention can step through the items to be counted. Klahr [7], Ullman [8], Trick and Pylyshyn [6] and others have sketched simple procedures that would enumerate items, relying on the basic ability to index targets one at a time. This indexing operation is seen as the same operator as that used to track moving targets among distractors in the Multiple Object Tracking paradigm

BOX 3.1

ATTENTION POINTERS

Physiological, fMRI, and behavioral studies have shown that the spatial allocation of attention is controlled by a map (e.g., salience map [27]; map of locations [28]) that is also the oculomotor map for eye movement planning [29,30]. Although the cortical and subcortical areas that are involved have been studied initially as saccade control areas, the activations on these maps do more than just indicate or point at a target's location for purposes of programming a saccade. Each activation also indexes the location of that target's feature information on other similarly organized retinotopic maps throughout the brain (Fig. 3.2). Overall, the link between these attention/saccade maps and spatial attention is compelling, indicating that activations on these maps provide the core function of spatial attention. In particular, attentional benefits follow causally from the effects these activations have on other levels of the visual system. The definitive evidence is given by a series of outstanding microstimulation studies. When delivering electric current to cells in saccade control areas with a movement field, for example, in the lower right quadrant, a high stimulating current triggers a saccade to that location. However, a slightly weaker stimulation that does not trigger a saccade generates either enhanced neural response for cells with receptive fields at that location (stimulating the Frontal Eye Fields and recording from cells in area V4 [31]) or lowered visual thresholds for visual tests at that location (shown for stimulation of superior colliculus [32]). These findings indicate that the attentional indexing system is realized in the activity patterns of these saccade/attention maps and the effects of their downward projections. A target to be counted needs to be individuated by an "attention pointer" in these maps. Once a new target is actively indexed, the item count can be incremented and a new target must then be selected among items not yet counted.

[14,15]. Although Pylyshyn attributed this indexing to a pre-attentive operator (a FINST), others, ourselves included, demonstrate that this operation is really the central function of attention: selecting and keeping track of an item of interest [16]. Although more than one of these "attention pointers" (see Box 3.1 and Fig. 3.2) may be deployed at a time, we will focus on counting in displays where it proceeds one by one (as in Fig. 3.1). It is easy to extend the same processes to counting two or three at a time, although not much more, but this leads to the same conclusions as those that we present here.

We will argue that the major bottleneck in enumeration is in the attention system that individuates and localizes targets [9]. In particular, counting is limited by the coarseness of attentional resolution (see Box 3.2). If the display is arranged in a way that prevents the attention system from accessing individual items, then counting is severely compromised. The error of the earlier studies was exactly this point: placing the items too close to be individuated by attention. On the other hand, if the items are arranged in a way that allows the

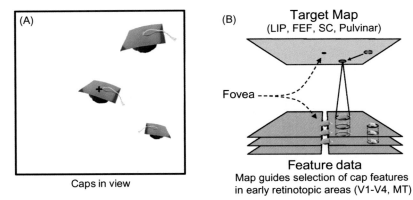

FIGURE 3.2 **Map of attention pointers.** A spatial map of attended locations directs the selection from early visual cortices (see Box 3.1). An attention pointer moves from one target to the next as one component of counting them. This map is not unlike Treisman's map of locations [28] except that it is attributed to specific anatomical structures: the sacacade control areas. Microstimulation in these areas has been shown to confer performance benefits (see [30] for a review) to corresponding retinotopic locations making these areas strong candidates for the core operations of spatial attention.

attention system to access each individual item, accurate counting can be achieved for many items without eye movements.

Our first study examines this indexing function, but counting involves both selecting the items and then, once counted, marking them as already processed. There are a number of strategies that could be considered for keeping track of already counted items. There might be a space-based strategy where counting progresses though the display from left to right, for example, always selecting the next item to the right. Or, there may be an object-based system of marking that tags counted items and where the tags stick to their items even if the items or the eyes move. Watson and Humphreys [17] claim that there are mobile markers that act to prevent the selection of a target for a second time and a similar claim is made for inhibition of return for moving items [18] or inhibitory tagging [19]. Pylyshyn [20] has demonstrated that there is indeed an inhibitory effect at the locations of moving distractors in the Multiple Object Tracking task and again this mobile inhibition might serve to mark processed items during counting. Our second study uses moving displays to test the claims of mobile object-based marking. However, we will find that explicit counting fails for moving displays. There does not appear to be any system that can tag already-processed items to prevent them from being counted again—other than attention pointers which can select and keep hold of items even as they move. However, these have a limit of about four and so are of no help for displays with more than four moving items. We conclude that explicit counting typically relies on a space-based marking of processed items.

Finally, we consider the evidence that for moving displays even subitizing is degraded. In these displays, with both explicit counting and subitizing disabled, only the approximate number system [1] remains and it makes surprising overestimates for small sets of moving items.

BOX 3.2

ATTENTIONAL RESOLUTION

An attentional focus (the downward projection from an attention pointer) selects a spatial region for processing benefits and engages surround suppression [33,34] to prevent nearby distractors from arriving at object recognition areas. However, if two objects are too close to be isolated in a single attentional selection region, the result is the loss of individuation of the two and an irretrievable mixing of both their features (Box 3.2 Fig. 1). This feature mixing and loss of access to individual items is the hallmark of crowding. We have proposed that the cause of crowding is this resolution limit of attention—the minimum possible size of the attentional selection region at a given eccentricity [15,35,36]. So when items are too close to be individuated—when they cannot be resolved by attention—they can no longer be counted either. This is easily noted in the linear arrays of Box 3.2 Fig. 2A when keeping your eye fixed at the central + sign. The first few items near fixation can be selected and counted but then next few seem inaccessible. Interestingly, the outermost item can be picked out, perhaps by a large selection region centered further out that only reaches in to the outer item.

Attentional resolution is finest at the fovea and coarser in the periphery, like visual resolution, but 10 times or so worse so that there are many textures where we can see the items, they are above visual resolution, but we cannot individuate or count them (as in Box 3.2 Fig. 2A). Our attentional resolution is so poor that if our visual resolution were that bad, we would be legally blind. In addition to being finer in the fovea, attention resolution is also better for items arrayed tangentially, around a circle

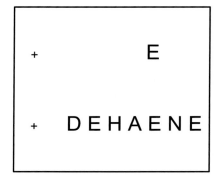

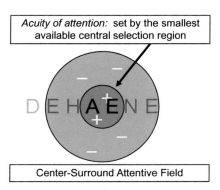

BOX 3.2 FIGURE 1 **Attentional resolution and crowding.** When fixating the + on the left, the "E" is easy to read on top, but hard on the bottom even though it is at the same eccentricity. This crowding effect has been attributed to the resolution of attention [35], the smallest selection region available at the eccentricity of the target (see Box 3.2). If more than one item is present in the selection region, they cannot be accessed individually, their features are mixed and it is no longer possible to tell how many there are [15].

BOX 3.2 *(cont'd)*

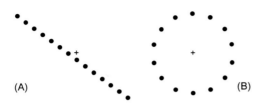

(A)   (B)

BOX 3.2 FIGURE 2 **Examples of linear and circular dot arrays.** While fixating on the + , try to move your attentional focus to select each dot in turn in A and then B, as you would if you were explicitly counting the dots. You may find this easier in B than in A, especially for the outer dots in A where the crowding effect becomes significant. Accurate counting without eye movements is possible for more items in configurations similar to B as compared to A.

centered at fixation, like a clock face, than radially, along lines passing through fixation [15,37]. This is part of the reason why the circular array in Box 3.2 Fig. 2B is easier to count than the linear array. The other reason is that the critical spacing at which crowding becomes significant is about ⅓ of the eccentricity [38] so the items around the circle can maintain a constant spacing, always greater than the critical spacing for their eccentricity. In the linear array, however, the fixed spacing between items will always at some point become closer than ⅓ their eccentricity. The linear, radial array guarantees crowding and failure of explicit counting when fixated in the center.

EXPERIMENT 1: WHAT IS THE LIMIT FOR EXPLICIT COUNTING IN AFTERIMAGES?

Many of the early studies on enumeration without eye movements were done with the stimuli arranged linearly, centered at the fovea like that in Box 3.2 Fig. 2a [3,10]. This leads to crowding of the outer items as the critical spacing for crowding is about ⅓ eccentricity and the fixed spacing of the previously used arrays will get too close quite rapidly. In this study, we again use an afterimage to stabilize the display on the retina, eliminating the effects of eye movements. We then demonstrate that with a circular arrangement counting in afterimages can be accurate for at least up to 16 items. This number is not the real upper limit of counting performance with afterimages as we did not explore arrays with more than 16 items. The performance is limited by the quality of afterimages, the duration they remain visible, but most importantly by attentional resolution itself (Box 3.2).

Methods

Observers

Four observers, three males and one female, aged between 21 and 34, participated in this experiment. All had normal or corrected to normal vision. Three of the four observers were naïve to the purpose of the experiment, one of the authors (SH) was the fourth observer.

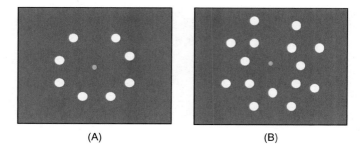

(A)   (B)

FIGURE 3.3 **Arrangements of bright discs used to generate afterimages.** (A) In the main experiment six to nine bright spots were used, placed around a circular ring with some jitter to avoid spacing cues. (B) In a second test, 14, 15, or 16 bright spots were arranged in two rings.

Apparatus and Stimuli

A large, thick, black cardboard screen was placed in front of a chin rest that could be switched between two positions to place the cardboard screen at 23 cm or 30 cm viewing distance. In the middle of the screen, an aperture was cut to expose a circular area (radius = 12.5 or 9.6 degrees, depending on the chin-rest position), where a ground glass diffuser was placed. Test cards were placed into a thin slot between the diffuser and the heavy black cardboard. The test cards were made of thin black cardboard with six, seven, eight, or nine holes punched in them using an ordinary paper hole puncher. The holes were arranged in a circular formation around the fixation. To make the configuration less regular, the spatial position of each hole was randomly perturbed from the imagined circle in a random direction (see Fig. 3.3A). This arrangement was used to prevent observers from making enumeration estimations based on regular inter-hole distances. To prevent possible familiarity from repeated exposures, four different cards were created for each number of holes yielding a total of 16 cards. The diffuser was illuminated very briefly (1 ms) by a camera flash unit (UNOMAT BC 32T) from behind so that the light was visible only through the holes, generating afterimages corresponding to the holes of the card. Figure 3.2 shows an example of the stimulus used.

Procedure

Observers were dark adapted for about 10 min before the start of the experiment. The experiment was run in a dark room. Test cards were randomly ordered and placed, one at a time, in the slot in front of the glass diffuser. When the observer was ready to begin a trial, he/she would place his/her chin on the chin rest, and fixate the small, photoluminescent dot in the center of the card. The discs on average were about 6 (or 8) degrees away from the fixation point when the chin rest was in the distant (or closer) position. After a verbal warning, the experimenter would trigger the camera flash. Following this exposure, observers were asked to count the number of discs in the resultant afterimage. To prolong their afterimage while they inspected it, they looked directly at a large, flickering uniform square that alternated between light (35 cd/m^2) and dark every 500 ms (1 Hz). Placing their afterimage on flickering background has been shown to significantly lengthen the visibility of the afterimage [21,22]. On average it usually took about 5 s for subjects to report the number of discs. There was a 2-min break before the next trial to allow the afterimage to dissipate. Each observer was tested on 16 trials, or four repetitions for each number of items. The position of the chin rest was changed between each trial (23 or 30 cm). This manipulation made the residual afterimage of the previous trial different both in size and in retinal position, hence minimized the possibility that any weak afterimage from the previous trial would be mistakenly counted in the present trial.

Results and Discussion

The results were clear. Three of the four subjects made no mistakes at all in any condition. The fourth subject made one mistake out of the 16 trials. In other words, in the combined performance of the four subjects (64 trials), only one mistake was made. The observers in our experiment could accurately count up to at least nine items when targets were presented as afterimages and eye movements were not a factor. This is twice the previously claimed limit.

Although the main purpose of this experiment was not to find the upper limit of counting without eye movements, all observers felt that they would be able to count more than nine discs. Consequently, we ran two of the four subjects (one author and one naïve subject) with 14, 15, and 16 discs. In this condition, the discs were arranged in two concentric rings (7 + 7, 7 + 8, or 8 + 8, see Fig. 3.3B). Each disc position was again randomly perturbed to avoid regularity. Each subject was tested four times for each condition. Together there were 24 trials, and both observers achieved 100% accuracy.

Although this experiment demonstrated that observers can count many items without eye movements when objects are presented as afterimages, the results were not entirely surprising to us. Earlier experiments have shown that the attention system is capable of indexing individual objects in visual space without eye movements [15,23] using only fixation instructions to control eye movements. Our current data support our belief that there is no fundamental difference between the fixating condition of our earlier attention experiments and the afterimage condition tested here. During the current experiment, observers had the sense of moving their focus of attention from one disc to the next, serving the purpose of indexing each item [6–8]. When the items were arranged in a way that minimized crowding, attentional indexing was not difficult for displays with many more items than the previously claimed limit of four [3].

Attentional resolution is not uniform across visual space being, like visual resolution, much finer in the fovea [15]. For this reason, eye movements are often required to bring fine details to the foveal area in dense displays in order for them to be selected and counted. However, we emphasize that the nature of these eye movements in facilitating counting is completely different from the claim of an obligatory role of eye movements in counting [10]. When all the display items are spaced so as to be resolvable without eye movements, counting can proceed based on movements of attention alone and the upper limit of counting performance is set by the resolution limits of attention. This attention limit is much coarser than the limits of visual resolution [15]. The scaling of attentional resolution with eccentricity predicts that the maximum number of individually accessible locations is in the range of 40 to 80 [15], an upper bound to counting which would require very long lasting afterimage or a stabilized but non-disappearing display to verify.

WHAT IS THE LIMIT FOR EXPLICIT COUNTING IN MOVING DISPLAYS?

Once an item in the display has been selected and counted, it needs to be marked so that it is not recounted. Certainly when counting using eye movements, the common experience is to use a space-based strategy, proceeding in an orderly fashion across the display, say, from left to right or from top to bottom so that the current location specifies the items remaining to be counted. In this way, counted items do not have to be actively marked as each item's status is given by the current position and the direction of progress across the display. Nevertheless, some authors propose object-based mechanisms where each previously attended item is marked "old" once attention moves away and this marking prevents attention from returning to the same location again. This object-based marking might be considered a purely local tag but Watson and Humphreys [17] claim that the mark can move with the object. Similar claims of mobile marking have been made for inhibition of return [18], inhibitory tagging [19], and distractor inhibition [20]. If this object-based tagging could really keep track of moving, already-processed items, explicit counting should be possible with arrays of moving items. If marking the already-counted items is purely space-based, however, it should fail with moving items and explicit counting should not be possible. Trick, Audet, and Dales [24] looked at counting in randomly changing displays and found that random motion did not preclude subitizing in the range of one to four items, whereas the motion did slow number discrimination above that range. In their study, however, subjects were unable to accurately discriminate numbers in the range from 6 to 9 even when they did not move and their accuracy did not get worse when the items were moving. So it remains to be seen if accurate enumeration is possible for moving displays under conditions where enumeration would be exact if the displays were static.

Methods

Observers

Ten observers, seven males and three females, aged between 24 and 45 participated in this experiment. All had normal or corrected to normal vision. The observers were naïve to the purpose of the experiment.

Apparatus and Stimuli

Between six and 18 high-contrast dots moved on a computer screen with a refresh rate of 60 Hz. The dots subtended about 0.5° and the screen 27.5° × 22.5°. Each dot followed a different circular path (7° radius), keeping all dots on the screen throughout the trial, with random centers, directions, and speeds (between 7.5° and 30° per second).

Procedure

After reading the task instruction, observers triggered each of 28 trials (four trials at each of seven numerosities: 6, 8, 10, 12, 14, 16, and 18) by clicking the computer mouse. The dots appeared in motion and continued for 10 s before disappearing. At the end of the trial subjects recorded their number judgment and clicked to proceed to the next trial.

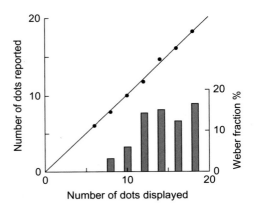

FIGURE 3.4 **Number estimation for moving dots.** With 10 observers, the average number estimated was quite close to the actual number. No errors were made in any of the 40 estimates for six items but for displays with more items, the Weber fraction of estimates steadily increased to about 15% of the number presented.

Results and Discussion

The results were straightforward (see Fig. 3.4). When the moving display had only six items, there were no errors. In this case, some subjects reported that they could track three of the items simultaneously and then rapidly "tell" that there were just three others. For more than six items, however, subjects' estimates became increasingly variable. They reported giving up on explicit counting and simply guessed. The estimates showed a Weber fraction that increased from eight to 12 items and then remained steady at about 15% (0.15, the mean absolute deviation divided by the mean estimate).

This experiment provided no evidence that there is any marking system that tags already-selected and counted items to prevent their recounting. We suggest that attentive tracking was able to individuate and facilitate groups of up to six and occasionally eight items by keeping track of three or four items and then quickly recognizing how many others there were in a glance. Beyond that number there was no obvious strategy that could track already-counted items and, as a consequence, counting depended on estimates. Note that unusually, the estimates here are quite accurate (although not precise). The mean reported number does not differ much from the actual number presented (slope = 1.07, intercept = −0.6, r^2 = 0.997). In contrast, numerical estimates are typically below the real value for randomly distributed static patterns [25].

CONCLUSIONS

We explored two components of explicit counting—selecting new items and marking old. The strategies used by our subjects draw on fundamental visual routines of spatial attention and help us understand the limits of these functions and how these limits constrain counting. We showed that eye movements are not obligatory for accurate counting

---

BOX 3.3

MOTION INDUCED OVERCOUNTING. MOTION DEFEATS SUBITIZING

In a recent paper, Afraz, Kiani, Varizi-Pashkam, and Esteky [26] report a breakdown of exact counting in displays with small numbers, three to six, of moving items. The items were equally spaced around a circular path and presented long enough for exact counting of these small numbers. Nevertheless, at higher rates of motion, the reports were reliably higher than the actual count, typically by one item even when there were only four items. Why would this happening?

We suggest two reasons. First, at the high speeds used by Afraz *et al.* [26], it is difficult or impossible to track more than a single item [39] making it hard to track a few targets and subitize the rest, a strategy we saw in our second experiment. Second, we suggest that in some conditions, rapid, accurate estimation like subitizing depends on perceiving the geometry of the dot array at a single glance [40]. Triangles and quadrilaterals can be recognized all-of-a-piece and the shape then defines the number without having to sequentially enumerate each vertex. We suggest that when a rigid dot array is rotating, the perception of its geometry breaks down and is no longer available to indicate the number of dots. Rather than triangles or squares, we just see dots moving along a circular motion path.

In the absence of the geometrical cue to number and the inability to track even three or four items at this speed, the only process available for enumerating is the approximate number system. These already-published data therefore suggest that the approximate number system overestimates for small numbers. This is an interesting observation as previously it has not been possible to evaluate the approximate number system for small number sets as other more accurate counting processes invariably intervene.

---

although, of course, they are useful for densely packed arrays of items where the extra resolution of central vision may be necessary. In our displays, accurate counting of up to 16 was possible in afterimages where eye movements are not possible. The actual limit with larger displays is undoubtedly much higher. The selection and individuation of items relies on a set of attention pointers [9] that are limited only by their spatial resolution. When inter-item spacing is closer than the size of the attentional selection regions, crowding prohibits access to individual items. We also found that there was no object-based marking operation that tagged items already attended and counted and that could then move if the objects were moving. Counting in moving displays even with long exposures cannot make use of a space-based strategy to keep track of counted items either. Judgments above six to eight items were likely based on guessing, calling on the approximate number system [1]. An earlier study [26] has shown that, at even higher speeds than we used in Experiment 2, exact counting is not even possible for small number sets (three to six). We argue that, at these speeds, the geometric cues to number are lost (see Box 3.3), so that even for small sets of items, only approximate judgments could be made. This is a range of numbers that has not been explored in adults with the approximate number system, and the results of Afraz *et al.* [26] show that judgments in this low range are overestimated as opposed to the classic underestimates seen for higher ranges.

Overall, the core component of explicit counting of items is the individuation of each item (or small groups of two or three) in turn, a process that is a central function of spatial attention (attention pointers [9]) matched with a space-based strategy for keeping track of counted items.

Acknowledgments

This work was supported by a Chaire d'Excellence and an NIH grant (EY09258) to P.C., by NSF grant BCS-0818588 to S.H. We thank Katherine Himes and James Intriligator for their invaluable contributions to the afterimage experiment.

References

[1] S. Dehaene, The Number Sense, Oxford University Press, New York, 1997.
[2] W. Jevons, The power of numerical discrimination, Nature 3 (1871) 281–282.
[3] J. Atkinson, F.W. Campbell, M.R. Francis, The Magic Number 4 ± 0: a new look at visual numerosity judgements, Perception 5 (3) (1976) 327–334.
[4] E.M. Jensen, E.P. Reese, T.W. Reese, The subitizing and counting of visually presented fields of dots, J. Psychol. 30 (1950) 363–392.
[5] E.L. Kaufman, M.W. Lord, T.W. Reese, J. Volkmann, The discrimination of visual number, Am. J. Psychol. 62 (1949) 498–525.
[6] L.M. Trick, Z.W. Pylyshyn, Why are small and large numbers enumerated differently? A limited-capacity preattentive stage in vision, Psychol. Rev. 101 (1) (1994) 80–102.
[7] D. Klahr, A production system for counting, subitizing, and adding, in: W.G. Chase (Ed.), Visual Information Processing, Academic Press, New York, 1973, pp. 527–546.
[8] S. Ullman, Visual routines, Cognition 18 (1–3) (1984) 97–159.
[9] P. Cavanagh, A. Hunt, A. Afraz, M. Rolfs, Visual stability based on remapping of attention pointers, Trends Cogn. Sci. 14 (2010) 147–153.
[10] T.J. Simon, S. Vaishnavi, Subitizing and counting depend on different attentional mechanisms: evidence from visual enumeration in afterimages, Percept. Psychophys. 58 (6) (1996) 915–926.
[11] X. Li, G.D. Logan, N.J. Zbrodoff, Where do we look when we count? The role of eye movements in enumeration. Atten, Percept. Psychophys. 72 (2) (2010) 409–426.
[12] J. Atkinson, M.R. Francis, F.W. Campbell, The dependence of the visual numerosity limit on orientation, colour, and grouping in the stimulus, Perception 5 (3) (1976) 335–342.
[13] M.P.V. Van Oeffelen, G. Peter, Enumeration of dots: an eye movement analysis, Mem. Cognit. 12 (6) (1984) 607–612.
[14] Z.W. Pylyshyn, R.W. Storm, Tracking multiple independent targets: evidence for a parallel tracking mechanism, Spat. Vis. 3 (1988) 179–197.
[15] J. Intriligator, P. Cavanagh, The spatial resolution of visual attention, Cognit. Psychol. 43 (2001) 171–216.
[16] P. Cavanagh, Attention-based motion perception, Science 257 (1992) 1563–1565.
[17] D.G. Watson, G.W. Humphreys, Visual marking of moving objects: a role for top-down feature-based inhibition in selection, J. Exp. Psychol. Hum. Percept. Perform. 24 (3) (1998) 946–962.
[18] S.P. Tipper, H. Jordan, B. Weaver, Scene-based and object-centered inhibition of return: evidence for dual orienting mechanisms, Percept. Psychophys. 61 (1999) 50–60.
[19] H. Ogawa, Y. Takeda, A. Yagi, Inhibitory tagging on randomly moving objects, Psychol. Sci. 13 (2002) 125–129.
[20] Z.W. Pylyshyn, Some puzzling findings in multiple object tracking (MOT): II. Inhibition of moving nontargets, Vis. cogn. 14 (2006) 175–198.

[21] S. Magnussen, T. Torjussen, Sustained visual afterimages, Vision Res. 14 (8) (1974) 743–744.

[22] B. Wallace, Prolongation of a visual afterimage with systematic alternation of room illumination, Bull. Psychon. Soc. 19 (6) (1982) 351–352.

[23] E. Kowler, R.M. Steinman, The role of small saccades in counting, Vision Res. 17 (1) (1977) 141–146.

[24] L.M. Trick, D. Audet, L. Dales, Age differences in enumerating things that move: implications for the development of multiple-object tracking, Mem. Cognit. 31 (8) (2003) 1229–1237.

[25] N. Ginsburg, Perceived numerosity, item arrangement, and expectancy, Am. J. Psychol. 91 (2) (1978) 267–273.

[26] S.R. Afraz, R. Kiani, M. Vaziri-Pashkam, H. Hossein Esteky, Motion-induced overestimation of the number of items in a display, Perception 33 (2004) 915–925.

[27] S. Treue, Visual attention: the where, what, how and why of saliency, Curr. Opin. Neurobiol. 13 (4) (2003) 428–432.

[28] A. Treisman, Features and objects: the fourteenth Bartlett memorial lecture, Q. J. Exp. Psychol. Section A 40 (1988) 201–237.

[29] G. Rizzolatti, L. Riggio, I. Dascola, C. Umiltá, Reorienting attention across the horizontal and vertical meridians: evidence in favor of a premotor theory of attention, Neuropsychologia 25 (1987) 31–40.

[30] E. Awh, K.M. Armstrong, T. Moore, Visual and oculomotor selection: links, causes and implications for spatial attention, Trends Cogn. Sci. 10 (2006) 124–130.

[31] T. Moore, K.M. Armstrong, Selective gating of visual signals by microstimulation of frontal cortex, Nature 421 (2003) 370–373.

[32] J.R. Muller, M.G. Philiastides, W.T. Newsome, Microstimulation of the superior colliculus focuses attention without moving the eyes, Proc. Natl. Acad. Sci. U. S. A. 102 (2005) 524–529.

[33] F. Cutzu, J.K. Tsotsos, The selective tuning model of attention: psychophysical evidence for a suppressive annulus around an attended item, Vision Res. 43 (2) (2003) 205–219.

[34] J.R. Mounts, Evidence for suppressive mechanisms in attentional selection: feature singletons produce inhibitory surrounds, Percept. Psychophys. 62 (2000) 969–983.

[35] S. He, P. Cavanagh, J. Intriligator, Attentional resolution and the locus of awareness, Nature 383 (1996) 334–338.

[36] P. Cavanagh, Attention routines and the architecture of selection, in: M. Posner, (Ed.), Cognitive Neuroscience of Attention, Guilford Press, New York, 2004, pp. 13–28.

[37] A. Toet, D.M. Levi, The two-dimensional shape of spatial interaction zones in the parafovea, Vision Res. 32 (7) (1992) 1349–1357.

[38] H. Bouma, Visual interference in the parafoveal recognition of initial and final letters of words, Vision Res. 13 (1973) 767–782.

[39] G.A. Alvarez, S.L. Franconeri, How many objects can you track? Evidence for a resource-limited attentive tracking mechanism, J. Vis. 7 (13) (2007) 1–10.

[40] G. Mandler, B.J. Shebo, Subitizing: an analysis of its component processes, J. Exp. Psychol. General 111 (1982) 1–22.

NEURAL CODES FOR SPACE, TIME AND NUMBER

Introduction, by Stanislas Dehaene

Although space, time and number are very abstract notions, they are well-defined from a mathematical point of view and, as noted by Randy Gallistel in the previous section, enter into formal operations that are easily captured by the standard laws of arithmetic. Thus, unlike other semantic domains such as the knowledge of animals, tools or actions, whose semantics are exceedingly hard to formalize, the domains of space, time and number offer a unique opportunity to study how, in a restricted semantic area, abstract conceptual notions are encoded and manipulated at the brain level. The question can be put very simply: how do populations of neurons encode a distance, a size, a location, a clock time, a duration, or a number? And how do these neural codes interact with each other to implement behaviorally relevant computations?

Historically, the first domain where a psycho-neural reduction of this kind was attempted was the sense of space. The discovery of place cells, and subsequent pioneering research led by John O'Keefe, Lynn Nadel and Bruce Naughton, among others, provided the first glimpse into the neural coding of spatial location. Historically the field was ripe for a neuronal exploration of space and this discovery was undoubtedly facilitated by the existence of numerous animal models of navigation behavior by Tolman and others which suggested that animals construct mental "maps" of their environment. In their chapter, **Dori Derdikman** and **Edvard I. Moser** concisely review the current state of affairs, concentrating solely on the hippocampus and neighboring areas of the entorhinal cortex and the pre- and parasubiculum. A panoply of space-sensitive neurons have been discovered, from head direction cells sensitive to where an animal is headed, to border cells reactive to the distance from a certain border in the environment, and finally to the remarkable grid cells in the entorhinal cortex whose firing periodically paves space according to a triangular metric. The authors suggest that these cells interact with each other multidirectionally to implement a highly flexible navigation system, capable of path integration but also of fast adjustments (remappings) in the face of environmental cues such as a sharp turn in a corridor. Thus, at the neural level, space appears to be fragmented into a manifold of maps, each coding the local spatial structure. Deredikman and Moser's novel proposal solves some problems and raises others. A positive side is that there is no need for the animal to maintain a constant, contradiction-free integrated coordinate system, which is computationally difficult in the twisted three-dimensional environment in which rodents typically live. However, it remains unclear how such a system provides the bearings between two distant locations, which are a prerequisite for many migrating or foraging animals—nor how it ever yields the highly integrated and formalized sense of Euclidean space experienced by humans.

The neural coding of time, which remains much more mysterious, is the subject of the next two chapters, by **Jennifer Coull** and by **Dean V. Buonomano** and **Rodrigo Laje**. Jennifer Coull uses functional magnetic resonance imaging (fMRI) in human subjects to map out the relevant areas of the cortex and underlying nuclei. She shows how the development of appropriate behavioral tasks is essential. With identical stimuli, participants may be asked to attend to duration, to develop expectancies of an event's onset, or to perform other temporal ordering tasks. Once these tasks are well separated, reproducible brain networks emerge: Supplementary Motor Area (SMA), right inferior frontal cortex and basal ganglia for duration judgment, parietal cortex for temporal order judgment, and left intraparietal sulcus for temporal expectation. All of these regions, several of which had been pioneered by other researchers such as Warren Meck and Richard Ivry, would thus appear to be potential candidates for finer-grained studies of how temporal parameters and processes are encoded at the single-cell level. Dean Buonamano and Rodrigo Laje review the various theoretical possibilities and the available data for how time might be encoded neuronally. In addition to the most obvious possibilities like neural oscillators, ramping units and delay lines, they introduce the interesting concept of a "population clock": the coding of time by the intrinsic, potentially chaotic dynamics of a recurrent network. The noisy and complex dynamics of neural networks, instead of being an obstacle, is harnessed and provides a simple mechanism by which a broad diversity of temporal basis functions, via simple learning mechanisms, can encode virtually any function of time.

Andreas Nieder then addresses the issue of the neural code for number. Interestingly, his work points to a brain network which overlaps with Jennifer Coull's timing system, inasmuch as it involves the intraparietal sulcus and the dorsolateral prefrontal cortex. Here, neurons can be recorded which are tuned to the particular number of objects that a monkey sees and attempts to remember. This remarkable observation is supplemented by Michael Platt, Elizabeth Brannon and Jamie Roitman's discovery of other neurons whose firing varies monotonically with the number of objects. Nieder describes an intermingled coding scheme, with some neurons specializing in concrete numerosities such as sets of objects, others in continuous quantities such as length, and others in symbols such as Arabic numerals. The latter finding, of course, is only found in monkeys trained to map these symbols onto the corresponding quantities. It is very exciting to see that the rudiments of a symbol-to-quantity mapping can begin to be explored at the single-neuron level in the macaque monkey.

Out of these pointillist studies, each focusing on a specific dimension of space, time or number, it remains hard to see whether overarching principles of neural coding or brain architecture for quantitative computation will ultimately emerge. Fortunately, this difficult issue is partially tackled in the final chapter by **Christopher Burgess, Nicolas Schuck** and **Neil Burgess**. Taking a resolutely theoretical stance, they show how many detailed properties of spatial grid cells can be explained by a process of integration based on membrane oscillations. Their model offers an elegant, if still tentative, solution to the problem of path integration—how do animals compute the integral of their motion vector in order to determine where they are at a given time? Furthermore, the proposed mechanism is so simple that it could exist in many if not all neurons, leading to the bold proposal that the computation of time integrals could be a basic computation for brain tissue. It might also account for some of the tuning properties of the number neurons studied by Andreas Nieder. Although the proposal remains highly speculative, and alternative models of grid cells have been presented by Ila Fiete and others, this model constitutes a first step towards the broader goal of identifying the neural mechanisms of general quantitative computations.

A Manifold of Spatial Maps in the Brain*

Dori Derdikman* and Edvard I. Moser†

*Department of Physiology, Faculty of Medicine, Technion, Haifa, Israel
†Kavli Institute for Systems Neuroscience and the Centre for the Biology
of Memory, Norwegian University of Science and Technology (NTNU),
Trondheim, Norway

Summary

Two neural systems are known to encode self-location in the brain: place cells in the hippocampus encode unique locations in unique environments, whereas grid cells, border cells and head-direction cells in the parahippocampal cortex provide a universal metric for mapping positions and directions in all environments. These systems have traditionally been studied in very simple environments; however, natural environments are compartmentalized, nested and variable in time. Recent studies indicate that hippocampal and entorhinal spatial maps reflect this complexity. The maps fragment into interconnected, rapidly changing and tightly coordinated submaps. Plurality, fast dynamics and dynamic grouping are optimal for a brain system thought to exploit large pools of stored information to guide behavior on a second-by-second time frame in the animal's natural habitat.

SPATIAL MAPS IN THE BRAIN

More than 60 years ago, Tolman proposed that animals form internal cognitive maps of their spatial environment [1]. Cognitive maps were thought to represent a mental knowledge base in which information is stored according to its relationship to locations in the

*Reprinted from Trends in Cognitive Sciences, Vol 14, Dori Derdikman, Edvard Moser, A manifold of spatial maps in the brain, pg 561–569, 2010, with permission from Elsevier.

environment. Following the discovery of place cells two decades later [2–4], O'Keefe and Nadel hypothesized that the location of the Tolmanian cognitive map of space was in the hippocampus [3]. They proposed that hippocampal cells represent the animal's location in an internal map of the local environment, with entity and event information linked to locations in the map, similar to Tolman's model. The view that animals form internal maps of the spatial environment continues to be supported; however, new research indicates that space is represented in several brain systems, each hosting a variety of representations involving functionally specialized cell types. These systems span wide regions of cortex, including not only the hippocampus but also the adjacent entorhinal cortex [5], pre- and parasubiculum [6], retrosplenial cortex [7,8], parietal cortex [9,10], frontal cortex [10,11] and other areas. The aim of the present review is to highlight how recent experimental work in the hippocampus and entorhinal cortex of the rat brain is revising and refining the concept of spatial maps. We will show that space is represented in these structures by a manifold of rapidly interacting maps generated in conjunction by functionally specific cell types such as place cells and grid cells.

HIPPOCAMPAL MAPS

Place cells are hippocampal pyramidal cells that fire when the animal is at specific positions in the environment (Fig. 4.1A; Box 4.1). Place cells are active both in light and dark, suggesting that a single modality such as vision is not responsible for their positional firing [12]. Different place cells fire at different positions; there is no apparent topography among their firing fields [13,14]. The brain can read out the activity of a local population of place cells to determine the position of the rat in the box. In experiments where activity is recorded from a large number of cells, the position of the rat can be reconstructed with considerable

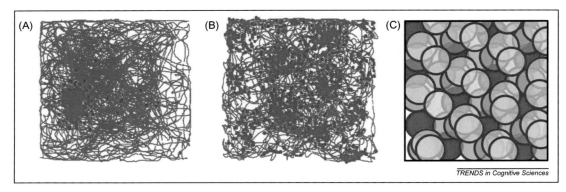

TRENDS in Cognitive Sciences

FIGURE 4.1   Place cells and grid cells form maps of the environment. (A) Example of a place cell in an open-field box. The trajectory of a rat is marked by a gray line and the positions where the cell fires are marked with a red dot. Most of the spikes of the cell occur when the rat is at a specific position inside the box. (B) Example of a grid cell in an open-field box. Positions of firing of grid cell are marked in red. The positions of firing form a hexagonal grid. (C) The population of grid cells forms a map of the environment. Firing vertices of different grid cells are marked with different colored circles. A specific position can be read out by determining what combination of grid cells fired at that position.

BOX 4.1

ANATOMY OF THE HIPPOCAMPAL FORMATION

We present here a simplified sketch of the connections between the neocortex, the parahippocampal regions (PHR) and the hippocampal formation (HF) (Box 4.1 Fig. 1). For a more comprehensive and detailed description see Witter and Amaral [88]. The neocortex is connected to the hippocampus mainly via two pathways through the para-hippocampal cortex. One projects through the perirhinal cortex (PER) and the lateral entorhinal cortex (LEC); the other projects through the postrhinal cortex (POR) and the MEC. Cells that carry information about the position of the animal, such as grid cells, head-direction cells, and border cells, are found in MEC but not in LEC [30]. MEC and LEC project to the same regions in the hippocampus, both via direct projections

to each hippocampal subfield and via the indirect trisynaptic circuit through dentate gyrus and CA3. While axons from MEC and LEC to dentate gyrus and CA3 tend to target the same cells, connections to CA1 are split, such that MEC is linked preferentially to the proximal part of CA1, and LEC preferentially to the distal part. This differential connectivity leads to stronger spatial modulation in proximal than distal CA1 [89]. The arrow from CA3 to itself stresses the abundance of recurrent connections within area CA3. Signals are routed back from CA1 to the entorhinal cortex either via direct projections, or via the subiculum (Sub), the presubiculum or the parasubiculum (not shown in Box 4.1 Fig. 1).

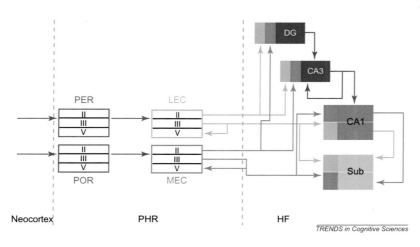

BOX 4.1 FIGURE 1   Major anatomical connections in the HF and PHR.
Reproduced with permission from [90].

BOX 4.2

DEVELOPMENT OF SPATIAL MAPS

Questions about whether spatial representations are innate or rather experience-dependent have a long history, dating back to the Greek philosophers, the British empiricists and Immanuel Kant. Two recent studies have addressed these old questions at the cellular level by asking if rudiments of the brain's spatial representation system are present at the time when rat pups make their first navigational movements at approximately 2.5 weeks of age [15,16]. The pups were implanted with tetrodes on P13, before the eyelids unsealed, and recordings were made a few days later when the animals explored an environment outside the nest for the first few times. Both studies show that a rudimentary brain map of space is present from the first day of outbound movement.

The most rapidly developing component of the brain map is the directional representation in the pre- and parasubiculum. Strong directional tuning was apparent already at P15 and P16 when activity was recorded from these regions for the first time (Box 4.2 Fig. 1A). The proportion of direction-tuned cells was similar to that of adult rats, and the degree of directional tuning was not different. Young animals exploring an open space for the first time also had place cells. The number of place cells in CA1 was only slightly lower at P16–P18 than at older ages, although the

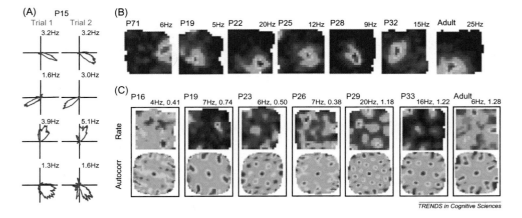

BOX 4.2 FIGURE 1   Rudiments of head-direction cells, place cells and grid cells in rat pups. (A) Strong directional tuning of presubiculum cells on P15. Traces show firing rate as a function of head direction on consecutive trials. Peak firing rate is indicated. (B) Firing fields of CA1 place cells between P17 and P35. Rate maps are color coded from blue to red; postnatal day and maximal rate are indicated. (C) Firing fields of entorhinal grid cells from P16 to P34 (top: rate maps, as in (B); bottom: spatial autocorrelations, color scale from blue ($r = -1$) to red ($r = +1$). Postnatal day, maximal rate and grid scores [15] are indicated. Adapted from [15].

BOX 4.2 *(cont'd)*

spatial tuning and stability of the cells continued to show some development (Box 4.2 Fig. 1B). Finally, young rats also had rudiments of grid cells. The number of grid cells was lower at P16–P19 than in older rats and the periodic structure of the grid fields was weaker than in the adults [15,16]. The number of grid cells, and their spatial periodicity, reached adult levels during the first week or two after the onset of navigation (Box 4.2 Fig. 1C). Therefore it seems that a rudimentary map of cells with directional and spatial firing correlates is present when animals navigate the outside world for the first time.

Although head-direction cells, place cells and grid cells show slightly different developmental profiles, these cells, or their predecessors, might interact from the outset.

The adult-like representation of direction in pre- and parasubiculum in the youngest animals could guide the development of spatial representations in entorhinal cortex and hippocampus, and rudimentary grid cells in entorhinal cortex might provide sufficiently patterned input to the hippocampus to generate place-specific responses in the hippocampal areas. It could also be that in young pups place cells are constructed by a larger proportion of head-direction cells and border cells, and that the contribution of grid cells to the construction of place cells grows with age. The evolution of functional intrinsic connections in MEC during the fourth week [15] could be an essential component for the generation of a combined entorhinal–hippocampal representation of space.

accuracy [13], indicating that the population of place cells forms a spatial map of the environment. This map could be innate, as is suggested by the fact that place cells are present as early as postnatal day 15 (P15) soon after young rats (pups) open their eyes [15,16] (Box 4.2). The same population of place cells can encode or retrieve different maps in different environments or different configurations of the same environment [17–19]. The process of switching to a different map is called remapping (Box 4.3) [17]. Place cells do not convey only spatial information. For example, place cells can be shown to encode conjunctions between spatial and olfactory information when this is relevant for the task [20–24]. When rats are rewarded in an odor discrimination task, in which they need to recognize odors that do not match a previously presented one, hippocampal neurons can encode not only position but also odor and training rule [20–22,24]. In some situations, the cells encode time intervals rather than positions, such as when the animal is using time to guide its behavior [22,25]. These examples suggest that place cells can link place to a variety of features in the environment. The capacity to associate locations with particular experiences could be useful for episodic memory encoding in the hippocampus [19,26–29].

ENTORHINAL MAPS

The brain contains another class of position-selective neurons: grid cells. These cells were recently discovered in the medial entorhinal cortex (MEC) [30,31] (Box 4.1) but are abundant

BOX 4.3

REMAPPING

Changes in the environment cause consistent changes in spatial maps in the hippocampus and the entorhinal cortex. These transformations are referred to as remapping [18].

Three main types of transformations can be considered:

1. **Place cell deformations**: squeezing or stretching the environment can cause a

systematic move of the position of the place fields relative to the surrounding boundaries (Box 4.3 Fig. 1A). Such deformation was reported in 2-D boxes [50] but also along linear tracks [65]. In situations where place cells undergo spatial deformation, grid cells deform too [91].

2. **Rate remapping**: in some cases, environmental transformations cause a

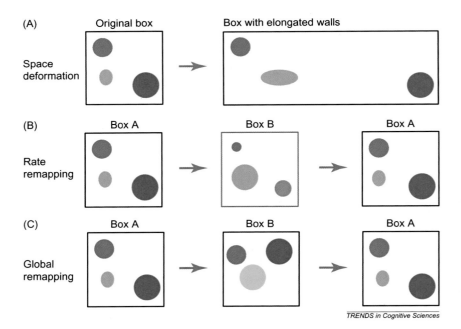

TRENDS in Cognitive Sciences

BOX 4.3 FIGURE 1   Transformation of place cell maps. (A) Illustration of a place cell deformation. When the box is elongated, different cells change their firing position to correspond to the deformation of the box. For example, the blue cell anchors its firing field to the left wall, the red cell anchors to the right wall, and the green cell elongates itself. (B) Illustration of rate remapping. The different cells in Box A continue to fire at a different firing rate in Box B but at similar positions. When returning to Box A the rates return to the original values. (C) Illustration of global remapping. Some cells fire in one room and not in another; other cells change the position of firing from one room to another in an unpredictable way.

BOX 4.3 *(cont'd)*

dramatic change in the distribution of firing rates among place cells without an accompanying change in firing positions (Box 4.3 Fig. 1B). An example of a manipulation of the environment that induces rate remapping is to change the wall color of the box the rat is in from black to white [92]. When place cells undergo rate remapping, simultaneously recorded grid cells do not change their firing in a consistent way [68].

3. **Global (place) remapping**: in some cases, environmental changes can change the position of the place fields in an unpredictable way. For example, when the rat is walking in a box in one room (room A) and then in a similar box in another room (room B), the positions and firing rates of the different place cells are apparently unrelated [93,94] (Box 4.3 Fig. 1C). Global remapping might also occur in the same location when the geometry or other salient properties of the environment change radically [18,68]. When place cells undergo global remapping, the firing vertices of grid cells undergo changes such as shifts in grid phase, grid orientation or grid scale [68]. Place cells do not preserve distance information during global remapping whereas grid cells do; that is, two place cells which had adjacent place fields in one environment might have very distant place fields in a second environment, whereas two grids with similar spacing will shift together such that the spatial phase relationships between the grid fields are conserved [30,68].

also in the presubiculum and the parasubiculum [6]. Grid cells are characterized by multiple firing locations that, in an open-field arena, collectively form a hexagonal grid over the entire space available to the animal (Fig. 4.1B). Grid cells can differ from each other in their grid spacing, grid phase and grid orientation [30,31]. It is known that the spacing of grid cells increases along the dorsal–ventral axis of the entorhinal cortex [30–32]. Similar to place cells, grid cells can be used to reconstruct the position of the rat in the environment [31] and so function as a map of the animal's position (Fig. 4.1C).

The same parahippocampal brain regions that accommodate grid cells [6] also contain two additional types of cells of potential relevance for spatial mapping: head-direction cells and border cells. Head-direction cells are cells that respond only when the animal is facing a specific azimuth [33,34]; different head-direction cells are tuned to different allocentric orientations. All directions are represented equally in the cell population. Head-direction cells were discovered in the presubiculum [33,34] but were later found also in MEC [35], as well as in several other brain regions [6,36,37]. Border cells respond when the animal is near a boundary of the local environment [38,39]. Boundary-related cells have been recorded also in the subiculum (Sub), which indirectly links the feedback from CA1 to the MEC, the presubiculum and the parasubiculum (Box 4.1) [40]. Grid, head-direction, and border cells might have strong innate components, given that rudiments of all three cell types are present when rat pups explore open spaces for the first time between P15 and P20 [15,16] (Box 4.2). Together, these cell types could be part of a metric navigation system able to map distances (grid cells), directions (head-direction cells), and vicinity to boundaries (border cells).

RELATION BETWEEN ENTORHINAL AND HIPPOCAMPAL MAPS

What are the relationships between place cells and the various cell types of the entorhinal cortex? Place cells in CA3 are contacted directly by axons from layer II cells in MEC (Box 4.1). Place cells in CA1 receive direct projections from layer III neurons in MEC. Both layers contain grid cells. Conversely, grid cells in layer V receive output from place cells in CA1. Thus it seems that grid cells and place cells are only one synapse apart, suggesting that there exists a simple transformation between grid and place representations. Several models have proposed that place cells, by use of a Fourier-like transformation, can emerge as a sum of inputs from many grid cells with different spatial phases and orientations [5,41–48]. Place cells could also depend on input from other entorhinal cell types, such as border cells [38,40,49,50]. Lesions of ventral MEC, where grid fields are larger, lead to a decrease in the size of place fields in the hippocampus [51]. This is consistent with the proposed grid-to-place cell transformation [5,41–48] because smaller place fields would be expected if inputs were restricted to grid cells with smaller grid fields. The view that place cells emerge from grid cell outputs is challenged by the finding that place cells mature earlier than grid cells during postnatal development of the nervous system [15,16]. The lag does not by itself exclude a role for grid cells in the formation of place cells because rudimentary grid fields can be sufficient to generate place fields (Box 2). However, if place cells can be constructed from a Fourier-like sum of grid cells, then it must also be possible to obtain the inverse transformation: the construction of grid cells as a Fourier-like sum of place cells [52]. Place-to-grid transformation models might not be able to explain the fact that grid structure persists for minutes after inactivation of the dorsal hippocampus (Bonnevie, Fyhn, Hafting, Derdikman, Moser and Moser, 2010, 40th Annual Meeting of the Society for Neuroscience, SfN, abstract 101.4); however, the gradual loss of stability and eventually all structure in grid fields of hippocampus-inactivated rats (ibid.) points to a role for hippocampal output in anchoring the grid fields to the local geometry and landmarks of the specific environment [48]. The reciprocal influences between grid cells and place cells will certainly remain a major target of study during the coming years.

THE MANIFOLD OF ENTORHINAL AND HIPPOCAMPAL MAPS

Most environments are more complex than the regular box and linear track environments in which most experiments on place cells and grid cells have been conducted. Environments such as a house with many rooms or a landscape with barriers such as rivers and fences are hard to describe purely in two-dimensional coordinates. An alternative way to represent such environments is to use a stack of maps where each subdivision of the environment has its own representation.

Several models have proposed that spatial environments are stored as large numbers of independent fragments or reference frames. Worden proposed that mammals store memories of their geographical environment as a collection of fragments each consisting of a small number of landmarks, their geometric relationship, and additional non-geometric properties [53]. In this model, fragments were rotated and pieced together to form a local map during navigation, in the same way that pieces are assembled in a jigsaw puzzle. Worden proposed that this geometric operation took place in the hippocampus and associated structures. The concept of multiple maps was further developed when McNaughton and colleagues introduced continuous attractor networks to understand translocation in hippocampal maps [54,55]. In their model, unique sets of place cells were active at different position coordinates in a virtual two-dimensional space called a chart. When the rat moved to a different position in the environment, its self-movement caused a movement of the place-cell activity bump to a different position in the chart, manifesting a neuronal implementation of path integration. Different spatial environments were associated with different, mutually exclusive charts. Redish and Touretzky provided additional theoretical support for a key role for path integration in the formation of hippocampal maps and proposed that the location of the path integrator involved regions both inside and outside the hippocampus, including the entorhinal cortex [56,57]. Different environments were suggested to be encoded by different spaces of path integrator coordinates reminiscent of the charts of McNaughton and colleagues [54,55].

The proposed multiplicity of the hippocampal–entorhinal map has received experimental verification. First, the presence of independent maps was supported by the fact that hippocampal place cells can undergo complete remapping even after small changes in the location or nature of the spatial environment [17–19]. Second, accumulating evidence indicates that hippocampal and entorhinal maps consist of fragmented submaps instead of a single universal representation. Frank and colleagues observed that entorhinal and hippocampal cells had similar firing patterns when rats were running along parallel corridors of the same complex maze [58]. Based on that, and to test whether entorhinal and hippocampal representations are decomposed into mosaics of connected maps, Derdikman *et al.* [59] recorded grid cells and place cells when rats were running in a square box of ten parallel corridors through which the animal had to run in a zigzag fashion to obtain reward at the ends (Fig. 4.2A). Grid cells did not exhibit periodic two-dimensional firing fields in this hairpin maze. Instead, the grid pattern broke up and similar maps were generated in every corridor where the rat was running in the same direction, creating repeating patterns across the alleys of the maze (Fig. 4.2C). Sharp transitions from one map to the next were observed whenever the rat turned from one corridor into the next. Because barriers could evoke local rate changes also in place cells [18,59] the fragmentation might apply across the grid and place map as a whole.

Are large natural spaces mapped in the same way as in the small confined space of a typical experimental study? Recordings from very large laboratory environments indicate that place cells extend in size from dorsal to ventral hippocampus [60,61]. The increase is finite, with an approximate field diameter of 10 meters at the ventral pole [60]. A similar finite scale expansion has been observed in entorhinal grid cells [32]. Therefore, the largest place fields and grid fields are probably substantially smaller than the largest environments visited by animals in their natural habitat. How are the latter environments then represented? One possibility would be to construct a more widely spaced representation based on interference between inputs from grid cells with different grid frequencies. The frequency of repetition of two grids with different

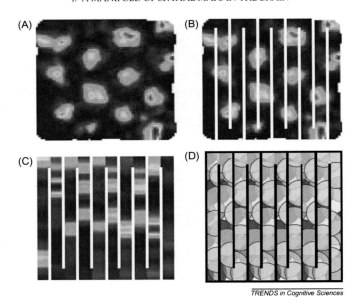

TRENDS in Cognitive Sciences

FIGURE 4.2   Grid pattern breaks up in a multi-compartment environment. (A) In the open-field box, a grid cell fires at multiple positions creating a hexagonal grid (red—high firing regions, blue—low firing regions). (B) When inserting walls into the same box, it could be hypothesized that the grid fields remain in the same positions. (C) However, what happens is that the grid breaks up, such that a similar map is expressed in every corridor with a similar running direction: every second corridor. (D) The multicompartment environment is composed of multiple fragmented maps, one for each corridor. Multiple grid cells fire in different locations (color coded in different colors) such that the ensemble of grid cells maps each corridor separately. Remapping occurs when the rat turns from one corridor to the next. This is different from the continuity of the grid map in the open field, as demonstrated in Fig. 4.1C. Adapted from [59].

spacing (the beat frequency) is equal to the least common multiplier of their spacing, which is generally larger than the spacing of each individual grid on its own [42,43]. The exploitation of beat frequencies would allow larger spaces to be represented but would not suffice to represent distances such as those covered during migration in animals or intercity travel in humans. A different solution would be to represent large environments as mosaics of smaller maps, breaking up along geometrical borders and landmarks, similar to the fragmentation described for the grid map the hairpin maze [59]. Representations of relationships between such map fragments might not use the metrics of grid and place cells but could rather depend on different mechanisms and brain systems.

DYNAMIC MAPS

The hippocampus hosts several maps, each anchored to a different reference frame or constellation of landmarks. Gothard and colleagues recorded place cells in an open-field task

[62] in which the rat ran from a small start-box to a small end-box in such a way that the relative positions of the start-box, end-box and goal in the arena were changed on every trial. Whereas some place cells seemed to fire anchored to the coordinates of the arena, other place cells changed their position when the goal or the start-/end-boxes were moved, apparently indicating that different cells were anchored to different reference frames (arena, start-box, end-box and goal). Place cells with different reference frames were never observed simultaneously; rather, different frames could be active in the population at different times, that is at any given time, the active map might be aligned with one frame and misaligned with another. Similar results were reproduced in a more recent study, in which a subset of the hippocampal cells were anchored to the reference frame of a local barrier, whereas other cells were locked to the external room frame [63].

Subsequent research has shown that the hippocampus can undergo remapping very rapidly, often within a few seconds or less [64]. In a second study, Gothard and colleagues [65] demonstrated that when the rat was running along a linear track from a start-box to an end-box, which was moved to various distances from the start box, place fields anchored to the start-box at the beginning of the track and to the end-box at the end of the track. When the end-box was moved to a new distance from the start-box, the position of the place fields nearer the end box moved accordingly, whereas the position of the fields near the start box remained constant. This meant that there was a relatively sharp realignment on the middle of the track from the start-box frame to the end-box frame. Derdikman and colleagues [59] demonstrated a similarly rapid transition between entorhinal maps as rats turned from one alley to the next in the hairpin maze (Fig. 4.2D). Such realignments seem to be coherent across the entire population of place cells, grid cells, head-direction cells and border cells, both within each population and between the populations [38,66–69]. Rotations of key landmarks cause coherent rotation of firing fields [38,66,67]. Remapping in place cells is accompanied by coherent changes in the phase and orientation of co-localized grid fields [68] and the orientation of direction fields and border fields [38]. The exact time scale or mechanisms of these global ensemble transitions has not been determined. It is not clear, for example, whether the transitions are all-or-none or pass smoothly through continua of intermediate network states. However, recordings from head-direction cells have shown that local ensembles can reset their firing preferences almost instantaneously, at a time scale of approximately 80 ms [70], and ongoing work in place cells, focusing specifically on the transition moment, indicates that hippocampal ensembles might switch from one map to another within less than a single theta cycle (Jezek, Treves, Moser and Moser, 2010, 40th Annual Meeting of the Society for Neuroscience, SfN, abstract 101.11). Such fast transitions are often followed by one or several discrete flashbacks to the original representation, before the network settles, but only one state is expressed at a time (ibid.).

Remapping can occur at a rapid rate also when there are no external constraints to induce the transition. Hippocampal place cells are known to be extremely variable in their firing rates, more than expected from a Poisson-like distribution of the firing rates [71,72]. The apparent overdispersion in the hippocampus place code could actually result from rapid remapping; for example the spatial map might alternate between a range of representations associated with the same place (Box 4.3)[73–76]. The fact that overdispersion in a given cell can be predicted from changes in the activity state of other simultaneously recorded cells [77] adds support to this suggestion. It follows from these findings that maps are dynamic entities that are loaded to and from working memory during the course of behavior. Alternations between reference frames could result from intrinsic properties of the network, such as when reference frames change several times per second [76–78], but at longer time scales, switches might also occur in response to more global inputs similar to those thought to be responsible for selective attention [75,79].

CAN SEVERAL MAPS BE ACTIVE SIMULTANEOUSLY?

The rapid time scale of hippocampal remapping raises the question whether hippocampal maps can co-occur completely simultaneously, or are always expressed in rapid succession. Early studies introduced the term partial remapping to characterize cases in which subsets of the place cell population remapped independently of each other [80]. In such cases, several maps, each associated with a different subpopulation of cells, were activated in the same trial. A paradigmatic example was the differential response of hippocampal place cells on trials on a circular track where proximal and distal cues were rotated in different directions [81–84]. A typical observation in such experiments was that one subset of the place cells rotated with the proximal cues in the environment, whereas another subset rotated with the distal cues. Similar to the cases described in the previous section, it could be hypothesized that there was a rapid alternation between a map anchored to the local cues and a map anchored to the distal cues, so the maps were not loaded simultaneously. Counter to this hypothesis, the authors of one of the studies [81] presented a single example in which the two maps were shown to be expressed completely simultaneously: Two different cells clearly belonging to different maps, one rotating with the proximal cues and another rotating with the distal cues, fired at the same time, as was evident from temporal cross-correlations between the two cells. In a conceptually similar set of studies in which rats were subjected to two shock-zones on a rotating arena, one rotating and one stationary, some place cells were anchored to the stationary shock-zone, whereas others were anchored to the rotating shock-zone [74,76]. Also in this case it is conceivable that the two maps, anchored to the two shock-zones, were never loaded simultaneously. However, the researchers reported a group of cells that was anchored to both shock-zones at once, firing only when the rat was at the same time at a certain position relative to both the stationary shock-zone and a the rotating shock-zone [76]. The presence of such cells would argue against temporal segmentation of stationary and rotating maps; however it should be noted that these cells appeared mostly near the centre of the disk where the difference between the reference frames was small. It therefore remains to be determined if discrete reference frames can be loaded simultaneously, or if conjunctions are always expressed by alternating expression of discrete representations.

CONCLUDING REMARKS

Studies of place cells and grid cells have led to the insight that there is more than one spatial map in the brain. These studies are based almost exclusively on rats; however, the probable presence of place cells [85] and grid cells [86] in humans as well as phylogenetically distant species, such as echolocating bats [87] (Yartsev, Witter and Ulanovsky, 2010, 40th Annual Meeting of the Society for Neuroscience, SfN, abstract 203.15), suggests that the mechanisms could be more general.

BOX 4.4

QUESTIONS FOR FUTURE RESEARCH

1. What is the nature of the transformation between place cells and grid cells?
2. If environments are mapped by fragmented representations, where are the fragments linked and how?
3. Can multiple maps be expressed simultaneously? If not, can different maps alternate and if so, at what frequencies and under which conditions?
4. How are very large environments represented?

5. How do neuronal oscillations and synchrony contribute to retrieval of distributed maps in the hippocampus?
6. Which components of spatial maps in the brain are genetically specified, and how are maps shaped by experience?
7. What are the cellular and network mechanisms responsible for transitions between spatial maps?
8. Do humans represent space in ways different from rodents?

The rat studies indicate that the brain hosts multiple maps representing different subsets of the environment at different times, in different brain regions, and at different scales. Spatial maps in the hippocampus and entorhinal cortex seem to be much more dynamic than previously appreciated. A map in these brain regions can be retrieved within a few hundred milli-seconds and replaced soon after if a different map is relevant to the goal of the behavior. A major objective for the next few years will be to determine how the plurality and variety of maps interacts and how different cell types and components of the circuit contribute to the rapid dynamics of spatial mapping (Box 4.4). This will hopefully lead us to a comprehensive theory about how the brain is used for navigation and for representing the space around us.

GLOSSARY

Allocentric coordinates

World-based coordinates. Opposite of egocentric coordinates.

Attractor dynamics

Attractor networks are neural networks with one or more stable states. These stable states are determined by the strengths of the recurrent connections between the individual neurons of the network. When the system is started from a location in state space other than the stable state, it will evolve until it arrives at one of the stable states and will then tend to stay there.

Azimuth

Orientation relative to world coordinates.

Fourier-like transform

A classical mathematical Fourier-transform transforms between the description of a signal in position terms to a description of the signal in spatial-frequency terms. The Fourier transform of a sine wave is a narrow pulse. In two dimensions, this resembles the transformation from grid cells (which are oscillatory sine waves) to place cells (which resemble a narrow pulse in space).

Grid orientation

The orientation of the grid pattern relative to an external reference orientation.

Grid phase

The position of one of the vertices of a grid cell in the x–y plane.

Grid spacing

The distance between adjacent grid vertices, expressed as the average distance from the central peak to any of the vertices of the inner hexagon in the spatial autocorrelogram.

Path integration

Position is the integral of velocity in time. Therefore one way to determine the current position is to sum up all momentary velocities and directions until the current moment. Path integration is a method to determine one's position from one's own self movement in this manner, without relying on external landmarks.

Reference frame

An external configuration of landmarks and geometry to which neuronal firing coordinates are associated.

Theta rhythm

A dominant regular ~8 Hz rhythm recorded in local-field potential signals in many brain areas, such as the hippocampus, the entorhinal cortex and the septum. Neuronal firing of individual cells is phase-modulated by this populaion rhythm. It occurs mostly when the rat is in movement.

Acknowledgments

We thank Laura Colgin for reading and commenting on the manuscript, and Menno Witter for advice about hippocampal anatomy.

References

[1] E.C. Tolman, Cognitive maps in rats and men, Psychol. Rev. 55 (1948) 189–208.
[2] J. O'Keefe, J. Dostrovsky, The hippocampus as a spatial map. Preliminary evidence from unit activity in the freely-moving rat, Brain Res. 34 (1971) 171–175.
[3] J. O'Keefe, L. Nadel, The Hippocampus as a Cognitive Map, Oxford University Press (Clarendon Press)
[4] R.U. Muller, Spatial firing patterns of hippocampal complex-spike cells in a fixed environment, J. Neurosci. 7 (1987) 1935–1950.

[5] E.I. Moser, Place cells, grid cells, and the brain's spatial representation system, Annu. Rev. Neurosci. 31 (2008) 69–89.

[6] C.N. Boccara, et al. Grid cells in pre- and parasubiculum, Nat. Neurosci. 13 (2010) 987–994.

[7] R.A. Epstein, Parahippocampal and retrosplenial contributions to human spatial navigation, Trends Cogn. Sci. 12 (2008) 388–396.

[8] S.D. Vann, et al. What does the retrosplenial cortex do?, Nat. Rev. Neurosci. 10 (2009) 792–802.

[9] J.R. Whitlock, et al. Navigating from hippocampus to parietal cortex, Proc. Natl. Acad. Sci. U. S. A. 105 (2008) 14755–14762.

[10] M.A. Silver, S. Kastner, Topographic maps in human frontal and parietal cortex, Trends Cogn. Sci. 13 (2009) 488–495.

[11] B. Poucet, et al. Spatial navigation and hippocampal place cell firing: the problem of goal encoding, Rev. Neurosci. 15 (2004) 89–107.

[12] G.J. Quirk, et al. The firing of hippocampal place cells in the dark depends on the rats recent experience, J. Neurosci. 10 (1990) 2008–2017.

[13] M.A. Wilson, B.L. McNaughton, Dynamics of the hippocampal ensemble code for space, Science 261 (1993) 1055–1058.

[14] A.D. Redish, et al. Independence of firing correlates of anatomically proximate hippocampal pyramidal cells, J. Neurosci. 21 (2001) RC134.

[15] R.F. Langston, et al. Development of the spatial representation system in the rat, Science 328 (2010) 1576–1580.

[16] T.J. Wills, et al. Development of the hippocampal cognitive map in preweanling rats, Science 328 (2010) 1573–1576.

[17] R.U. Muller, et al. Spatial firing correlates of neurons in the hippocampal formation of freely moving rats, in: J. Paillard, (Ed.), Brain and Space, Oxford University Press, pp. 296–333.

[18] R.U. Muller, J.L. Kubie, The effects of changes in the environment on the spatial firing of hippocampal complex-spike cells, J. Neurosci. 7 (1987) 1951–1968.

[19] L.L. Colgin, et al. Understanding memory through hippocampal remapping, Trends Neurosci. 31 (2008) 469–477.

[20] E.R. Wood, et al. The global record of memory in hippocampal neuronal activity, Nature 397 (1999) 613–616.

[21] S.P. Wiebe, U.V. Staubli, Dynamic filtering of recognition memory codes in the hippocampus, J. Neurosci. 19 (1999) 10562–10574.

[22] R.E. Hampson, et al. Hippocampal cell firing correlates of delayed-match-to-sample performance in the rat, Behav. Neurosci. 107 (1993) 715–739.

[23] R.W. Komorowski, et al. Robust conjunctive item-place coding by hippocampal neurons parallels learning what happens where, J. Neurosci. 29 (2009) 9918–9929.

[24] J. Manns, H. Eichenbaum, A cognitive map for object memory in the hippocampus, Learn. Mem. 16 (2009) 616–624.

[25] E. Pastalkova, et al. Internally generated cell assembly sequences in the rat hippocampus, Science 321 (2008) 1322–1327.

[26] L.R. Squire, Memory and the hippocampus: a synthesis from findings with rats, monkeys, and humans, Psychol. Rev. 99 (1992) 195–231.

[27] E. Tulving, H.J. Markowitsch, Episodic and declarative memory: role of the hippocampus, Hippocampus 8 (1998) 198–204.

[28] H. Eichenbaum, N.J. Cohen, From Conditioning to Conscious Recollection, Oxford University Press

[29] D. Tse, et al. Schemas and memory consolidation, Science 316 (2007) 76–82.

[30] T. Hafting, et al. Microstructure of a spatial map in the entorhinal cortex, Nature 436 (2005) 801–806.

[31] M. Fyhn, Spatial representation in the entorhinal cortex, Science 305 (2004) 1258–1264.

[32] V.H. Brun, et al. Progressive increase in grid scale from dorsal to ventral medial entorhinal cortex, Hippocampus 18 (2008) 1200–1212.

[33] J.B. Ranck, Head-direction cells in the deep cell layer of dorsal presubiculum in freely moving rats, in: G. Buzsaki, C.H. Vanderwolf, (Eds.), Electrical Activity of the Archicortex, Akademiai Kiado, (1985), pp. 217–220.

[34] J.S. Taube, et al. Head-direction cells recorded from the postsubiculum in freely moving rats. 1. description and quantitative analysis, J. Neurosci. 10 (1990) 420–435.

[35] F. Sargolini, Conjunctive representation of position, direction, and velocity in entorhinal cortex, Science 312 (2006) 758–762.

[36] S.I. Wiener, J.S. Taube, Head-direction cells and the Neural Mechanisms of Spatial Orientation, (2005), The MIT Press

[37] J.S. Taube, The head direction signal: origins and sensory-motor integration, Annu. Rev. Neurosci. 30 (2007) 181–207.

[38] T. Solstad, et al. Representation of geometric borders in the entorhinal cortex, Science 322 (2008) 1865–1868.

[39] F. Savelli, et al. Influence of boundary removal on the spatial representations of the medial entorhinal cortex, Hippocampus 18 (2008) 1270–1282.

[40] C. Lever, et al. Boundary vector cells in the subiculum of the hippocampal formation, J. Neurosci. 29 (2009) 9771–9777.

[41] T. Solstad, et al. From grid cells to place cells: a mathematical model, Hippocampus 16 (2006) 1026–1031.

[42] M.C. Fuhs, D.S. Touretzky, A spin glass model of path integration in rat medial entorhinal cortex, J. Neurosci. 26 (2006) 4266–4276.

[43] B.L. McNaughton, et al. Path integration and the neural basis of the 'cognitive map', Nat. Rev. Neurosci. 7 (2006) 663–678.

[44] C. Molter, Y. Yamaguchi, Entorhinal theta phase precession sculpts dentate gyrus place fields, Hippocampus 18 (2008) 919–930.

[45] E.T. Rolls, et al. Entorhinal cortex grid cells can map to hippocampal place cells by competitive learning, Network 17 (2006) 447–465.

[46] E.T. Rolls, An attractor network in the hippocampus: theory and neurophysiology, Learn. Mem. 14 (2007) 714–731.

[47] L. de Almeida, et al. The input–output transformation of the hippocampal granule cells: from grid cells to place fields, J. Neurosci. 29 (2009) 7504–7512.

[48] J. O'Keefe, N. Burgess, Dual phase and rate coding in hippocampal place cells: theoretical significance and relationship to entorhinal grid cells, Hippocampus 15 (2005) 853–866.

[49] T. Hartley, et al. Modeling place fields in terms of the cortical inputs to the hippocampus, Hippocampus 10 (2000) 369–379.

[50] J. O'Keefe, N. Burgess, Geometric determinants of the place fields of hippocampal neurons, Nature 381 (1996) 425–428.

[51] T. Van Cauter, Unstable CA1 place cell representation in rats with entorhinal cortex lesions, Eur. J. Neurosci. 27 (2008) 1933–1946.

[52] E. Kropff, A. Treves, The emergence of grid cells: intelligent design or just adaptation?, Hippocampus 18 (2008) 1256–1269.

[53] R. Worden, Navigation by fragment fitting: a theory of hippocampal function, Hippocampus 2 (1992) 165–187.

[54] A. Samsonovich, B.L. McNaughton, Path integration and cognitive mapping in a continuous attractor neural network model, J. Neurosci. 17 (1997) 5900–5920.

[55] B.L. McNaughton, et al. Deciphering the hippocampal polyglot: the hippocampus as a path integration system, J. Exp. Biol. 199 (1996) 173–185.

[56] D.S. Touretzky, A.D. Redish, Theory of rodent navigation based on interacting representations of space, Hippocampus 6 (1996) 247–270.

[57] A.D. Redish, D.S. Touretzky, Cognitive maps beyond the hippocampus, Hippocampus 7 (1997) 15–35.

[58] L.M. Frank, et al. Trajectory encoding in the hippocampus and entorhinal cortex, Neuron 27 (2000) 169–178.

[59] D. Derdikman, et al. Fragmentation of grid cell maps in a multicompartment environment, Nat. Neurosci. 12 (2009) 1325–1332.

[60] K.B. Kjelstrup, et al. Finite scale of spatial representation in the hippocampus, Science 321 (2008) 140–143.

[61] M.W. Jung, et al. Comparison of spatial firing characteristics of units in dorsal and ventral hippocampus of the rat, J. Neurosci. 14 (1994) 7347–7356.

[62] K.M. Gothard, et al. Binding of hippocampal CA1 neural activity to multiple reference frames in a landmark-based navigation task, J. Neurosci. 16 (1996) 823–835.

[63] B. Rivard, et al. Representation of objects in space by two classes of hippocampal pyramidal cells, J. Gen. Physiol. 124 (2004) 9–25.

[64] A.D. Redish, Dynamics of hippocampal ensemble activity realignment: time versus space, J. Neurosci. 20 (2000) 9298–9309.

[65] K.M. Gothard, et al. Dynamics of mismatch correction in the hippocampal ensemble code for space: interaction between path integration and environmental cues, J. Neurosci. 16 (1996) 8027–8040.

[66] J.J. Knierim, et al. Place cells, head-direction cells, and the learning of landmark stability, J. Neurosci. 15 (1995) 1648–1659.

[67] J.J. Knierim, et al. Interactions between idiothetic cues and external landmarks in the control of place cells and head-direction cells, J. Neurophysiol. 80 (1998) 425–446.

[68] M. Fyhn, et al. Hippocampal remapping and grid realignment in entorhinal cortex, Nature 446 (2007) 190–194.

[69] E.L. Hargreaves, et al. Cohesiveness of spatial and directional representations recorded from neural ensembles in the anterior thalamus, parasubiculum, medial entorhinal cortex, and hippocampus, Hippocampus 17 (2007) 826–841.

[70] M.B. Zugaro, et al. Rapid spatial reorientation and head direction cells, J. Neurosci. 23 (2003) 3478–3482.

[71] A.V. Olypher, et al. Properties of the extra-positional signal in hippocampal place cell discharge derived from the overdispersion in location-specific firing, Neuroscience 111 (2002) 553–566.

[72] A.A. Fenton, R.U. Muller, Place cell discharge is extremely variable during individual passes of the rat through the firing field, Proc. Natl. Acad. Sci. U. S. A 95 (1998) 3182–3187.

[73] J.K. Leutgeb, et al. Progressive transformation of hippocampal neuronal representations in "morphed" environments. Neuron 48 (2005) 345–358.

[74] A.A. Fenton, et al. Both here and there: simultaneous expression of autonomous spatial memories in rats, Proc. Natl. Acad. Sci. U. S. A. 95 (1998) 11493–11498.

[75] A.A. Fenton, et al. Attention-like modulation of hippocampus place cell discharge, J. Neurosci. 30 (2010) 4613–4625.

[76] E. Kelemen, A.A. Fenton, Dynamic grouping of hippocampal neural activity during cognitive control of two spatial frames, PLoS Biol. 8 (2010) e1000403.

[77] J. Jackson, A.D. Redish, Network dynamics of hippocampal cell-assemblies resemble multiple spatial maps within single tasks, Hippocampus 17 (2007) 1209–1229.

[78] L.L. Colgin, et al. Frequency of gamma oscillations routes flow of information in the hippocampus, Nature 462 (2009) 353–357.

[79] C.G. Kentros, et al. Increased attention to spatial context increases both place field stability and spatial memory, Neuron 42 (2004) 283–295.

[80] W.E. Skaggs, B.L. McNaughton, Spatial firing properties of hippocampal CA1 populations in an environment containing two visually identical regions, J. Neurosci. 18 (1998) 8455–8466.

[81] J.J. Knierim, Dynamic interactions between local surface cues, distal landmarks, and intrinsic circuitry in hippocampal place cells, J. Neurosci. 22 (2002) 6254–6264.

[82] I. Lee, et al. A double dissociation between hippocampal subfields: differential time course of CA3 and CA1 place cells for processing changed environments, Neuron 42 (2004) 803–815.

[83] M.L. Shapiro, et al. Cues that hippocampal place cells encode: dynamic and hierarchical representation of local and distal stimuli, Hippocampus 7 (1997) 624–642.

[84] H. Tanila, et al. Discordance of spatial representation in ensembles of hippocampal place cells, Hippocampus 7 (1997) 613–623.

[85] A.D. Ekstrom, et al. Cellular networks underlying human spatial navigation, Nature 425 (2003) 184–187.

[86] C.F. Doeller, et al. Evidence for grid cells in a human memory network, Nature 463 (2010) 657–661.

[87] N. Ulanovsky, C.F. Moss, Hippocampal cellular and network activity in freely moving echolocating bats, Nat. Neurosci. 10 (2007) 224–233.

[88] M.P. Witter, D.G. Amaral, Hippocampal Formation, in: G. Paxinos, (Ed.), The Rat Nervous System, third ed., Elsevier Academic Press, (2004), pp. 635–704.

[89] E.J. Henriksen, et al. Spatial representation along the proximodistal axis of CA1, Neuron 68 (2010) 127–137.

[90] M.P. Witter, Connectivity of the Hippocampus, in: V. Cutsuridis et al. (Ed.), Hippocampal Microcircuits, Springer, (2010) pp. 5–26.

[91] C. Barry, et al. Experience-dependent rescaling of entorhinal grids, Nat. Neurosci. 10 (2007) 682–684.

[92] S. Leutgeb, et al. Independent codes for spatial and episodic memory in hippocampal neuronal ensembles, Science 309 (2005) 619–623.

[93] S. Leutgeb, et al. Distinct ensemble codes in hippocampal areas CA3 and CA1, Science 305 (2004) 1295–1298.

[94] J. O'Keefe, D.H. Conway, Hippocampal place units in freely moving rat—why they fire where they fire, Exp. Brain Res. 31 (1978) 573–590.

Temporal Neuronal Oscillations can Produce Spatial Phase Codes

Christopher Burgess*, Nicolas W. Schuck[†],
Neil Burgess*

*UCL Institute of Cognitive Neuroscience and UCL Institute of Neurology,
University College London, London, UK
[†]Department of Psychology, Humboldt Universität zu Berlin, Berlin, Germany

Summary

The ability to integrate information over time is a fundamental operation of the brain, but the neuronal mechanisms underlying it are poorly understood. Here we describe how rhythmic variation in the activity of neurons—a common observation in neural recordings—could provide one such mechanism. In particular, we review a model that uses interference between neuronal oscillations to account for the spatio-temporal firing patterns of place cells in the hippocampus and grid cells in entorhinal cortex. The mechanism integrates movement information by varying the frequencies of the oscillations according to running velocity, thus mapping temporal oscillations into phase codes for *distance traveled* and, in combination with environmental information, *spatial location*. This provides a specific model of path integration and spatial orientation, but also provides an example of how, more generally, dynamic neural oscillations could be used to integrate and encode information. In this vein, we suggest how representations of sequential (or "rank") order and numerosity could also be generated using such a system.

The idea of related processing mechanisms in the brain for spatial and temporal information enjoys increasing popularity among researchers, as reflected in some of the chapters in this volume (see also [1,2]). Here we discuss how subthreshold membrane potential oscillations (MPOs) could encode representations of the animal's spatial location in their phase relationship with other oscillations. The oscillatory interference model of how the spatial firing patterns of grid cells in the entorhinal cortex [3] could result from motion-related

© 2011 Elsevier Inc. All rights reserved.

information on speed and direction of movement is reviewed. We discuss how, in principle, similar models could also account for representations of sequential order [4,5].

Our starting point is the observation of "theta phase precession" in the firing of "place cells" in the hippocampi of freely moving rats [6]. Place cells embody a representation of space: each cell firing whenever the animal enters a specific portion of its environment (the corresponding "place field", see [7]). In parallel to this firing rate code for location, a temporal or phase code has also been observed relating to the theta rhythm: a large-amplitude oscillation in the local field potential of navigating rats, at 6–10 Hz in adult rats [8,9]. As the rat runs through a place field, the corresponding place cell fires bursts of spikes at systematically earlier phases of the theta rhythm such that the firing phase corresponds to the location of the rat within the place field. O'Keefe and Recce [6] suggested that this firing pattern reflected an intrinsic MPO in place cells which has a slightly higher frequency than the theta rhythm when the rat is in the place field (see also [10]). Subsequent research has confirmed the independence of the phase code from the firing rate code [11] and verified the link between firing phase and an intrinsic MPO in place cells [12].

An interesting aspect of place cell phase precession is that the phase of firing correlates with the distance traveled through the place field whether the rat runs quickly or slowly [6,11]. This suggests that the MPO frequency must increase with running speed so that the *temporal* oscillation can produce a phase code for *distance* [10]. Here we review the potential for neuronal oscillations to produce a representation of spatial location by integrating the animal's velocity (i.e. speed and direction of running)—a process often referred to as "path integration". Such a mechanism has been proposed to explain the spatial firing pattern of "grid cells" in the entorhinal cortex of freely moving rats [3] (see [13,14]). In addition, we examine the potential for neuronal oscillations to produce a representation of the serial order of stimuli, such as seen in recordings from primates [4,5].

A FUNCTIONAL ROLE FOR INTERFERENCE BETWEEN NEURONAL OSCILLATIONS

Oscillatory behavior of single neurons or groups of neurons is a common finding in a variety of brain areas. On a single-cell level, this dynamic is likely linked to voltage-sensitive membrane currents (e.g., [15]). In the review below, we focus on potential functional mechanisms that utilize interference between neuronal oscillations, and leave out many of the biological details and constraints that have been discussed elsewhere [14,16,17]. The general principle of phase coding and oscillatory interference can be understood by considering a pair of oscillations, initially matched in phase and frequency, that experience a transient frequency difference (see Fig. 5.1A). Undisturbed, they will remain in phase indefinitely as long as their frequencies remain equal. However, a change in one of their frequencies will cause a drift in their phases relative to one another for the duration of the change (with a rate of drift proportional to the frequency difference). Crucially, once the oscillation frequencies become equal again, any acquired phase advance will be maintained until another frequency change should further modify it. Mathematically, the phase difference between the two oscillations, $\phi_{ab}(t) = \phi_a(t) - \phi_b(t)$, is the time integral of their frequency difference, i.e.

$$\phi_{ab}(t) = \phi_{ab}(0) + \int_0^t 2\pi[f_a(\tau) - f_b(\tau)]d\tau \qquad (5.1)$$

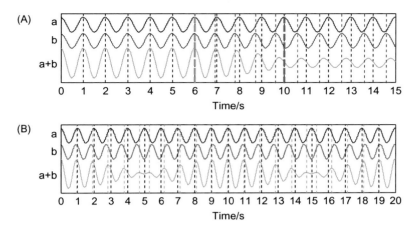

FIGURE 5.1   The amplitude of interference patterns between oscillations reveals the difference between their phase, which, in turn reflects their history of past frequency differences. (A) Oscillations a and b (blue) begin matched in frequency and phase. A transient frequency increase in oscillation a (beginning at the green vertical dashed line) causes it to drift ahead in phase relative to a. Once oscillation a returns to baseline (vertical red dashed line), the acquired phase difference is preserved. The amplitude of the interference pattern produced by their addition (green plot) reflects their phase difference. Peak times of oscillations a and b are indicated by black and blue vertical dashed lines respectively. (B) Oscillations a and b (blue and red, respectively) each have constant frequency but b is slightly faster (A: 1 Hz, B: 1.1 Hz), causing a cyclical advance in relative phase. The amplitude of their interference delineates an oscillating envelope with a wavelength of their frequency difference (i.e. 0.1 Hz). Peak times of oscillation a are indicated by black vertical dashed lines, while the peaks of the interference pattern are indicated by green vertical dashed lines.

where ϕ_a and ϕ_b are the phases of the two oscillations, and $f_a(t)$ and $f_b(t)$ are their time-varying frequencies. The relationship between oscillatory phase and frequency offers a potential mechanism for neuronal oscillations to integrate information arriving over extended periods of time. Although such protracted integration of information is a fundamental property of memory, its neuronal implementation is non-trivial. Hence one of the features of the oscillatory interference model is to offer a plausible account of how this could be achieved by neurons whose membrane potential or firing rate undergoes rhythmic variation.

If the frequency difference between two oscillations varies according to some variable X, at any given moment, the relative phase between the two oscillations will reflect the time integral of X. Since oscillatory phase is periodic, such an encoding scheme will also be cyclic; e.g., under a sustained frequency difference, two oscillations will move steadily into and out of phase with one another. When two such oscillations are combined, e.g., by addition, to generate an interference pattern, the amplitude of the resulting oscillation waxes and wanes as the two oscillations transition between constructive and destructive interference (see Fig. 5.1B). The amplitude profile is referred to as the envelope of the interference pattern, and varies with a frequency equal to the difference between the frequencies of the two oscillations. The amplitude of the envelope is proportional to the phase difference at that moment, and therefore also proportional to the time integral of X. Furthermore, the peaks of the interference pattern occur between the peaks of the two oscillations. This is an important property for phase coding discussed later since, as a consequence, the interference peaks always advance relative to those of the slower oscillation and regress relative to the faster oscillation (see Fig. 5.1B).

In this way, oscillatory interference offers a potential mechanism to retrieve information dynamically integrated over time. First we consider how these principles have been applied to models of grid cell firing and later we describe a new potential model for the firing of rank-order cells [4].

AN OSCILLATORY INTERFERENCE MODEL OF GRID CELL FIRING

Grid cells recorded in the medial entorhinal cortex of freely moving rats fire whenever the animal is located within one of a number of spatially defined regions or "firing fields". The firing fields of individual cells define the vertices of a remarkably regular triangular or hexagonal array mapped onto the environment surface, providing a very specific representation of the animal's location within the environment (see Box 5.1 and Fig. 5.2). In the

---

BOX 5.1

NEURAL BASIS OF SPATIAL NAVIGATION: ENTORHINAL GRID-CELLS

Grid cells, first discovered in the medial entorhinal cortex (MEC) of freely moving rats exhibit spatially modulated firing fields, much like the hippocampal place cells discovered before them. However, unlike place cells, a grid cell fires in multiple firing fields that are repeated across the environment, arranged in a regular triangular structure. Within individual fields, the firing rate of cells is center-peaked, diminishing with distance relative to the field center. Their spatial stability in the face of variation in the animal's speed and direction intimate that they are performing a path integrative function, i.e. using self-movement information to continually update the animal's estimate of its position. Furthermore, a prominent feature of the hippocampal-entorhinal brain region is the prevalence of local field potential oscillations in the theta band.

Like place cells, the majority of grid cells show a spatial organization in the phase of firing relative to the theta oscillation; firing occurs at progressively earlier phases of subsequent theta cycles as the animal passes through the field [22]. Such phase precession can be explained if grid cell firing reflects interference between oscillations with shifting relative phases. Indeed, the oscillatory interference model was originally proposed to explain the same phenomenon in the firing of place cells [6].

The firing patterns of grid cells appear to provide a metric of space: compellingly, the grid scale of cells varies systematically along the dorsoventral axis of the MEC [35]. The activity of a few cells with different scales could unambiguously encode an animal's location. Intriguingly, while grid cells have so far only been recorded in rats and mice, there is also evidence for grid cells in the human MEC, as well as grid-like firing in other regions putatively involved in spatial navigation and memory [25].

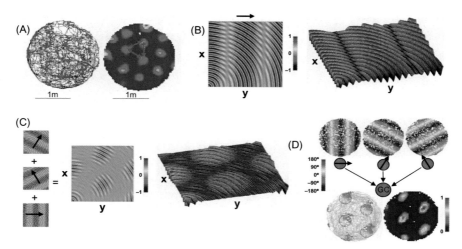

FIGURE 5.2 An oscillatory interference model can explain the spatial firing patterns of grid cells. (A) Spatial firing maps of a grid cell recorded from a rat during a 30-min run in a circular environment (2 m diameter; scale bars shown). Left: Spike locations (red) superimposed onto the trajectory of the animal in the enclosure (black). Note how the spikes occur within an array of distinct "firing fields". Right: Spatial rate map showing the mean firing rate of the cell across the environment. The triangular structure of the field array is emphasized by the red arrows. Adapted, with permission, from Moser and Moser, *Hippocampus* 18: 1142–1156 (2008). (B) The spatial interference pattern between two oscillations with a velocity-modulated frequency difference, during constant velocity runs from the origin (bottom left). Amplitude modulation of the envelope occurs only along the preferred direction (arrow). Left: Flat amplitude color-coded map. Right: 3-D plot showing amplitude on the z-axis. Note the clear interference profile along the bottom edge. (C) Spatial interference patterns produced with preferred directions differing by multiples of 60° (left: flat patterns) can be summed to produce 2-D amplitude modulation (middle: flat spatial pattern; right: 3-D map as in B). (D) Spatial firing maps of a model grid cell (below) and its velocity-controlled oscillator inputs (VCOs, above, preferred directions shown by arrows) during a simulated 5-min run using real trajectory data in a circular environment (gray line bottom left plot). Above plots show the locations at which spikes were fired, color-coded according to their phase relative to the baseline oscillation. Bottom left: Grid cell spike phase map. Bottom right: Color-coded spatial firing rate map for the same cell. Note the equivalent baseline phase range of VCO and grid cell spikes within the field locations (circled).

oscillatory interference model of grid cell firing [13,14], the phase relationship between neuronal oscillations in the theta band encodes the animal's current allocentric position. This is achieved in the model using so-called velocity-controlled oscillators (VCOs), which are subject to a frequency modulation from a common baseline according to the velocity of the animal. The VCOs are assumed to be direction-specific such that a VCO's frequency varies in proportion to the component of the animal's velocity along the VCO's "preferred direction". Thus, if $f_b(t)$ is the baseline frequency, $f_a(t)$ is the VCO's (active) frequency, $s(t)$ is the animal's speed, $\theta(t)$ is its running direction and φ_d is the preferred direction of the VCO then:

$$f_a(t) = f(t)_b + \beta s(t) \cos(\theta(t) - \varphi_d) \qquad (5.2)$$

where β is a scaling constant. As described above, this produces a difference between the VCO phase ϕ_a and the baseline oscillation phase ϕ_b that is the time integral of the component of the animal's velocity along the preferred direction. Thus the phase difference ϕ_{ab}

reflects distance traveled by the animal along the VCO's preferred direction in the time t since the phases were aligned, which we refer to as $d(t)$:

$$\phi_{ab}(t) - \phi_{ab}(0) = \int_0^t 2\pi[f_a(\tau) - f_b(\tau)]\,d\tau = \int_0^t 2\pi\beta[s(\tau)\cos(\theta(\tau) - \varphi_d)]\,d\tau = 2\pi\beta d(t) \quad (5.3)$$

The interference pattern formed by adding the two oscillations manifests the mapping between relative phase and environmental position with a smooth and periodic variation of its amplitude along the VCOs preferred direction (see Fig. 5.2B). Since the phase difference cycles every 2π, the spatial period of this variation along the preferred direction is $1/\beta$. The amplitude modulation is one-dimensional, however, as movement perpendicular to the preferred direction elicits no frequency modulation, producing bands of equal amplitude across the environment perpendicular to the preferred direction.

A neuron's firing could be driven by such an interference pattern if both oscillations are summed at the soma (see [14,16]). In this case, the firing rate would reflect the amplitude of the interference pattern, with peak firing occurring at the locations where the phases of the contributing oscillations coincide. An extension to a two-dimensional spatial modulation of firing, as it is the case for grid cells, can be accomplished by assuming modulation from two or more VCOs with non-parallel preferred directions. Moreover, the characteristic tessellated triangle motif of grid fields can be reproduced from a cell receiving input from VCOs with preferred directions that differ by multiples of 60° (see Fig. 5.2C, D). This configuration produces grid nodes aligned 30° to the preferred directions. Since completing a VCO spatial period when traveling 30° (or 150°) to its preferred direction requires traveling $2/\sqrt{3}$ (i.e. $1/\cos 30°$) times the period, the spacing between grid nodes is $2/\sqrt{3}\beta$, see also [18].

The above-described VCOs are proposed to be implemented as MPOs, either occurring in dendritic subunits of the grid cell itself [13] or in individual neurons that form the driving inputs to the grid cell ([14], see also [16]). In the model, the oscillators share a common intrinsic frequency in the theta band that is modulated by velocity-dependent depolarizing inputs. Such inputs could be provided by speed-modulated head direction cells. Head direction cells [19] co-localize with grid cells in the MEC, and the pre- and parasubiculum [20,21] and only fire when the animal is facing a particular direction (regardless of their location). The firing rates of a subset of head-direction cells are further modulated by running speed ("speed-modulated head direction cells") thus offering a viable potential input to VCOs.

The implementation of VCOs in different dendritic subunits of grid cells may be ruled out by biophysical constraints. Modeling studies have suggested that multiple dendritic oscillations within the same neuron phase lock within a timescale that may rule out their use for integration ([17], but also see [36]). In the neuronal VCO implementation, however, each VCO is implemented by a distinct neuron and forms the inputs to the grid cell [14,16]. In this implementation, the VCO neurons spike periodically at the peaks of their MPO. Hence, the *phase* at which VCO spikes occur relative to the baseline oscillation shows the spatial pattern of bands perpendicular to the VCO's preferred direction (see VCO spike phase plots in Fig. 5.2D). The spikes from VCOs elicit EPSPs in the target grid cell enabling temporal integration between VCO inputs over the timescale of the decay constant of the EPSPs. Thus, the grid cell effectively operates as a coincidence detector of its VCO inputs: when the VCO phases are sufficiently aligned, their spikes will arrive close together in time and the cell can reach threshold. The grid cell membrane potential is further modulated by the baseline oscillation to select spikes that coincide with a range of its phases. With an appropriate membrane potential spike threshold, the model produces firing patterns matching those of real grid cells (see grid cell spike phase and rate maps in Fig. 5.2D). Firing fields are arranged in a triangular structure (as expected from the interference runs in Fig. 5.2B), with spacing dependent on the scale of the velocity-modulation (i.e. the β parameter in Equation 5.2).

The ideas behind this model can be implemented in various ways (e.g., with different numbers of VCOs and different preferred directions). Burgess [14] proposes that the baseline oscillation frequency is actually the mean frequency of all of the VCOs, and that only those VCOs aligned with the current running direction contribute to the firing of the grid cell. This allows the input to VCOs to be solely depolarizing, rather than changing sign with running direction, as implied by Equation 5.2 (and thus not violating Dale's law). It also allows the grid cell to show theta phase precession, as seen experimentally [22]. This specific implementation of the model allows quantitative predictions to be made regarding the relationships between the frequency of the local field potential theta rhythm, the frequency of modulation of the grid cell's firing rate, the animal's running speed and the spatial scale of the grid-like firing pattern. These predictions have been broadly confirmed [23].

An important consideration for this model is its ability to maintain stable grids when more realistic noisy oscillators are used. In slice recordings, the variability of interspike intervals of persistent spiking cells in the entorhinal cortex is too high to produce stable grids over the timescales expected from grid cell recordings [37]. However, these slice preparations may eliminate stabilizing properties of networks *in vivo*, as intimated by their lack of the typical *in vivo* theta rhythm. Coupling the activity of populations of grid cells (or VCOs directly) could enable individually unstable oscillations to become more stable collectively [37]. Along these lines, an alternative model of grid cells firing, the continuous attractor model, utilizes recurrent connections between populations of cells to maintain a stable bump of activity [38,39]. In this model however, intricate asymmetric interactions between grid cells that are dependent on running velocity are required to allow the activity bump (and therefore the grid cell firing patterns) to track the movement of the animal. Furthermore, the model does not predict theta phase precession. However, a mechanism which combines oscillatory interference at the cellular level with recurrent connections could improve the stability of the population. The oscillatory interference mechanism would enable activity to track animal movement and provide a natural mechanism for theta phase precession.

OSCILLATORY INTERFERENCE AND REPRESENTATIONS OF SEQUENTIAL ORDER?

In the previous section we have shown how the oscillatory interference model of grid cell firing utilizes velocity-driven variations in frequency to produce a phase code for position that, in turn, can create a spatially modulated firing pattern. Now we consider how the same principles could be applied to findings in primate parietal cortex, specifically cells in

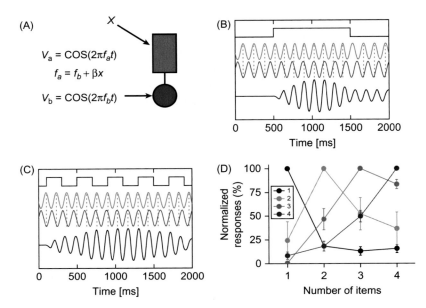

FIGURE 5.3   Oscillatory interference mechanisms for temporal integration and rank order. (A) Basic architecture of an oscillatory interference model. A baseline oscillation vb of constant frequency fb (illustrated as a somatic input, blue) is initially out of phase with an active oscillation va of similar frequency fa (illustrated as a dendritic membrane potential, red). Synaptic input x causes a proportional increase in the active frequency fa proportional to that input. When the two oscillations are combined, an interference pattern is produced (B-C, black line). (B) Interference pattern caused by a transient input x (upper line, black). This causes a transient increase in the frequency of the active oscillation (red) relative to that of the baseline oscillation (blue), resulting in a successively increasing phase difference between the two oscillations (see vertical red dotted lines) consequent interference pattern (lower line, black). (C) If the perception of individual items each causes a similar transient input x (upper line, black), the phase difference between an active oscillation (red) and the baseline oscillation (blue) will track the number of items perceived so far. This will be reflected in an interference pattern (lower line, black) which will peak for a specific number of items, according to the initial phase difference between the oscillations, and the gain of the increase of the active oscillation with synaptic input (β see main text, peak after three items shown here). (D) Normalized responses from cells recorded in intra-parietal sulcus of primates are shown, adapted, with permission, from [4]. Neurons were grouped according to the rank order of the event during which they fired most and averaged separately. Different lines show firing behavior of neurons selective for different rank-order values. The neurons show graded firing rates, tuned to specific values of rank order, with substantial activity for neighboring rank order values.

the intraparietal sulcus whose firing rates show tuning to specific values of the rank order of stimuli ([4,24], see Fig. 5.3 and Chapter 8 in this volume). We note that the intraparietal sulcus has been proposed to be the locus of the interaction between number- and space-related representations [1,2]. It is perhaps of interest that fMRI data from human participants suggesting the presence of grid-like representations in entorhinal cortex also detected a similar signal in the human intraparietal sulcus [25]. This area, and its homolog in rodents, is the subject of current investigations regarding the neural mechanisms of spatial navigation, given its close connectivity to parahippocampal cortices [26,27], and the presence of representations of spatial locations relative to the body [28].

As noted above, the oscillatory interference model works as an integrator: if the perception of each item causes a transient increase in the input to the active oscillation, it will produce a phase shift relative to the baseline oscillation, see Fig. 5.3. In this way, the phase code used for distance in the model of theta phase precession in place cells, or for spatial location in the model for grid cell firing, might encode the number of items presented so far, i.e. a rank order code. Evidence for the phase coding of the sequential order of two items has been found in primate prefrontal cortex [5]. If such a phase code is read out via the interference mechanism (i.e. summing the active and baseline oscillations) it can produce neuronal responses tuned to specific values of rank order, see Fig. 5.3. In the case of sequential foveation of multiple stimuli, such a mechanism could also produce neurons tuned to specific values of numerosity. A single pair of oscillators would produce a repeating representation of number (as the oscillations go cyclically in and out of phase with each other). More generally, by analogy with Fourier analysis, one can see that populations of neurons with appropriately chosen initial phase relationships and values of β could be combined to approximate a single-peaked representation of number, or indeed represent any function of the temporal integration of a given input. Interestingly, the two-dimensional firing patterns of grid cells can also be seen as spatial Fourier components contributing to the single-peaked responses of place cells [40], and combinations of grids with different spatial scales could be used to encode location over extremely large areas [41,42].

Such a representation of order information, where the ordinal position of an event within a sequence is signaled, has also attracted much interest in the context of working memory for serially ordered items. There, representations of serial order information resembling rank order coding have been proposed to drive various models of working memory for serial order (e.g., [29–32]). Reasonably accurate models of human performance in working memory for serial order can be produced by associating item information with these representations of serial order during encoding, reactivating the sequence of activity across them during retrieval, and using a "competitive queuing" mechanism [33,34] for output selection.

SUMMARY AND CONCLUSIONS

We have reviewed the potential for neuronal oscillations to produce phase codes for information that can be derived from simple sensory/motor inputs by a process of temporal integration. Thus it is possible that distance traveled through a place cell's firing field is encoded by its phase of firing relative to the ongoing theta rhythm, given an input that codes for running speed [6,10]. Equally the spatial pattern of firing of grid cells may reflect temporal integration of inputs reflecting running velocity along specific directions [13,14]. More speculatively, we have suggested that representations of serial order and numerosity might be derived in a similar manner from inputs signaling the perception of each new item. Although conclusive proof has yet to be found, these models are at least capable of generating experimentally testable predictions, and have done so in the spatial domain [18,23].

Acknowledgments

We gratefully acknowledge the support of the UK Medical Research Council and the SpaceBrain project of the EU, an MRC Biomedicine PhD studentship to CB and a fellowship of the International Max Planck Research School "The Life Course: Evolutionary and Ontogenetic Dynamics" (LIFE, www.imprs-life.mpg.de) to NS.

References

[1] E.M. Hubbard, et al., Interactions between number and space in parietal cortex, Nature Neurosci. Rev. 6 (2005) 435–448.

[2] V. Walsh., A theory of magnitude: common cortical metrics of time, space and quantity, Trends Cogn. Sci. 7 (2003) 483–488.

[3] T. Hafting, et al., Microstructure of a spatial map in the entorhinal cortex, Nature 436 (2005) 801–806.

[4] A. Nieder, et al., Temporal and spatial enumeration processes in the primate parietal cortex, Science 313 (2006) 1431–1435.

[5] M. Siegel, et al., Phase-dependent neuronal coding of objects in short-term memory, PNAS 106 (2009) 21341–21346.

[6] J. O'Keefe, M.L. Recce, Phase relationship between hippocampal place units and the EEG theta rhythm, Hippocampus 3 (1993) 317–330.

[7] J. O'Keefe, Place units in the hippocampus of the freely moving rat, Exp. neurol. 51 (1976) 78–109.

[8] C.H. Vanderwolf, Hippocampal electrical activity and voluntary movement in the rat, Electroencephalogr. Clin. Neurophysiol. 26 (1969) 407–418.

[9] J. O'Keefe, L. Nadel, The Hippocampus as a Cognitive Map, Oxford University Press

[10] M. Lengyel, et al., Dynamically detuned oscillations account for the coupled rate and temporal code of place cell firing, Hippocampus 13 (2003) 700–714.

[11] J. Huxter, et al., Independent rate and temporal coding in hippocampal pyramidal cells, Nature 425 (2003) 828–832.

[12] C.D. Harvey, et al., Intracellular dynamics of hippocampal place cells during virtual navigation, Nature 461 (2009) 941–946.

[13] N. Burgess, et al., An oscillatory interference model of grid cell firing, Hippocampus 17 (2007) 801–812.

[14] N. Burgess, Grid cells and theta as oscillatory interference: theory and predictions, Hippocampus 18 (2008) 1157–1174.

[15] E. Fransén, et al., Ionic mechanisms in the generation of subthreshold oscillations and action potential clustering in entorhinal layer II stellate neurons, Hippocampus 14 (2004) 368–384.

[16] M.E. Hasselmo, Grid cell mechanisms and function: contributions of entorhinal persistent spiking and phase resetting, Hippocampus 18 (2008) 1213–1229.

[17] M.W. Remme, et al., Democracy-independence trade-off in oscillating dendrites and its implications for grid cells, Neuron 66 (2010) 429–437.

[18] L.M. Giocomo, et al., Temporal frequency of subthreshold oscillations scales with entorhinal grid cell field spacing, Science 315 (2007) 1719–1722.

[19] J.S. Taube, et al., Head-direction cells recorded from the postsubiculum in freely moving rats. I. Description and quantitative analysis, J. Neurosci. 10 (1990) 420–435.

[20] F. Sargolini, et al., Conjunctive representation of position, direction, and velocity in entorhinal cortex, Science 312 (2006) 758–762.

[21] C.N. Boccara, et al., Grid cells in pre- and parasubiculum, Nat. Neurosci. 13 (2010) 987–994.

[22] T. Hafting, et al., Hippocampus-independent phase precession in entorhinal grid cells, Nature 453 (2008) 1248–1252.

[23] A. Jeewajee, et al., Grid cells and theta as oscillatory interference: electrophysiological data from freely moving rats, Hippocampus 18 (2008) 1175–1185.

[24] Sawamura, et al., Numerical representation for action in the parietal cortex of the monkey, Nature 415 (2002) 918–922.

[25] C.F. Doeller, et al., Evidence for grid cells in a human memory network, Nature 463 (2010) 657–661.

[26] P. Byrne, et al., Remembering the past and imagining the future: a neural model of spatial memory and imagery, Psychol. Rev. 114 (2007) 340–375.

[27] J.R. Whitlock, et al., Navigating from hippocampus to parietal cortex, Proc. Natl. Acad. Sci. USA 105 (2008) 14755–14762.

[28] R.A. Anderson, et al., Encoding of spatial location by posterior parietal neurons, Science 230 (1985) 456–458.

[29] N. Burgess, G. Hitch, A revised model of short-term memory and long-term learning of verbal sequences, J. Mem. Lang. 55 (2006) 627–652.

[30] N. Burgess, G. Hitch, Memory for serial order: A network model of the phonological loop and its timing, Psych. Rev. 106 (1999) 551–581.

[31] G.D.A. Brown, et al., Oscillator-based memory for serial order, Psych. Rev. 107 (2000) 127–181.

[32] M. Botvinick, T. Watanabe, From numerosity to ordinal rank: a gain-field model of serial order representation in cortical working memory, J. Neurosci. 27 (2007) 8636–8642.

[33] D. Bullock, Adaptive neural models of queuing and timing in fluent action, Trends Cogn. Sci. 8 (2004) 426–433.

[34] G. Houghton, The problem of serial order: A neural network model of sequence learning and recall, in: R. Dale, C. Mellish, M. Zock, (Eds.), Current Research in Natural Language Generation, Academic Press, pp. 287–319.

[35] V.H. Brun, et al., Progressive increase in grid scale from dorsal to ventral medial entorhinal cortex, Hippocampus 18 (2008) 1200–1212.

[36] H. Hu, et al., Complementary theta resonance filtering by two spatially segregated mechanisms in CA1 pyramidal neurons, J. Neurosci. 29 (2009) 14472–14483.

[37] E.A. Zilli, M.E. Hasselmo, Coupled noisy spiking neurons as velocity-controlled oscillators in a model of grid cell spatial firing, J. Neurosci. 30 (2010) 13850–13860.

[38] M.C. Fuhs, D.S. Touretzky, A spin glass model of path integration in rat medial entorhinal cortex, J. Neurosci. 26 (2006) 4266–4276.

[39] B.L. McNaughton, F.P. Battaglia, O. Jensen, E.I. Moser, M.B. Moser, Path integration and the neural basis of the 'cognitive map', Nature Reviews Neurosci. 7 (2006) 663–678.

[40] T. Solstad, E.I. Moser, G.T. Einevoll, From grid cells to place cells: a mathematical model, Hippocampus 16 (2006) 1026–1031.

[41] I.R. Fiete, Y. Burak, T. Brookings, What grid cells convey about rat location, J. Neurosci. 28 (2008) 6858–6871.

[42] A. Gorchetchnikov, S. Grossberg, Space, time and learning in the hippocampus: how fine spatial and temporal scales are expanded into population codes for behavioral control, Neural Netw. 20 (2007) 182–193.

Population Clocks: Motor Timing with Neural Dynamics*

Dean V. Buonomano*,
Rodrigo Laje*†

*Departments of Neurobiology and Psychology and Brain Research
Institute, University of California, Los Angeles, USA
†Departamento de Ciencia y Tecnología, Universidad Nacional de Quilmes,
Bernal, Argentina

Summary

An understanding of sensory and motor processing will require elucidation of the mechanisms by which the brain tells time. Open questions relate to whether timing relies on dedicated or intrinsic mechanisms and whether distinct mechanisms underlie timing across scales and modalities. Although experimental and theoretical studies support the notion that neural circuits are intrinsically capable of sensory timing on short scales, few general models of motor timing have been proposed. For one class of models, population clocks, it is proposed that time is encoded in the time-varying patterns of activity of a population of neurons. We argue that population clocks emerge from the internal dynamics of recurrently connected networks, are biologically realistic and account for many aspects of motor timing.

THE PROBLEM OF TIME

The fact that people can communicate using a purely temporal code—as occurs when two individuals are receiving and sending messages in Morse code—is one of many pieces of evidence that the nervous system has evolved sophisticated mechanisms to tell time and

*Reprinted from Trends in Cognitive Sciences, Vol 14, Dean V. Buonomano, Rodrigo Laje, Population Clocks: motor timing with neural dynamics, pg 520–527, 2010, with permission from Elsevier.

BOX 6.1

DEDICATED *VS* INTRINSIC NEURAL MECHANISMS OF TIMING

Central to the issue of the neural basis of timing and temporal processing is the question of whether the brain uses dedicated or intrinsic neural mechanisms to tell time [3]. This distinction in many ways revolves around whether there are 'clocks' in the brain, that is, whether there are specialized systems that were 'designed' to tell time and are exclusively devoted to the problem of timing, or whether timing is a general and intrinsic ability of neurons and neural circuits. In this view the same circuits responsible for timing can process other aspects of sensory stimuli simultaneously in a multiplex fashion.

The classic internal clock model, composed of a pacemaker and accumulator, is an instantiation of a dedicated and centralized mechanism of timing [74,75]. By contrast, an example of an intrinsic model is a state-dependent network; in this class of models, sensory timing emerges from the interaction of the time-varying internal state of neural networks with incoming stimuli [13,14]. Although the notion that subsecond timing is performed locally has recently received experimental support [10–12,76], there is still little direct evidence of whether the brain relies on dedicated or intrinsic mechanisms.

---

process temporal information. Indeed, the sheer diversity of time scales and computational problems that rely on temporal processing suggests that multiple mechanisms are in place to tell time. The neural bases of timing have been the subject of a number of recent reviews [1–6] and one critical question addressed in these reviews is whether timing relies on dedicated (specialized) neural mechanisms or on an intrinsic and general ability of networks of neurons (Box 6.1). An equally important and related unanswered question is whether sensory and motor forms of timing share mechanisms and circuits. For example, does the discrimination of a 400- or 500-ms tone rely on the same neural circuitry as that required to generate a 400- or 500-ms depression of a piano key?

Here we focus on the problem of motor timing and, although the issue of whether motor and sensory timing rely on the same circuitry remains open [7–12], we take the position that they generally rely on nonoverlapping networks. Specifically, we argue that motor timing relies on the internal dynamics that arise from the ability of recurrent neural networks to generate self-sustained, complex, time-varying patterns of neural activity, whereas, as previously proposed, sensory timing depends on the interaction between incoming stimuli and time-dependent changes in the internal state of recurrent networks [13,14]. A key distinction between models is the regime of recurrent networks. Motor timing would rely on regimes with strong internal connections capable of self-sustained activity, whereas sensory timing depends on weak connections regimes, which do not support self-perpetuating dynamics. One consequence of these differences is that the circuits involved in motor timing can encompass longer time scales of many seconds.

MOTOR TIMING

Motor control, from catching a ball to playing the piano, requires the production of complex spatiotemporal patterns of muscle activity. The spatial dimension refers to which muscle groups are activated, and the temporal dimension to the timing of activity in relation to other muscle groups or to external sensory stimuli. Most motor tasks, including speech production and playing a musical instrument, require carefully orchestrated movements timed on the order of tens of milliseconds to a few seconds. In the following discussion we focus on motor problems that explicitly require timing, as opposed to the production of any sequence of movements, such as touching different points on a computer screen (which should not be taken to imply that we view the mechanisms as different).

Localization of Motor Timing

Many different neural structures are known to contribute to motor control. Most movements require a precise temporal structure, so it is not surprising that many of these areas have also been implicated in motor timing. One area known to be important for motor coordination, the cerebellum, was one of the first structures hypothesized to contribute to timing [15] and decades of research have provided compelling evidence that the cerebellum is critical to some forms of motor timing. For example, human studies have revealed that patients with cerebellar lesions exhibit a range of general motor coordination deficits [16,17]. In addition, this patient population has impairments in pure motor timing tasks, including the precision (standard deviation) of finger tapping ([18,19], but see [20]). More directly, animal studies have established that the appropriate timing of conditioned eyeblink responses, which are learned as a function of the conditioned stimulus–unconditioned stimulus interval, are abolished by localized cerebellar lesions [21,22].

Other areas also play an important role in timing, particularly in the timing of complex movements associated with recently learned motor tasks. Numerous studies indicate that the basal ganglia are involved in motor timing. Such a role has been inferred in part from pharmacological and Parkinson's disease studies that point to alteration in motor timing on a scale of seconds [23–25]. In addition, imaging studies have revealed changes in activity in the basal ganglia during motor production tasks [5,26–28].

Different neocortical areas have also been implicated in motor timing. Imaging studies have revealed a large, and as yet not agreed on, network of cortical areas that are activated during implicit and explicit timing tasks [5,26]. In addition, electrophysiological studies have revealed time-sensitive neuronal responses during motor timing tasks in many different cortical areas [29–32]. But converging evidence supports the role of pre- and supplementary motor areas [30,33], which are also known to contribute to sequence generation [34]. In subsequent sections, we argue that many aspects of motor timing can be addressed by models based on the internal dynamics of excitatory recurrent networks characteristic of neocortical circuits; for this reason, our discussion focuses primarily on timing in neocortical areas.

MODELS OF TIMING

Timing has long been incorporated into abstract models of motor control [35]. However, relatively few biologically realistic neuron-based models of motor timing have been proposed. The internal clock model (Glossary), for instance, assumes the presence of a pacemaker and accumulator in the brain; however, evidence on the location of the pacemaker or nature of the accumulator has been elusive after several decades of research. Other models of motor control and sequence generation either have simply assumed that there is a population of neurons that fires selectively at different points in time, or have limited their focus to sequence generation [36–38].

Multiple Oscillator Models

Some models are based on the hypothesis that timing arises from a population of elements oscillating at different frequencies [39,40]. These multiple-oscillator models do not require integration or counting of pulses in any of the oscillators, but rely on detecting specific beats or synchronous patterns among the population of oscillators. This detection process can be performed by readout neurons that detect the coincident activity of a subset of oscillators corresponding to a specific point in time.

Labeled-Line Models

Other biologically inspired models have proposed that motor timing might rely on an array of neuronal elements that exhibit a spectrum of different time constants of some neuronal or synaptic property, implementing what is commonly referred to as a labeled line [37,41]. Biologically plausible implementations of such spectral, or delay line, models have been proposed, including the time constants of neurotransmitter receptors [42], the time constant of slow membrane conductances [43,44] and the decay time of inhibitory postsynaptic potentials [45,46]. In these models all elements share a common implementation, but at least one of the variables is set to a different value, which endows each unit with the ability to respond selectively to a different interval. In specialized domains, such as the auditory system of the bat, there is evidence that the duration of inhibitory postsynaptic potentials contributes to the detection of temporal windows of <50 ms. However, it seems unlikely that such mechanisms can be generalized to complex forms of temporal processing that require discrimination of the patterns generated by consecutive intervals and there is little evidence that they are involved in motor timing.

Population Clock Models

A distinct class of neural-based models proposes that time is both generated and represented in a population of essentially identical neurons [47]. Here timing emerges from the dynamics of the entire network and is encoded in the population vector of neurons that are active at any specific point in time (Box 6.2). Critical to the notion of a population clock is that the activity of neurons in the network is time-varying and that output units can be trained to recognize specific patterns of activity within the population clock network and thus serve as a readout of time. Note that as with multiple oscillator or labeled-line models, time can ultimately be read by a single output neuron; importantly, however, timing per se

BOX 6.2

POPULATION CLOCKS

For a population clock it is assumed that a group of neurons exhibit time-varying activity and that each point in time is coded by a unique pattern of activity in the network [47–49]. Consider a group of three neurons (N1–N3) that in response to a start signal (t = 0) reliably produce a specific pattern of firing (represented as the number of spikes in a time bin, Box 6.2 Fig. 1). In this example, each time step can be identified by a unique combination of the number of spikes in each cell: bin t1 has the spike signature [0,3,1], whereas bin t3 has the signature [3,0,3]. Time can be read by output units that receive synapses from all the neurons in the population clock network if the synaptic weights are adjusted appropriately. For example, to generate a motor response at time bin 3, the synapses onto the output neuron from N1 and N3 should be fairly strong, because both these neurons are strongly active at this time bin and not at the others (note that the synapses cannot be too strong because then the output would fire at other time points as well). In a network in which thousands of neurons fire in a time-varying manner, it is easy to establish a population code for time. A simple instantiation of a population clock consists of a chain of neural activity in a population of neurons. In this case, each point in time would be represented by the activity of a single or a small population of neurons [52,53,77,78]. This sparse code (which is essentially a labeled line) for time has been observed experimentally [79].

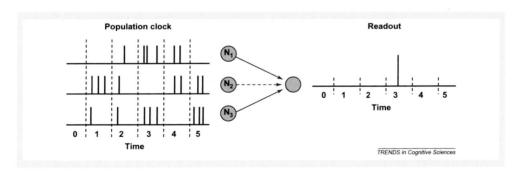

BOX 6.2 FIGURE 1   Reading a population clock.

(the clock) is an emergent property of the network; in other words, it relies on the interaction between many units, and the time scale over which a network can time far exceeds the longest time constant of the individual elements.

The critical challenge to any population clock model is how a dynamic population of active neurons would be generated. In principle, any recurrent neural network (Glossary) can produce time-varying activity, which can be thought of as a neural trajectory (Box 6.3). Assuming

BOX 6.3

NEURAL TRAJECTORY

A complex and time-varying pattern of activity in a population of neurons can be thought of as a neural trajectory in neural space. In a network with three neurons, all possible patterns of activity can be represented in three-dimensional space, where each axis corresponds to the instantaneous firing rate of each neuron (or the presence or absence of a spike at each point in time). In a network composed of 1500 neurons, the trajectory takes place in a 1500-dimensional space that can nevertheless be visualized using dimension reduction methods. Figure 1 illustrates the simulated activity of 10 units from the network shown in Box 6.3 Fig. 1. In this simulation the activity of each unit is bounded between −1 and 1. The activity of the entire network can be visualized as a 3D neural trajectory by plotting the first three components of a principal component (PC) analysis on the activity of the entire network. Note that in the neural trajectory time is represented as a color gradient. Thus, the rate of color change provides information about the speed of the trajectory or the rate of change of the firing pattern. The same point in time could be represented by many nearby points in state space, and the output or downstream neurons that would fire with the network is somewhere within this cloud of points. The effect of both the input pulse and the output pulse (fed back) on the network activity is evident as large excursions in PC space.

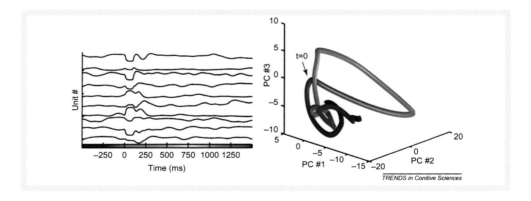

BOX 6.3 FIGURE 1   Low-dimensional representation of a high-dimensional neural trajectory. Left: Activity of 10 sample units in a network of 1500 units. Right: Plot of the first three components of a Principal Component analysis on the activity of the whole network.

that a network is in the appropriate regime, a given population of active neurons A could activate population B and so on, leading to the pattern A→B→C→. . ., in which each letter corresponds to a distinct but possibly overlapping population of neurons. The second challenge to population clock models is that the trajectory must be able to be elicited in a robust and reproducible manner. We address these two issues below and show that the dynamics of a recurrently connected neural network can subserve a population clock in neocortical circuits.

DYNAMICS IN RECURRENT NETWORKS

The first population clock model was proposed by Michael Mauk in the context of the cerebellum [48–50]. In his model, a continuously changing population of granule cells encodes time, and specific time points are read by Purkinje cells that detect distinct patterns of granule cell activity. It is proposed that the evolving trajectory of granule cells arises from the interaction between a tonic input into the cerebellum and the internal state defined by the granule and Golgi cells. Granule cells excite, and are inhibited by, Golgi cells, thus creating a negative feedback loop that can result in a dynamic pattern of granule cell activity and implement a population clock. Realistic large-scale simulations based on spiking neurons have revealed that it accounts for many of the experimental observations on timing of eyeblink conditioning [50,51].

The cerebellar circuitry is unique for its absence of recurrent excitatory activity. Consequently, the cerebellum cannot sustain a self-maintaining and dynamic pattern of activity in the absence of an external input. By contrast, neocortical networks are characterized by robust excitatory connections capable of sustaining internal dynamics.

Critical to the dynamics of recurrent neural networks, and whether they support self-maintaining activity, is the average strength of the recurrent synaptic weights. It is evident that if the internal weights are on average very weak, there is little coupling between the units and in response to a brief input (or start signal) network activity will quickly fade away (this is generally the regime a state-dependent network model operates in for sensory timing). By contrast, if the recurrent weights are strong, it is easy to imagine that in response to a brief input the network could potentially enter a self-maintaining activity regime (which could be steady state, periodic or non-periodic in nature). Thus, the weights within the recurrent network are critical to the behavior of the circuits. Yet setting these weights in theoretical models has proven challenging because of the highly nonlinear nature of the internal dynamics. It has recently been shown that biologically plausible learning rules facilitate the development of spatiotemporal patterns that can be used for motor timing, although the patterns are simple and limited in time scale [52,53].

It seems likely that the brain harnesses the computational potential of recurrent networks by using the complex dynamic regimes that are ideally suited to generate population clocks. However, these regimes are precisely those that lead to chaotic dynamics [54]. In a system with chaotic activity, there is a critical dependence on the initial conditions and noise: tiny perturbations to the system will make the trajectory of a system diverge exponentially in time. It has been shown that feedback is a powerful tool for controlling the chaotic dynamics of nonlinear systems [55,56] and advances have provided insights into how recurrent networks can both generate complex patterns—that could be used for a population clock—and not be dominated by chaos. In the context of artificial networks, Jaeger and Haas [57] demonstrated that carefully controlled feedback can be used to generate complex

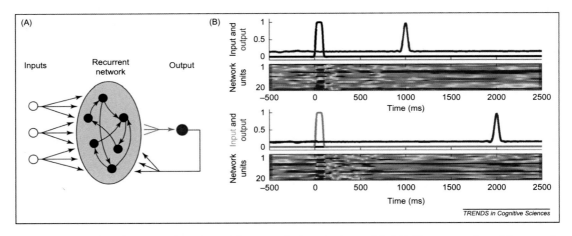

FIGURE 6.1   Simple interval timing with a population clock model. (A) The network architecture is composed of a population of 1500 firing-rate units (time constant 10 ms), all of which are connected to a single output unit that also provides feedback to the network. Each target output pattern (blue traces in panels b and c) is triggered by a combination of the three inputs to the network. Tonic input 3 sets the network to a ready state (not shown) and then pulses at inputs 1 or 2 are used to elicit either of two different trained output patterns. Training consists of adjusting the weights from the recurrent units onto the output unit (red arrows). Network architecture and the learning rule used to train the weights onto the output units were similar to those reported by Sussillo and Abbott [58]. The network connectivity matrix was sparse with probability of connection p = 0.1 and synaptic strength factor g of 1.35. A noise 'current' from a uniform distribution with a maximal amplitude of 0.001 was present in all the units. It should be stressed that although these simulations are biologically realistic in the sense that they rely on the interaction of neuron-like units, future work must use spiking units with realistic synaptic dynamics. In addition, the precise role of feedback when using non-periodic targets must be examined; indeed, similar results can be obtained in the absence of feedback. (B) The upper panel shows the activity of the output unit trained to generate a delayed pulse-like response at 1 s to input 1 at time zero (traces from three different trials are overlaid). The lower panel shows a sample of the activity of the units in the recurrent network. The activity level of the recurrent units is color-coded and bounded between −1 (blue) and 1 (red). Input and output activity is normalized to the corresponding maximum value. (c) The same network shown in panel b generates an output pulse at 2 s in response to a pulse in input 2 at time zero (three traces overlaid).

yet reproducible patterns. Sussillo and Abbott [58] recently extended this approach and demonstrated how it can be used for networks that are spontaneously active (strong internal connections). The recurrent weights in these networks are set at random (with specific distributions), avoiding the need to carefully set them. Pivotal, however, are the weights of the recurrent network onto the output unit, because they define the output and feedback (if present). Different supervised learning rules have been used to effectively adjust these weights, and using both firing-rate and spiking models it has been shown that recurrent networks with feedback can generate time-varying outputs [57–60].

Recurrent networks with strong internal coupling, with or without feedback, are potentially well suited for timing tasks. Consider a psychophysical task that requires a subject to press a button 1 s after stimulus 1 and 2 s after stimulus 2. As shown in Fig. 6.1, a recurrent network can be trained to solve this task; in response to a brief input representing stimulus 1,

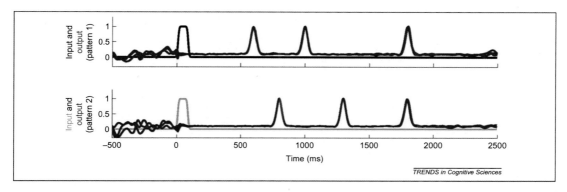

FIGURE 6.2 Production of two different complex temporal patterns. The same type of network as shown in Figure 1 was trained to produce two different temporal patterns, each consisting of three pulses. When pattern 1 is elicited, the output unit pulses at 600, 1000 and 1800 ms, whereas in pattern 2 the output pulses at 800, 1300 and 1800 ms. Pattern 1(2) is triggered by input 1(2). Three traces for each input are overlaid. Input and output are normalized to the corresponding maximum value. The synaptic strength factor was 1.4.

a well-timed response is generated with a delay of 1 s (the time constant of the elements in this circuit was 10 ms, which, along with the size of the network, determines the upper limit that can be timed [61]). Importantly, in response to a different input (stimulus 2) the same network can be trained to generate a response at 2 s. Specifically, different input patterns will set the network along different neural trajectories, and thus the same points in absolute time can be encoded in different network states, depending on the task. An inherent strength of this approach is that it provides a general and robust model of motor timing. As shown in Fig. 6.2, it is easy to use the same network to generate temporal patterns (multiple time responses from the same output unit), each triggered by different inputs. Thus, the same network can be used to generate multiple distinct temporal or spatiotemporal output patterns [58].

NEURAL CORRELATES OF TIMING

In vivo electrophysiology studies have revealed neural correlates of time in animals when performing tasks involving implicit or explicit timing tasks. One robust observation is that some neurons exhibit a more or less linear change in firing rate as time elapses (increasing or decreasing). Such ramping activity has been observed in different parts of the brain, including the prefrontal, parietal and motor areas [30,33,62,63]. Typically, graded firing rates that peak at the time of an anticipated response are observed. Although activity in ramping neurons correlates with time, these neurons might not be keeping track of absolute time, but might reflect temporal expectation of or preparation for a motor response, which in most tasks is linearly related to absolute time. In a study in which the delay before an expected event was drawn from a bimodal distribution, the firing rate of ramping neurons did not increase monotonically with time, but increased and decreased according to expected likelihood [64]. Thus, ramping neurons might not be telling time, but using temporal information from other areas to anticipate or react to events [5].

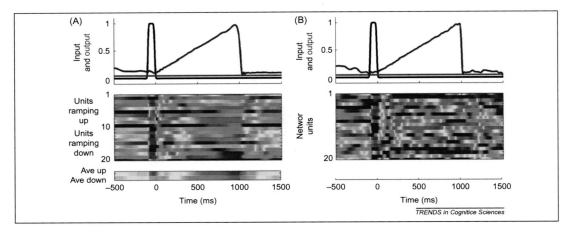

FIGURE 6.3 Ramping output. Dynamics or the regime in the network is governed in part by the synaptic strength factor g that scales the weights in the recurrent network. A value of g < 1 leads to decaying activity, whereas values greater than 1 make the network increasingly chaotic. (A) In this simulation, the internal synaptic strength factor was at the low end of the g > 1 regime (g = 1.25) and the output unit was trained to ramp linearly from 0 to 1000 ms. In this regime, many of the neurons in the recurrent network exhibit approximately linear (graded color transitions) responses during the trained interval (raster plot shows selected units grouped according to whether they exhibit a positive or negative slope; average of ramping up and ramping down units shown below). Input and output are normalized to the corresponding maximum value. (B) When the internal synaptic coupling is increased (g = 1.5) the internal dynamics of the network becomes more complex and most recurrent units do not ramp in a linear fashion; however, the output unit can still be trained to exhibit a linear ramp. The weights of the output to recurrent units were bounded between −0.5 and 0.5 in these simulations.

It has been proposed that the linear ramping of neuronal firing rate is a result of neuronal or network mechanisms [65–67]. Importantly, the population clock model based on recurrent networks with feedback can account for the experimentally observed ramping responses. Specifically, the readout units of these networks can be trained to exhibit ramping behavior. As shown in Fig. 6.3, when the strength of the coupling within the recurrent network is relatively weak (but still self-sustaining), the activities of neurons in the population clock can themselves be positively or negatively ramping. On the other hand, with strong internal coupling (rich internal dynamics), activity in the population clock is highly variable. In both cases, however, the weights of synapses onto the readout unit can be set so that it fires in a linear manner.

In addition to linearly ramping neurons, electrophysiological studies have revealed a rich diversity of time varying firing rate profiles, including neurons that fire at select time intervals or in a complex aperiodic manner [31,68–70]. These observations are what would be expected for a population clock. Indeed, some of these studies have shown that a linear classifier (readout unit) can be used to decode time based on the profiles of the experimentally recorded neurons, thus effectively implementing a population clock.

CONCLUDING REMARKS

Population clock models propose that motor timing arises from the time-varying activity of a population of neurons. We suggest that the dynamics required for a population clock arises naturally in recurrent cortical networks as a result of the internally generated dynamics, but many critical issues regarding the control and regimes of neural dynamics in these networks remain to be resolved. Importantly, a given network can embark on different neural trajectories depending on the task at hand; this provides a powerful mechanism to generate a large number of timed motor patterns (Figs 6.1, 6.2). Thus, in principle, different well-timed sequences of key presses on a piano can be generated by triggering different sets of inputs to the recurrent network and appropriately adjusting the weights from the recurrent units to a small set of output units.

The population clock framework falls into the category of intrinsic models, and thus many of its predictions require resolution of whether different forms of timing rely on distinct circuits. Recent psychophysical experiments have suggested that sensory timing is local, which indirectly supports the notion that sensory and motor timing are distinct [10–12], but future research must further examine this issue. Population clocks predict that the spatial and temporal components of motor patterns can be inextricably linked; once a spatiotemporal motor pattern is learned, it could be difficult to transfer the learned temporal structure to a new spatial pattern (e.g., a different sequence of finger movements). This is because both the spatial and temporal patterns are jointly encoded in the internal dynamics of the network (although population clocks could be used to code for absolute time if different external stimuli triggered a master neural trajectory). Whereas some psychophysical data are consistent with this suggestion [71,72], it remains an unresolved issue [73]. Ultimately, however, validation of the population clock model will require electrophysiological confirmation of the predicted complex neural trajectories and demonstration that modification of these trajectories alters behavioral timing.

GLOSSARY

Dedicated Models of Timing

Models in which timing relies on specialized and modular neural mechanisms that are primarily dedicated to temporal processing. Man-made clocks are examples of dedicated timers, as is the internal clock model of timing (Box 6.1).

Internal clock model

One of the first models of timing. The pulses of a central oscillator or a pacemaker are integrated by an accumulator, thus providing an explicit and linear metric of time (Box 6.1).

Intrinsic models of timing

Models in which timing is a general and inherent ability of neural networks. In these models the same neural circuit processes temporal information and other feature dimensions of stimuli. An example of an intrinsic mechanism for timing is the state-dependent network model (Box 6.1).

Labeled-line model

Phenomenological model in which it is assumed that different cells represent different time periods or delays. Labeled lines are often used in models that require timing but that are agnostic as to the neural mechanisms of timing.

Motor timing

Production of timed motor actions or responses, ranging from a simple timed motor response to complex spatiotemporal patterns of muscle activation. Examples of motor timing include self-paced finger tapping, interval reproduction, sending a message in Morse code and playing the piano.

Population clock model

Models in which a given point in time is represented by a unique spatial pattern of activity within a neural network. Distinct patterns of activity in the network unfold over time (Box 6.2).

Recurrently connected neural networks

Networks in which the connections can form a loop; thus, activity in a single unit could indirectly feedback onto itself. Most neocortical circuits exhibit robust recurrent connectivity and many theoretical models, including state-dependent networks, rely on recurrent connectivity. Recurrent networks stand in contrast to feed-forward models such as a standard multilayer perceptron.

Sensory timing

Processing or discrimination of stimuli based on temporal features. A typical sensory timing task is discrimination of the duration or interval of auditory or visual stimuli.

Spatiotemporal pattern

Pattern of neural activation that unfolds both in time and space, where space refers to different neurons in a circuit.

State-dependent network model

Model that proposes that cortical networks are inherently capable of processing spatial and temporal information in the range of hundreds of milliseconds as a result of state-dependent network properties imposed by ongoing activity (the active state) and time-dependent cellular and synaptic properties (the hidden state).

Acknowledgments

The authors are supported by the NIMH (DVB) and the Fulbright Foundation and CONICET (RL).

References

[1]   M.D. Mauk, D.V. Buonomano, The neural basis of temporal processing, Annu. Rev. Neurosci. 27 (2004) 307–340.

[2] C.V. Buhusi, W.H. Meck, What makes us tick? Functional and neural mechanisms of interval timing, Nat. Rev. Neurosci. 6 (2005) 755–765.

[3] R.B. Ivry, J.E. Schlerf, Dedicated and intrinsic models of time perception, Trends Cogn. Sci. 12 (2008) 273–280.

[4] V. van Wassenhove, Minding time—an amodal representational space for time perception, Phil. Trans. R. Soc. B 364 (2009) 1815–1830.

[5] J. Coull, A. Nobre, Dissociating explicit timing from temporal expectation with fMRI, Curr. Opin. Neurobiol. 18 (2008) 137–144.

[6] R.B. Ivry, R.M.C. Spencer, The neural representation of time, Curr. Opin. Neurobiol. 14 (2004) 225–232.

[7] R.B. Ivry, R.E. Hazeltine, Perception and production of temporal intervals across a range of durations—evidence for a common timing mechanism, J. Exp. Psychol. Hum. Percept. Perform. 21 (1995) 3–18.

[8] S.W. Keele, R.B. Pokorny, D.M. Corcos, R. Ivry, Do perception and motor production share common timing mechanisms: a correctional analysis, Acta Psychol. (Amst.) 60 (1985) 173–191.

[9] H. Merchant, et al., Do we have a common mechanism for measuring time in the hundreds of millisecond range? Evidence from multiple-interval timing tasks, J. Neurophysiol. 99 (2008) 939–949.

[10] A. Johnston, et al., Spatially localized distortions of event time, Curr. Biol. 16 (2006) 472–479.

[11] D. Burr, et al., Neural mechanisms for timing visual events are spatially selective in real-world coordinates, Nat. Neurosci. 10 (2007) 423–425.

[12] U.R. Karmarkar, D.V. Buonomano, Timing in the absence of clocks: encoding time in neural network states, Neuron 53 (2007) 427–438.

[13] D.V. Buonomano, W. Maass, State-dependent computations: spatiotemporal processing in cortical networks, Nat. Rev. Neurosci. 10 (2009) 113–125.

[14] D.V. Buonomano, M.M. Merzenich, Temporal information transformed into a spatial code by a neural network with realistic properties, Science 267 (1995) 1028–1030.

[15] V. Braitenberg, Is the cerebellar cortex a biological clock in the millisecond range? Prog. Brain Res. 25 (1967) 334–346.

[16] J. Hore, et al., Cerebellar dysmetria at the elbow, wrist, and fingers, J. Neurophysiol. 65 (1991) 563–571.

[17] D. Timmann, et al., Failure of cerebellar patients to time finger opening precisely causes ball high–low inaccuracy in overarm throws, J. Neurophysiol. 82 (1999) 103–114.

[18] R.B. Ivry, S.W. Keele, Timing functions of the cerebellum, J. Cogn. Neurosci. 1 (1989) 136–152.

[19] R. Spencer, et al., Disrupted timing of discontinuous but not continuous movements by cerebellar lesions, Science 300 (2003) 1437–1439.

[20] D.L. Harrington, et al., Does the representation of time depend on the cerebellum? Effect of cerebellar stroke, Brain 127 (2004) 561–574.

[21] S.P. Perrett, et al., Cerebellar cortex lesions disrupt learning dependent timing of conditioned eyelid responses, J. Neurosci. 13 (1993) 1708–1718.

[22] J. Raymond, et al., The cerebellum: a neuronal learning machine? Science 272 (1996) 1126–1132.

[23] W.H. Meck, Neuropharmacology of timing and time perception, Brain Res. Cogn. Brain Res. 3 (1996) 227–242.

[24] C.V. Buhusi, W.H. Meck, Differential effects of methamphetamine and haloperidol on the control of an internal clock, Behav. Neurosci. 116 (2002) 291–297.

[25] C.R. Jones, et al., Basal ganglia, dopamine and temporal processing: performance on three timing tasks on and off medication in Parkinson's disease, Brain Cogn. 68 (2008) 30–41.

[26] P.A. Lewis, R.C. Miall, Distinct systems for automatic and cognitively controlled time measurements: evidence from neuroimaging, Curr. Opin. Neurobiol. 13 (2003) 250–255.

[27] M. Jahanshahi, et al., The substantia nigra pars compacta and temporal processing, J. Neurosci. 26 (2006) 12266–12273.

[28] D.L. Harrington, et al., Temporal processing in the basal ganglia, Neuropsychology 12 (1998) 3–12.

[29] D.J. Crammond, J.F. Kalaska, Prior information in motor and premotor cortex: activity during the delay period and effect on premovement activity, J. Neurophysiol. 84 (2000) 986–1005.

[30] S. Roux, et al., Context-related representation of timing processes in monkey motor cortex, Eur. J. Neurosci. 18 (2003) 1011–1016.

[31] M.A. Lebedev, et al., Decoding of temporal intervals from cortical ensemble activity, J. Neurophysiol. 99 (2008) 166–186.

[32] D. Schoppik, et al., Cortical mechanisms of smooth eye movements revealed by dynamic covariations of neural and behavioral responses, Neuron 58 (2008) 248–260.

[33] A. Mita, et al., Interval time coding by neurons in the presupplementary and supplementary motor areas, Nat. Neurosci. 12 (2009) 502–507.

[34] J. Tanji, Sequential organization of multiple movements: involvement of cortical motor areas, Annu. Rev. Neurosci. 24 (2001) 631–651.

[35] D.R. Gentner, Timing of skilled motor-performance—tests of the proportional duration model, Psychol. Rev. 94 (1987) 255–276.

[36] E. Salinas, Rank–order–selective neurons form a temporal basis set for the generation of motor sequences, J. Neurosci. 29 (2009) 4369–4380.

[37] J.E. Desmond, J.W. Moore, Adaptive timing in neural networks: the conditioned response, Biol. Cybern. 58 (1988) 405–415.

[38] M.M. Botvinick, D.C. Plaut, Short-term memory for serial order: a recurrent neural network model, Psychol. Rev. 113 (2006) 201–233.

[39] C. Miall, The storage of time intervals using oscillating neurons, Neural Comput. 1 (1989) 359–371.

[40] M.S. Matell, W.H. Meck, Cortico-striatal circuits and interval timing: coincidence detection of oscillatory processes, Cogn. Brain Res. 21 (2004) 139–170.

[41] S. Grossberg, N.A. Schmajuk, Neural dynamics of adaptive timing and temporal discrimination during associative learning, Neural Netw. 2 (1989) 79–102.

[42] J.C. Fiala, et al., Metabotropic glutamate receptor activation in cerebellar Purkinje cells as substrate for adaptive timing of the classically conditioned eye-blink response, J. Neurosci. 16 (1996) 3760–3774.

[43] S.L. Hooper, et al., A computational role for slow conductances: single-neuron models that measure duration, Nat. Neurosci. 5 (2002) 552–556.

[44] J.M. Beggs, et al., Prolonged synaptic integration in perirhinal cortical neurons, J. Neurophys. 83 (2000) 3294–3298.

[45] W.E. Sullivan, Possible neural mechanisms of target distance coding in the auditory system of the echolocating bat *Myotis lucifugus*, J. Neurophysiol. 48 (1982) 1033–1047.

[46] B. Aubie, et al., Computational models of millisecond level duration tuning in neural circuits, J. Neurosci. 29 (2009) 9255–9270.

[47] D.V. Buonomano, U.R. Karmarkar, How do we tell time? Neuroscientist 8 (2002) 42–51.

[48] D.V. Buonomano, M.D. Mauk, Neural network model of the cerebellum: temporal discrimination and the timing of motor responses, Neural Comput. 6 (1994) 38–55.

[49] M.D. Mauk, N.H. Donegan, A model of Pavlovian eyelid conditioning based on the synaptic organization of the cerebellum, Learn. Mem. 4 (1997) 130–158.

[50] J.F. Medina, et al., Timing mechanisms in the cerebellum: testing predictions of a large-scale computer simulation, J Neurosci. 20 (2000) 5516–5525.

[51] J.F. Medina, M.D. Mauk, Simulations of cerebellar motor learning: computational analysis of plasticity at the mossy fiber to deep nucleus synapse, J Neurosci. 19 (1999) 7140–7151.

[52] J.K. Liu, D.V. Buonomano, Embedding multiple trajectories in simulated recurrent neural networks in a self-organizing manner, J. Neurosci. 29 (2009) 13172–13181.

[53] I.R. Fiete, et al., Spike-time-dependent plasticity and heterosynaptic competition organize networks to produce long scale free sequences of neural activity, Neuron 65 (2010) 563–576.

[54] H. Sompolinsky, et al., Chaos in random neural networks, Phys. Rev. E 61 (1988) 259–262.

[55] K. Pyragas, Continuous control of chaos by self-controlling feedback, Phys. Lett. A 170 (1992) 421–428.

[56] S. Boccaletti, et al., The control of chaos: theory and applications, Phys. Rep. 329 (2000) 103–197.

[57] H. Jaeger, H. Haas, Harnessing nonlinearity: predicting chaotic systems and saving energy in wireless communication, Science 304 (2004) 78–80.

[58] D. Sussillo, L.F. Abbott, Generating coherent patterns of activity from chaotic neural networks, Neuron 63 (2009) 544–557.

[59] W. Maass, et al., Computational aspects of feedback in neural circuits, PLoS Comput. Biol. 3 (2007) e165.

[60] H. Jaeger, et al., Special issue on echo state networks and liquid state machines, Neural Netw. 20 (2007) 287–289.

[61] S. Ganguli, et al., Memory traces in dynamical systems, Proc. Natl. Acad. Sci. U. S. A. 105 (2008) 18970–18975.

[62] C.D. Brody, et al., Timing and neural encoding of somatosensory parametric working memory in macaque prefrontal cortex, Cereb. Cortex 13 (2003) 1196–1207.

[63] M.I. Leon, M.N. Shadlen, Representation of time by neurons in the posterior parietal cortex of the macaque, Neuron 38 (2003) 317–327.

[64] P. Janssen, M.N. Shadlen, A representation of the hazard rate of elapsed time in the macaque area LIP, Nat. Neurosci. 8 (2005) 234–241.

[65] D. Durstewitz, Self-organizing neural integrator predicts interval times through climbing activity, J Neurosci. 23 (2003) 5342–5353.

[66] D. Durstewitz, G. Deco, Computational significance of transient dynamics in cortical networks, Eur. J. Neurosci. 27 (2008) 217–227.

[67] C.K. Machens, et al., Flexible control of mutual inhibition: a neural model of two-interval discrimination, Science 307 (2005) 1121–1124.

[68] D.Z. Jin, et al., Neural representation of time in cortico-basal ganglia circuits, Proc. Natl. Acad. Sci. U. S. A. 106 (2009) 19156–19161.

[69] M.S. Matell, et al., Interval timing and the encoding of signal duration by ensembles of cortical and striatal neurons, Behav. Neurosci. 117 (2003) 760–773.

[70] E. Pastalkova, et al., Internally generated cell assembly sequences in the rat hippocampus, Science 321 (2008) 1322–1327.

[71] J.X. O'Reilly, et al., Acquisition of the temporal and ordinal structure of movement sequences in incidental learning, J. Neurophysiol. 99 (2008) 2731–2735.

[72] J.C. Shin, R.B. Ivry, Concurrent learning of temporal and spatial sequences, J. Exp. Psychol. Learn. Mem. Cogn. 28 (2002) 445–457.

[73] F. Ullen, S.L. Bengtsson, Independent processing of the temporal and ordinal structure of movement sequences, J Neurophysiol. 90 (2003) 3725–3735.

[74] C.D. Creelman, Human discrimination of auditory duration, J. Acoust. Soc. Am. 34 (1962) 582–593.

[75] M. Treisman, Temporal discrimination and the indifference interval: implications for a model of the 'internal clock', Psychol. Monogr. 77 (1963) 1–31.

[76] M.G. Shuler, M.F. Bear, Reward timing in the primary visual cortex, Science 311 (2006) 1606–1609.

[77] D.V. Buonomano, A learning rule for the emergence of stable dynamics and timing in recurrent networks, J. Neurophysiol. 94 (2005) 2275–2283.

[78] M.S. Goldman, Memory without feedback in a neural network, Neuron 61 (2009) 621–634.

[79] R.H.R. Hahnloser, et al., An ultra-sparse code underlies the generation of neural sequence in a songbird, Nature 419 (2002) 65–70.

7

Discrete Neuroanatomical Substrates for Generating and Updating Temporal Expectations

Laboratoire de Neurobiologie de la Cognition, Université de Provence and
CNRS, Marseille, France

Summary

Being able to predict when relevant events are likely to occur improves speed and accuracy of information processing. In a series of fMRI investigations, we have found that temporally informative cues consistently activate the left intraparietal sulcus. This activation was independent of the laterality (left/right) or type (hand/eye) of motor response and was observed equally during non-motor perceptual tasks, whether temporal expectation was established endogenously via temporal cues or exogenously via stimulus speed. Yet temporally predictive information can also be conveyed by the unidirectional nature of time's flow. As the objective probability, and hence subjective expectancy, of event onset increases with increased waiting time ("hazard function"), activity in the right prefrontal cortex increases. Taken together, these data reveal distinct neural substrates for the initial generation of a temporal expectation (left intraparietal sulcus) *vs* subsequent updating of the expectation as a function of time itself (right prefrontal).

Time, the fourth dimension, surrounds us. We know how long events lasted in the past and can use this to predict how long they should last in the future. Moreover, accurate estimates of time are integral to a wide range of cognitive processes, from motion perception to action planning. Given this ubiquity, the term "timing" is, perhaps unsurprisingly, used

Space, Time and Number in the Brain.
DOI: 10.1016/B978-0-12-385948-8.00007-4

© 2011 Elsevier Inc. All rights reserved.

to cover a number of quite distinct cognitive processes [1–5]. For instance, it can be used to refer to *how long* an event lasts (estimation of duration), *when* an event is likely to occur (expectation of event onset or offset) or the relative *order* of successive events (temporal order judgement).[1]

Yet despite this "sense" of time, we have no sensory receptors that are specifically dedicated for perceiving time. It is an almost uniquely intangible sensation: we do not perceive time in the same way that we perceive sound, color, or even spatial location. So how is time represented in the brain? The past decade has witnessed an exponential increase in the number of neuroscientific investigations of time. However, the ambiguity of the term "timing" has given rise to some confusion in the literature. While some authors report a cortico-striatal network for timing (Box 7.1), others specifically highlight right prefrontal [31–33] or right parietal [34] cortices, whereas still others report activation of left parietal cortex [35,36]. However, by functionally characterizing the timing processes measured in each of these studies, it becomes clear that there is, in fact, some degree of consistency within the literature. For example, Supplementary Motor Area (SMA), right inferior frontal cortex, and basal ganglia are most often recruited when estimating stimulus *duration* (Box 7.1), parietal cortex in left [37] or right [34] hemisphere is implicated in judging the temporal *order* of consecutive events, whereas left intraparietal sulcus (IPS) more particularly is activated by the temporal *expectation* that an event will occur at a particular moment in time [35,38], before the temporal interval has even started to elapse.

In this chapter, I will focus specifically on the last of these temporal processes: temporal expectation. In fact, temporal expectation has been associated not only with activity in parietal cortex [35,39], but also with activity in right prefrontal cortex [33,40,41], visual cortex [42,43], premotor cortex [44,45], primary motor cortex [46,47] and temporal cortex [48]. By functionally decomposing the notion of "temporal expectation", I hope to demonstrate that apparent inconsistencies in the neuroscientific literature are simply the result of an insufficient level of cognitive specification. By distinguishing the metric of time from the *use* of this metric to generate and/or update expectations and, furthermore, by differentiating different ways in which temporal expectations can be established (e.g., by learned associations or by the very passage of time itself), the neuroanatomical differences across different experimental paradigms can, in fact, be plausibly reconciled.

TEMPORAL ORIENTING OF ATTENTION: TEMPORAL EXPECTATIONS DERIVED FROM LEARNED CUES

In everyday life we rarely time events without recourse to a prior temporal context. Instead, we frequently use previously acquired temporal information, collated over repeated presentations, to determine whether a particular event is shorter or longer, or

---

[1] Making a distinction between ordinal and metrical characteristics of time may provide a useful guiding principle for studying the potential overlap [6] between time, space and number. On the one hand, temporal order appears akin to ordinal number properties or spatial direction (e.g., left-right, up-down), while on the other temporal duration appears more analogous to cardinal number properties or spatial distance (e.g., near-far) or extent (e.g., small-big).

BOX 7.1

WHERE IS STIMULUS DURATION REPRESENTED IN THE BRAIN?

Explicit estimates of stimulus duration can be measured by motor timing tasks, in which the timed duration is indexed by a sustained, delayed or periodic motor act, or by perceptual timing tasks, in which one stimulus duration is judged to be shorter or longer than another. Functional neuroimaging studies have particularly highlighted the role of preSMA and the dorsal striatum of the BG, during both motor timing (e.g., [7–11]) and perceptual timing tasks (e.g., [12–16]). Furthermore, activity in either region is independent of the effector used to register a motor timing estimate [17] or the sensory modality of a perceptual timing estimate [15], suggesting a context-independent representation of time. Although durations in the tens to hundreds of milliseconds range are likely to be represented locally in a variety of context-specific processing areas [18–21], timing of longer durations, necessitating attentional and mnemonic resources, additionally

engage a more context-independent co-operative timing network [4]. Psychological models of timing usually comprise several discrete functional components: a sensory signal is timed, its value is stored in working memory, where it can then be compared to previous, or subsequent, values. These discrete functional components appear to map onto distinct anatomical nodes of a timing network. Timing a currently elapsing duration activates SMA (a) [22–24], storing this duration into working memory engages BG (b) [12,16,22,25], while later comparison processes activate right prefrontal and superior temporal cortices (c) [12,16,22,23]. Although the cerebellum has also often been implicated in timing, it appears to play a more context-dependent role [26], being activated principally by motor timing tasks [7–9,17,27,28] but only rarely by perceptual timing tasks and then, only when these implicate sub-second durations [15,23,29,30].

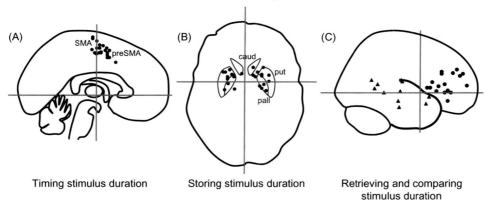

| Timing stimulus duration | Storing stimulus duration | Retrieving and comparing stimulus duration |

BOX 7.1 FIGURE 1 Each point represents the site of peak amplitude of a timing-induced activation cluster taken from a representative sample of motor and perceptual timing studies in healthy volunteers (see J.T. Coull, R.K. Cheng, W.H. Meck, The neuroanatomical and neurochemical substrates of timing. Neuropsychopharmacology, 36 (2011) 3–25, for details). These templates should be considered as "glass" brains and activations were actually spread in either the (A, C) medial/lateral or (B) dorsal/ventral direction.

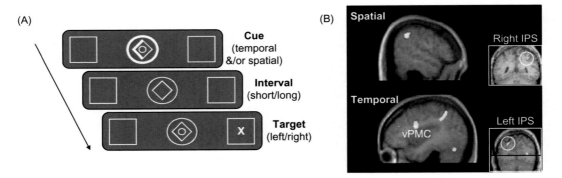

FIGURE 7.1 **Temporal orienting of attention activates left IPS.** (A) Subjects detected targets appearing in one of two peripheral locations (left/right) after one of two inter-stimulus intervals (short/long). Prior to target presentation, one of four attentional cues manipulated subjects' expectations of where and/or when the target would appear by predicting its eventual spatial location and/or the temporal delay before it appears. In the example illustrated here, the SPACE–TIME cue directs subjects' attention to the left location and to a long cue-target interval. The target appears unexpectedly on the right (i.e. spatially invalid) but, as expected, after 1500 ms (i.e. temporally valid). (B) A direct comparison of spatial to temporal orienting revealed hemispheric lateralization in posterior parietal cortex, centered around the IPS. Spatial orienting preferentially activated right IPS whereas temporal orienting preferentially activated left IPS. When subjects made use of spatially and temporally informative cues simultaneously, both right and left parietal cortices were preferentially activated. In addition to the parietal activation, temporal orienting also selectively activated left ventral premotor cortex (vPMC). Adapted from [35], Coull and Nobre (1998) Where and When to Pay Attention: The Neural Systems for Directing Attention to Spatial Locations and to Time Intervals as Revealed by Both PET and fMRI, Journal of Neuroscience 18, 7426-7435, with permission from Society for Neuroscience.

occurs sooner or later, than expected [49]. Imagine approaching an amber traffic light. If it has not turned red within 2 or 3 s, we would estimate it as lasting longer than expected, and so may assume it is faulty. Essentially, current duration is compared to a template of expected duration that is held in long-term memory. Yet, temporal expectations not only inform us as to the relative duration of current events, but can also actively optimize behavior. In our example, expectation of the moment at which the amber traffic light will turn red is established through repeated association of visual cues with event timing, with color essentially acting as a temporally informative cue. Such temporal cues allow us to predict when an imminent event is likely to occur, thus optimizing behavior (e.g., by adjusting driving/braking behavior accordingly).

Behavior is optimized not only by knowing when an event will appear, but also by knowing *where* it will appear. The beneficial effects of spatially informative cues have been extensively studied with variants of the spatial orienting paradigm developed by Posner *et al.* [50], in which a pre-cue predicts the spatial location of an upcoming target. Inspired by the success and ubiquity of this paradigm, my colleague Kia Nobre and I devised a temporal analog of Posner's task, in which pre-cues predicted the temporal interval at which a target would be presented (Fig. 7.1a). We found a behavioral advantage for temporal cues that was qualitatively similar to that for spatial cues (e.g., [35,51–53]). We hypothesized that similar attentional mechanisms operated in both domains, such that resources were directed in an anticipatory way to the location in space *or the moment in time* at which the event was predicted to happen, thus enhancing selectivity of processing at that point. However, although these processes appeared mechanistically similar, they had quite distinct neural substrates. Comparing spatial to temporal orienting directly, functional neuroimaging data revealed a hemispheric lateralization in parietal cortex for directing attention within the spatial *vs* temporal domain. Spatial orienting activated right inferior parietal cortex, confirming numerous previous studies, whereas temporal orienting preferentially activated left inferior parietal cortex, specifically around the IPS [35].

However, a very similar region of left parietal cortex has also been implicated in directing attention towards a particular motor effector [54,55]. Therefore, the left parietal activation in our study could potentially reflect incidental motor attentional processes that were differentially recruited during the temporal *vs* spatial orienting tasks.[2] To explore this possibility, we designed a variation of the Posner task in which motor and temporal components of response preparation were independently cued within the same experimental paradigm [56] (Fig. 7.2A). Temporal orienting activated left IPS even when the motor effector used to respond to target onset could not be prepared in advance, and did so whether the target required a manual or saccadic response and whether this response was left- or right-sided (Fig. 7.2A). We therefore concluded that left IPS represents an effector-independent substrate for temporal orienting and does not simply represent a motor attention confound during the temporal orienting task. The functional significance of the neural overlap in left IPS for temporal and motor cueing remains unclear, but may reflect "neural recycling" of motor circuits for representations of time (see also Box 7.2).

If left IPS plays a fundamental role in temporal orienting, whatever the ontogenetic roots of this activation are, it should be activated even when temporal cues are being used to optimize *non-motor* task goals. Prior behavioral studies have confirmed that temporal orienting not only confers faster responses [35,52] but also enables faster and more accurate stimulus perception [64–66]. We therefore designed a perceptual version of the temporal orienting task (Fig. 7.2B) and compared its neural correlates directly to those of the motor version used previously [67]. As hypothesized, temporal orienting activated left IPS whether temporal cues were being used to react more quickly or, critically, to enhance perceptual sensitivity (Fig. 7.2B).

Yet demonstrating that left IPS is consistently activated by temporal cues does not reveal *how* these cues exert their performance-enhancing effects. In the attentional literature, it has long been known that simply attending to a specific stimulus feature, even in the absence of physical change, modulates activity in basic feature-specific processing areas (e.g., [68–70]). Spatial attention in particular is known to affect neural activity via top-down inputs, and to bias information processing for stimuli appearing at attended locations [69]. Analogous attentional control mechanisms could also be activated during directed *temporal* orienting. For example, left IPS could modulate activity in task-specific sensorimotor areas so as to bias information processing for stimuli appearing at the cued time. To test this hypothesis, we examined how the functional connectivity of left IPS changed as a function of task context [67]. During the motor version of the temporal orienting task, left IPS activity covaried with premotor activity, but during the perceptual version it covaried with visual extrastriate

[2]Although this is unlikely since response preparation requirements were matched across the temporal and spatial tasks.

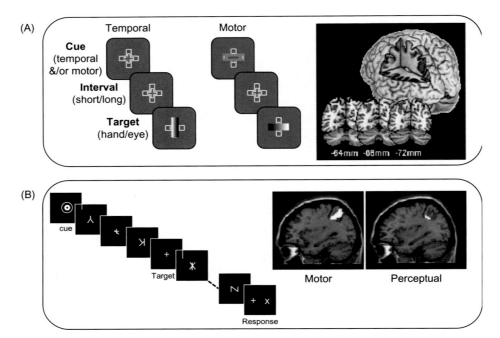

FIGURE 7.2 **Left IPS activation is effector- and task-independent.** (A) A temporal and/or motor cue predicted that a target would appear after a short/long delay and/or would require a manual/saccadic response. Target orientation specified the type of motor response to be given: vertical targets specified button-presses and horizontal targets specified saccades. Target shading specified the side of response, such that left/right responses corresponded to the lighter side of the target. Two example trials are illustrated. In the temporal condition, the cue predicts a short delay but with no indication of whether a manual or saccadic response will be required. After the cued delay, the target appears and specifies a leftward manual response. In the motor condition, the cue predicts a saccadic response then, after a variable delay, the target specifies a rightward saccadic response. Temporal orienting activated left IPS, whether the target was eventually detected with a manual button-press or an ocular saccade and whether responses were lateralized to the left or right side. Spatial co-ordinates (mm) define the anatomical location of each slice in the y-dimension. Adapted from [56], Cotti *et al.* (2011) Functionally dissociating temporal and motor components of response preparation in left intraparietal sulcus, *Neuroimage* 54:1221–1230, with permission from Elsevier. (B) A temporal cue predicted that a target (+ or ×) would appear after a short (illustrated here) or long temporal delay whereas neutral cues provided no temporally predictive information. Targets could appear after an empty interval, in which case a speeded motor response was required (Motor Detection task), or embedded within a serial stream of rapidly presented visual distractors (illustrated here), in which case a delayed perceptual discrimination was required (Perceptual Discrimination task). Left IPS was activated by temporal orienting during both Motor Detection and Perceptual Discrimination tasks (adapted from [67], Davranche *et al.*, in press).

activity. Such task-specificity supports the proposition that left IPS could exert a top-down attentional influence on context-specific processing areas.

Yet in order to bias information processing at the cued time, left IPS would first require a representation of elapsed time. How does it get this representation? One possibility is that time is encoded directly within parietal cortex. While this may be true for tasks requiring spatial saccades in particular (e.g., [39]), a process known to depend upon parietal functioning, it is unlikely to provide a general, context-independent representation of time. First,

---

BOX 7.2

NEURONAL RECYCLING OF ACTION CIRCUITS FOR TIME

Why would SMA and basal ganglia, which are traditionally regarded as action structures, be recruited during timing? This neuroanatomical overlap is especially intriguing given that these structures are engaged even during perceptual timing tasks, for which the timing process is independent of the motor response. Moreover, perturbation of the dopaminergic D2 receptor system, commonly associated with motor function, has also been associated with both motor and perceptual timing [57,58], therefore suggesting a further neurochemical overlap between the two processes. One possibility for such neural overlap is that of "neuronal recycling", with action circuits being recruited to estimate time in much the same way that, for example, spatial areas are recruited to estimate number [59]. Indeed, from a developmental point of view, our sense of time may be acquired via motor strategies. For example, when told "Dinner in 15 minutes" a young child may ask "How long's 15 minutes"? A common reply might be "The time it takes to walk to school". Such an everyday scenario illustrates how a sense of time may be instantiated with a sense of time may be instantiated with a reference to a motor act. This has been tested more formally in the laboratory, where it has been shown that three-year-old infants are unable to reproduce the duration of one action (e.g., "press the button for 3 seconds") with another action (e.g., "squeeze the bulb for the same amount of time"), though by the age of five years such temporal abstraction from the motor act is possible [60]. Moreover, three-year-olds' production of relative time intervals (shorter/longer) is more accurate when instructed implicitly via action instructions ("press harder than before") than explicitly via timing instructions ("press longer than before") [61]. Children have also been shown to display "collateral" motor activity, such as following a path in the experimental room or producing rhythmic finger movements, to help them accurately mark time [62]. These data suggest that action circuits are engaged early in development in order to build up and acquire representations of time, a "recycling" idea that was first suggested by Guyau as long ago as 1890 [63]. The ontogenetic roots of our notion of time could therefore be embedded within action circuits.

---

numerous electrophysiological studies have demonstrated similar indices of elapsed time in a variety of other (task-specific) cortical regions (e.g., [42,46]). Second, fMRI data show that left parietal cortex is not differentially activated as a function of duration, but instead responds to whether a temporal prediction can be made, or not [71].

An alternative, more likely explanation, is that time is encoded within patterns of neural activity in context-specific processing areas (e.g., [3,72]). In our perceptual temporal orienting task, for example, the neural signature of elapsed time could be instantiated in visual cortex [42,43]. Then, when the cued time was reached, a bottom-up signal from visual cortex to IPS would activate attentional mechanisms in parietal cortex which would, in turn, feedback into visual cortex so as to bias information processing. Since functional connectivity analysis does not specify the direction of influence, we cannot yet conclude whether our data represent a bottom-up or top-down mechanism, or indeed some combination of the two.

RHYTHM AND SPEED: TEMPORAL EXPECTATIONS DERIVED FROM REGULAR STIMULUS DYNAMICS

Spatial and temporal information can also be integrated to predict the time of a certain event at a particular location in space. For example, speed and distance to an amber traffic light can be used to estimate the time at which we are likely to reach it (and therefore to judge whether we will get there before it turns red). However, in contrast to the endogenous pre-cues used in the temporal orienting task (described above), temporal expectation is established in a more exogenous manner here, by the dynamics of stimulus motion itself. In the laboratory, this process has often been simulated by collision judgement tasks. Assmus et al.[36,73] asked subjects to estimate whether two balls, moving in perpendicular directions, would eventually collide. Essentially subjects were predicting object position at particular moments in time. fMRI data revealed that collision judgements selectively activated left-lateralized inferior parietal cortex, in an area similar to that activated by our temporal orienting studies.

We investigated this further using an ecologically valid Time to Contact (TTC) task [74], in which subjects viewed a braking car approaching a wall from either an allocentric (bird's eye view) or egocentric (driver's point of view) perspective. The constant speed of deceleration allowed subjects to predict where and when the car would stop, and so to judge whether the car was braking sufficiently to avoid a collision. Whether the scenario was seen from an allocentric or egocentric viewpoint, TTC estimates selectively activated left-lateralized inferior parietal and ventral premotor cortex, a result strongly reminiscent of our temporal attentional orienting findings. Despite widely differing visual and task demands, both the temporal orienting and collision judgment paradigms encouraged subjects to use temporal information (attentional cues or stimulus motion) to predict what would happen at a precise moment in time. Mechanistically, we suggested that the inherent temporal structure of the moving stimulus generated a temporal expectation, which could then be used to deploy attentional resources to the moment in time the target was expected to appear. In support of this, prior studies have repeatedly demonstrated that targets appearing at the time predicted by a prior visuospatial [75,76] or auditory [77] rhythmic context are processed more quickly and accurately than targets appearing before the entrained time.

THE HAZARD FUNCTION: TEMPORAL EXPECTATIONS DERIVED FROM THE FLOW OF TIME ITSELF

Temporal expectations can be formed not only by sensory stimuli, such as arbitrary pre-cues or the speed of stimulus motion, but also by the very passage of time itself. Imagine arriving at a red traffic light. The longer you wait, the more you expect the light to change color sometime soon. This ever-heightening temporal expectation illustrates the experimental phenomenon of the "hazard function": the increasing conditional probability over time that an event will occur given that it has not already occurred [78,79]. The hazard function relies on the predictive power of the unidirectional flow of time: since time flows inexorably forward an event that we expect to occur, but has not yet occurred, must do so at some time in the future.

Several electrophysiological studies in monkeys have used hazard functions to index temporal expectancies at the neuronal level. Neural activity has been shown to vary dynamically as a function of the hazard function in early visual [42], primary motor [80] or parietal cortices [39] during tasks of visual discrimination, pointing or spatial saccades, respectively. A variety of different brain regions can therefore represent temporal expectancies, with anatomical localization depending upon the specific characteristics of the task in question. Yet whole-brain functional neuroimaging in humans has allowed a broader picture to be revealed. Although activity in task-specific primary visual cortex varied in line with the hazard function during a visual speeded detection task [43], thus confirming the electrophysiological data, so too did activity in a variety of higher association areas, comprising SMA (see also [81]) and right prefrontal and parietal cortices.

Right prefrontal cortex in particular has previously been implicated in the hazard function in a series of methodologically diverse studies of the variable foreperiod paradigm. In this paradigm, the delay (or "'foreperiod'") between a warning cue and a response signal varies from one trial to the next within a block of trials. Empirically, as the foreperiod gets longer, signal reaction times get faster [82,83] due to the hazard function. Using TMS and neuropsychological approaches, Vallesi and colleagues [40,41] demonstrated that right prefrontal cortex was necessarily implicated in the monitoring or updating of conditional probabilities over time, with fMRI data confirming that the magnitude of prefrontal activation correlated with the size of the behavioral benefit afforded by longer foreperiods [33]. In fact, these results confirmed and extended an earlier fMRI finding of our own, in which we compared the neural substrates of premature *vs* delayed targets in the temporal orienting task [71]. In this task, a target that does not appear at the short delay as expected, must appear at the long one. Subjects therefore have the opportunity to voluntarily shift their attention to the later time-point, rendering the behavioral costs of unexpectedly delayed trials negligible (Fig. 7.3A) [35,52]. Whereas premature targets were accompanied by increased activation in visual cortex, consistent with automatic capture of attention by unexpected sensory events (bottom-up attentional mechanism), delayed targets were accompanied by increased activation of right ventrolateral and dorsolateral prefrontal cortex (Fig. 7.3B), consistent with processes of response inhibition and voluntary control of attention respectively (top-down attentional mechanism). Our results, together with those of Vallesi *et al.* [33,40,41,84], suggest that right prefrontal cortex may be critical specifically for the *updating* of temporal expectancies, as conditional probabilities change over time throughout the course of a trial, rather than being critical for their deployment in the first place. This hypothesis fits well with the monitoring role of the right prefrontal cortex in working memory [85,86].

CONCLUSIONS: GENERATING *VS* UPDATING TEMPORAL EXPECTATIONS

In this chapter, I have distinguished temporal expectations established by memorized cues, by the regularity of stimulus dynamics or by the predictive nature of the flow of time itself.

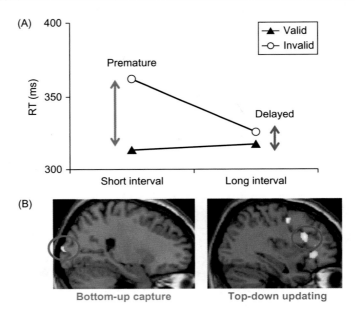

FIGURE 7.3 **The hazard function activates right PFC.** (A) The behavioral benefits of temporal orienting (speeded RTs for validly *vs* invalidly cued targets) are far greater at short intervals than at long ones. If a target has not yet appeared at the short interval when expected (i.e. a delayed target) then the unidirectional flow of time itself provides temporally predictive information (i.e. the hazard function) that allows attentional resources to be redirected towards the later time-point, thus removing the cost of being invalidly cued. (Data from [35].) (B) Targets appearing earlier than expected (i.e. premature targets) activate posterior visual cortex, suggesting bottom-up, reflexive attentional capture. Conversely, delayed targets (for which the hazard function reduced the behavioral cost of invalid cueing) activate a cluster of right frontal areas, suggesting the involvement of a top-down, voluntary attentional mechanism. Adapted from [71], Coull *et al.* (2000) Orienting attention in time: behavioural and neuro-anatomical distinction between exogenous and endogenous shifts, *Neuropsychologia* 38, 808–819, with permission from Elsevier.

I propose that temporal cues, or a regular temporal structure, make use of learned associations to *generate* initial expectations about the time of stimulus onset. By contrast, the hazard function makes use of the flow of time itself to *update* these expectations on-line. In the former, an input (e.g., a learned temporal cue) provokes a stereotyped, pre-defined output (e.g., expectation that an event will occur at time *t*), and is therefore akin to a *feedforward* anticipatory mechanism (see also [87]). In the latter, sensory *feedback* from the environment (i.e. the presence or absence of the target) is integrated with the flow of time itself allowing these expectations to be updated on a moment-by-moment basis. Taken as a whole, the neuroscientific results outlined above indicate that fixed temporal expectations are initially generated in a feedforward manner by left parietal cortex but are then monitored, and potentially updated on-line as a function of elapsing time and sensory feedback, by right prefrontal cortex (Fig. 7.4). Although these two temporal mechanisms can be distinguished, both functionally and neuroanatomically, most temporal expectation tasks will comprise a combination of both processes: an initial expectation will be generated (based on a learned cue or prior stimulus timing) but then modified as a result of time on task and incoming information.

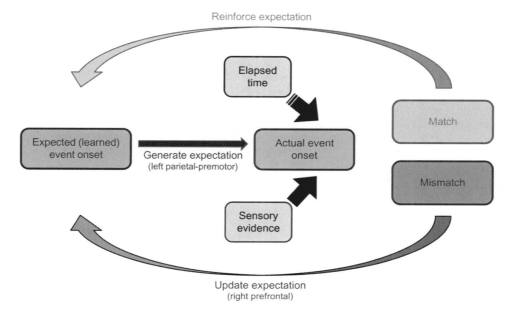

FIGURE 7.4 Generating and updating temporal expectations. Learned temporal cues (e.g., temporal orienting paradigms) or stimulus dynamics (e.g., rhythmic stimulus presentation) allow the time of onset of an event to be predicted, thus *generating* temporal expectations. A representation of elapsed time can be integrated with the sensory evidence that the event occurred to determine whether the event occurred at the expected time. If the event occurred when expected (match), the learned temporal expectation is reinforced. If however, the event did not occur when expected (mismatch), temporal expectations can be *updated* to create a new expectation for the next possible time-point. Even when there is no learned temporal expectation (e.g., a variable foreperiod paradigm) expectations can still be continuously generated and updated due to the predictive nature of the unidirectional flow of time (the "hazard function"). Neuroimaging evidence demonstrates that fixed temporal expectations are initially generated by left parietal cortex but are monitored, and potentially updated on-line, by right prefrontal cortex. Sensory evidence would be provided by activity in feature-specific processing areas whereas elapsed time may be represented in both context-dependent (e.g., visual cortex) and context-independent (e.g., preSMA) brain areas.

Electroencephalographic (EEG) recordings of the Contingent Negative Variation (CNV), a slow wave indexing temporal preparation, further support a hemispheric dissociation for these two mechanisms. When CNV was measured over right frontocentral electrodes, it increased steadily with elapsing duration until the offset of stimulus presentation [88]. By contrast, if measured over left frontal [88], parietal [89] or premotor [90] electrodes, the CNV increased only up until the memorized or learned duration had been reached, even though stimulus presentation actually continued beyond this point. Interestingly, Serrien *et al.* [91] have proposed a very similar hemispheric dissociation in the control of action, with left and right hemispheres differentially contributing to feedforward (planning of future limb dynamics) *vs* feedback (use of sensory input to control final limb position) aspects of motor control, respectively. This mirrors the results outlined above for temporal expectations: left parietal cortex is implicated when prior temporal information (e.g., cues or a rhythmic context) is used to generate an initial expectation of stimulus onset or duration, but right prefrontal cortex is recruited when sensory feedback is used to modify this expectation.

However, in order for right prefrontal cortex to monitor whether the initial temporal expectation has been verified, an estimate of elapsing time is needed. While many studies suggest that elapsed time is represented in context-specific processing areas [19,21,39,42,43,46], at least for durations of a few hundred milliseconds or less [19,92,93], many others (see Box 7.1) suggest time engages certain key areas, such as SMA or basal ganglia, in a more context-*independent* manner. Intriguingly, SMA, in particular, has also recently been implicated in the hazard function [43,81]. Cui *et al.* [81] reported a phasic increase in SMA activity at expected target durations, the amplitude of which varied as a function of temporal expectation. Notably, the SMA activity did not evolve dynamically as the duration unfolded, but instead momentarily indexed the *integrated* temporal expectancy that the target would have occurred at that particular moment. It is therefore possible that the SMA activity typically observed during duration estimation does not simply reflect an estimate of time-in-passing, but rather a more complex integration of elapsing time with expected time. It may be that whenever we time an event we simultaneously invoke an appropriate temporal context, meaning that rather than blindly accumulating temporal pulses as they occur, with no end-point in sight, instead we time events by constantly comparing current duration to expected duration [49].

In conclusion, the neural substrates for temporal expectation differ depending upon the nature of the predictive mechanism being measured. Left parietal cortex makes use of previously learned information to generate a fixed expectation of the timing of future events (feedforward), whereas right prefrontal cortex uses current sensory information to update these expectations on-line as a function of the flow of time itself (feedback). Future studies should aim to fully parse this temporal control system into its constituent functional and neural components. This may shed light onto the more conceptual issue of whether perceptual timing ever occurs without the influence of temporal expectation. It is possible that accurately timing an event's duration may necessarily activate a temporal context or representation that provides an implicit expectation of the event's likely duration.

References

[1] J.A. Michon, The complete time experiencer, in: J.A. Michon, J.L.J. Jackson, (Eds.), Time, Mind and Behavior, Springer, Berlin, Germany, (1985).

[2] E. Poppel, A hierarchical model of temporal perception, Trends Cog. Sci. 1 (1997) 56–61.

[3] D.V. Buonomano, UR Karmarkar, How do we tell time? Neuroscientist 8 (2002) 42–51.

[4] R.B. Ivry, J.E. Schlerf, Dedicated and intrinsic models of time perception, Trends Cogn. Sci. 12 (7) (2008) 273–280.

[5] V. van Wassenhove, Minding time in an amodal representational space, Philos. Trans. R. Soc. Lond. B. Biol. Sci. 364 (2009) 1815–1830.

[6] V. Walsh, A theory of magnitude: common cortical metrics of time, space and quantity, Trends Cogn. Sci. 7 (2003) 483–488.

[7] D. Bueti, V. Walsh, C. Frith, G. Rees, Different brain circuits underlie motor and perceptual representations of temporal intervals, J. Cogn. Neurosci. 20 (2) (2008) 204–214.

[8] M. Jahanshahi, C.R. Jones, G. Dirnberger, C.D. Frith, The substantia nigra pars compacta and temporal processing, J. Neurosci. 26 (47) (2006) 12266–12273.

[9] K.J. Jantzen, F.L. Steinberg, J.A. Kelso, Brain networks underlying human timing behavior are influenced by prior context, Proc. Natl. Acad. Sci. USA 101 (17) (2004) 6815–6820.

[10] P.A. Lewis, A.M. Wing, P.A. Pope, P. Praamstra, R.C. Miall, Brain activity correlates differentially with increasing temporal complexity of rhythms during initialisation, synchronisation, and continuation phases of paced finger tapping, Neuropsychologia 42 (10) (2004) 1301–1312.

[11] S.M. Rao, D.L. Harrington, K.Y. Haaland, J.A. Bobholz, R.W. Cox, J.R. Binder, Distributed neural systems underlying the timing of movements, J. Neurosci. 17 (14) (1997) 5528–5535.

[12] S.M. Rao, A.R. Mayer, D.L. Harrington, The evolution of brain activation during temporal processing, Nat. Neurosci. 4 (3) (2001) 317–323.

[13] A.M. Ferrandez, L. Hugueville, S. Lehericy, J.B. Poline, C. Marsault, V. Pouthas, Basal ganglia and supplementary motor area subtend duration perception: an fMRI study, Neuroimage 19 (4) (2003) 1532–1544.

[14] J.T. Coull, F. Vidal, B. Nazarian, F. Macar, Functional anatomy of the attentional modulation of time estimation, Science 303 (5663) (2004) 1506–1508.

[15] L.Y. Shih, W.J. Kuo, T.C. Yeh, O.J. Tzeng, J.C. Hsieh, Common neural mechanisms for explicit timing in the sub-second range, Neuroreport 20 (10) (2009) 897–901.

[16] D.L. Harrington, J.L. Zimbelman, S.C. Hinton, S.M. Rao, Neural modulation of temporal encoding, maintenance, and decision processes, Cereb Cortex (2010). doi:10.1093/cercor/bhp194

[17] S.L. Bengtsson, H.H. Ehrsson, H. Forssberg, F. Ullen, Effector-independent voluntary timing: behavioural and neuroimaging evidence, Eur. J. Neurosci. 22 (12) (2005) 3255–3265.

[18] D. Bueti, B. Bahrami, V. Walsh, The sensory and association cortex in time perception, J. Cogn. Neurosci. 20 (6) (2008) 1054–1062.

[19] A. Johnston, D.H. Arnold, S. Nishida, Spatially localized distortions of event time, Curr. Biol. 16 (5) (2006) 472–479.

[20] U.R. Karmarkar, D.V. Buonomano, Timing in the absence of clocks: encoding time in neural network states, Neuron 53 (3) (2007) 427–438.

[21] M.C. Morrone, J. Ross, D. Burr, Saccadic eye movements cause compression of time as well as space, Nat. Neurosci. 8 (7) (2005) 950–954.

[22] J.T. Coull, B. Nazarian, F. Vidal, Timing, storage, and comparison of stimulus duration engage discrete anatomical components of a perceptual timing network, J. Cogn. Neurosci. 20 (12) (2008) 2185–2197.

[23] B. Morillon, C.A. Kell, A.L. Giraud, Three stages and four neural systems in time estimation, J. Neurosci. 29 (47) (2009) 14803–14811.

[24] F. Macar, F. Vidal, L. Casini, The supplementary motor area in motor and sensory timing: evidence from slow brain potential changes, Exp. Brain Res. 125 (1999) 271–280.

[25] D.L. Harrington, L.A. Boyd, A.R. Mayer, D.M. Sheltraw, R.R. Lee, M. Huang, et al., Neural representation of interval encoding and decision making, Cogn. Brain Res. 21 (2) (2004) 193–205.

[26] P.A. Lewis, R.C. Miall, Distinct systems for automatic and cognitively controlled time measurement: evidence from neuroimaging, Curr. Opin. Neurobiol. 13 (2) (2003) 250–255.

[27] V.B. Penhune, R.J. Zattore, A.C. Evans, Cerebellar contributions to motor timing: a PET study of auditory and visual rhythm reproduction, J. Cogn. Neurosci. 10 (6) (1998) 752–765.

[28] L. Jancke, R. Loose, K. Lutz, K. Specht, N.J. Shah, Cortical activations during paced finger-tapping applying visual and auditory pacing stimuli, Cogn. Brain Res. 10 (1–2) (2000) 51–66.

[29] P.A. Lewis, R.C. Miall, Brain activation patterns during measurement of sub- and supra-second intervals, Neuropsychologia 41 (12) (2003) 1583–1592.

[30] J.R. Tregellas, D.B. Davalos, D.C. Rojas, Effect of task difficulty on the functional anatomy of temporal processing, Neuroimage 32 (1) (2006) 307–315.

[31] M. Wiener, P. Turkeltaub, H.B. Coslett, The image of time: a voxel-wise meta-analysis. Neuroimage 49 (2010) 1728–1740.

[32] P.A. Lewis, R.C. Miall, Remembering the time: a continuous clock. Trends Cogn. 10 (2006) 401–406.

[33] A. Vallesi, A.R. McIntosh, T. Shallice, D.T. Stuss, When time shapes behavior: fMRI evidence of brain correlates of temporal monitoring, J. Cogn. Neurosci. 21 (6) (2009) 1116–1126.

[34] L. Battelli, A. Pascual-Leone, P. Cavanagh, The 'when' pathway of the right parietal lobe, Trends Cogn. Sci. 11 (5) (2007) 204–210.

[35] J.T. Coull, A.C. Nobre, Where and when to pay attention: the neural systems for directing attention to spatial locations and to time intervals as revealed by both PET and fMRI, J. Neurosci. 18 (18) (1998) 7426–7435.

[36] A. Assmus, J.C. Marshall, A. Ritzl, J. Noth, K. Zilles, G.R. Fink, Left inferior parietal cortex integrates time and space during collision judgments, Neuroimage 20 (Suppl 1) (2003) S82–88.

[37] B. Davis, J. Christie, C. Rorden, Temporal Order Judgments Activate Temporal Parietal Junction, J. Neurosci. 29 (2009) 3182–3188.

[38] M. Wiener, P. Turkeltaub, H.B. Coslett, Implicit timing activates the left inferior parietal cortex. Neuropsychologia 48 (2010) 3967–3971.

[39] P. Janssen, M.N. Shadlen, A representation of the hazard rate of elapsed time in macaque area LIP, Nat. Neurosci. 8 (2) (2005) 234–241.

[40] A. Vallesi, A. Mussoni, M. Mondani, R. Budai, M. Skrap, T. Shallice, The neural basis of temporal preparation: insights from brain tumor patients, Neuropsychologia 45 (12) (2007a) 2755–2763.

[41] A. Vallesi, T. Shallice, V. Walsh, Role of the prefrontal cortex in the foreperiod effect: TMS evidence for dual mechanisms in temporal preparation, Cereb Cortex 17 (2) (2007b) 466–474.

[42] G.M. Ghose, J.H.R. Maunsell, Attentional modulation in visual cortex depends on task timing, Nature 419 (2002) 616–620.

[43] D. Bueti, B. Bahrami, V. Walsh, G. Rees, Encoding of temporal probabilities in the human brain, J. Neurosci. 30 (12) (2010) 4343–4352.

[44] K.H. Mauritz, S.P. Wise, Premotor cortex of the rhesus monkey: neuronal activity in anticipation of predictable environmental events, Exp. Brain Res. 61 (1986) 229–244.

[45] C. Lucchetti, L. Bon, Time-modulated neuronal activity in the premotor cortex of macaque monkeys, Exp. Brain Res. 141 (2001) 254–260.

[46] L. Renoult, S. Roux, A. Riehle, Time is a rubberband: neuronal activity in monkey motor cortex in relation to time estimation, Eur. J. Neurosci. 23 (2006) 3098–3108.

[47] B.E. Kilavik, J. Confais, A. Ponce-Alvarez, M. Diesmann, A. Riehle, Evoked potentials in motor cortical LFPs reflect task timing and behavioral performance, J. Neurophysiol. (2010). in press

[48] B. Anderson, D.L. Sheinberg, Effects of temporal context and temporal expectancy on neural activity in inferior temporal cortex, Neuropsychologia 46 (2008) 947–957.

[49] J.T. Coull, Neural substrates of mounting temporal expectation, PLoS Biol. 7 (8) (2009) e1000166.

[50] M.I. Posner, C. Snyder, B.J. Davidson, Attention and the detection of signals, J. Exp. Psychol. 109 (1980) 160–174.

[51] J.T. Coull, A.C. Nobre, C.D. Frith, The noradrenergic alpha2 agonist clonidine modulates behavioural and neuroanatomical correlates of human attentional orienting and alerting. Careb Cortex 11 (2011) 73–84.

[52] I.C. Griffin, C. Miniussi, A.C. Nobre, Orienting attention in time, Front Biosci. 6 (2001) D660–71.

[53] I.C. Griffin, C. Miniussi, A.C. Nobre, Multiple mechanisms of selective attention differential modulation of stimulus processing by attention to space or time. Neuropsychologia. 40 (2002) 2325–2346.

[54] M.F.S. Rushworth, P.D. Nixon, S. Renowden, D.T. Wade, R.E. Passingham, The left parietal cortex and motor attention, Neuropsychologia 35 (1997) 1261–1273.

[55] M.F. Rushworth, H. Johansen-Berg, S.M. Gobel, J.T. Devlin, The left parietal and premotor cortices: motor attention and selection, Neuroimage. 20 (S1) (2003) S89–100.

[56] J. Cotti, G. Rohenkohl, M. Stokes, A.C. Nobre, J.T. Coull (2010) Functionally dissociating temporal and motor components of response preparation in left intraparietal sulcus. Neuroimage. 54 (2011) 1221–1230.

[57] W.H. Meck, Neuropharmacology of timing and time perception, Cogn Brain Res 3 (3–4) (1996) 227–242.

[58] T.H. Rammsayer, Are there dissociable roles of the mesostriatal and mesolimbocortical dopamine systems on temporal information processing in humans? Neuropsychobiology 35 (1) (1997) 36–45.

[59] S. Dehaene, L. Cohen, Cultural recycling of cortical maps, Neuron 56 (2007) 384–398.

[60] S. Droit-Volet, A.-C. Rattat, Are time and action dissociated in young children's time estimation? Cog. Dev. 14 (1999) 573–595.

[61] S. Droit-Volet, Time estimation in young children: an initial force rule governing time production, J. Exp. Child Psychol. 68 (1998) 236–249.

[62] Pouthas V. (1985) Timing behaviour in young children: A developmental approach to conditioned speed responding. In: Michon JA and

[63] J.A. Michon, V. Pouthas, J.L. Jackson (eds) Guyau and the idea of time. Elsevier: Amsterdam (1989).

[64] Á. Correa, J. Lupiáñez, B. Milliken, P. Tudela, Endogenous temporal orienting of attention in detection and discrimination tasks, Percept Psychophys. 66 (2) (2004) 264–278.

[65] A. Correa, J. Lupianez, P. Tudela, Attentional preparation based on temporal expectancy modulates processing at the perceptual level, Psychon. Bull. Rev. 12 (2) (2005) 328–334.

[66] S. Martens, A. Johnson, Timing attention: Cuing target onset interval attenuates the attentional blink, Mem Cognit. 33 (2) (2005) 234–240.

[67] K. Davranche, B. Nazarian, F. Vidal, J.T. Coull, Orienting attention in time activates left intraparietal sulcus for perceptual, as well as, motor task goals. J. Cog. Neuro. (in press).

[68] M. Corbetta, F.M. Miezin, S. Dobmeyer, G.L. Shulman, S.E. Petersen, Attentional modulation of neural processing of shape, color, and velocity in humans, Science 248 (4962) (1990) 1556–1559.

[69] S. Kastner, L.G. Ungerleider, The neural basis of biased competition in human visual cortex, Neuropsychologia 39 (12) (2001) 1263–1276.

[70] L. Pessoa, S. Kastner, L.G. Ungerleider, Neuroimaging studies of attention: from modulation of sensory processing to top-down control, J, Neurosci. 23 (10) (2003) 3990–3998.

[71] J.T. Coull, C.D. Frith, C. Buchel, A.C. Nobre, Orienting attention in time: behavioural and neuroanatomical distinction between exogenous and endogenous shifts, Neuropsychologia 38 (6) (2000) 808–819.

[72] M.D. Mauk, D.V. Buonomano, The neural basis of temporal processing, Annu. Rev. Neurosci. 27 (2004) 307–340.

[73] A. Assmus, J.C. Marshall, J. Noth, K. Zilles, G.R. Fink, Difficulty of perceptual spatiotemporal integration modulates the neural activity of left inferior parietal cortex, Neuroscience 132 (4) (2005) 923–927.

[74] J.T. Coull, F. Vidal, C. Goulon, B. Nazarian, C. Craig, Using time-to-contact information to assess potential collision modulates both visual and temporal prediction networks, Front Hum. Neurosci. 2 (2008) 10. doi: 10.3389/neuro.09.010.2008

[75] J.R. Doherty, A. Rao, M.M. Mesulam, A.C. Nobre, Synergistic effect of combined temporal and spatial expectations on visual attention, J. Neurosci. 25 (2005) 8259–8266.

[76] A. Correa, A.C. Nobre, Neural modulation by regularity and passage of time, J. Neurophysiol. 100 (2008) 1649–1655.

[77] R. Barnes, M.R. Jones, Expectancy, attention, and time, Cognit. Psychol. 41 (3) (2000) 254–311.

[78] A. Elithorn, C. Lawrence, Central inhibition—some refractory observations, Quart. J. Exp. Psychol. 11 (1955) 211–220.

[79] R.D. Luce, Response Times: Their Role in Inferring Elementary Mental Organization, Oxford University Press, New York, 1986.

[80] A. Riehle, S. Grun, M. Diesmann, A. Aertsen, Spike synchronization and rate modulation differentially involved in motor cortical function, Science 278 (1997) 1950–1953.

[81] X. Cui, C. Stetson, P.R. Montague, D.M. Eagleman, Ready...Go: Amplitude of the fMRI Signal Encodes Expectation of Cue Arrival Time, PLOS Biol. 7 (2009) e1000167.

[82] H. Woodrow, The measurement of attention. Psychol. Monographs. 17 (1914) 5.

[83] P. Niemi, R. Näätänen, Foreperiod and simple reaction time, Psychol. Bull. 89 (1981) 133–162.

[84] A. Vallesi, A.R. McIntosh, D.T. Stoss, Temporal preparation in aging: a functional MRI study. Neuropsychologia 47 (2009) 2876–2881.

[85] R.N. Henson, T. Shallice, R.J. Dolan, Right prefrontal cortex and episodic memory retrieval: a functional MRI test of the monitoring hypothesis, Brain 122 (1999) 1367–1381 Pt 7

[86] M. Petrides, Specialized systems for the processing of mnemonic information within the primate frontal cortex, Phil. Trans. R. Soc. Lond. B. Biol. Sci. 351 (1346) (1996) 1455–1461 discussion 1461–1452.

[87] J.X. O'Reilly, M.M. Mesulam, A.C. Nobre, The cerebellum predicts the timing of perceptual events, J. Neurosci. 28 (9) (2008) 2252–2260.

[88] M. Pfeuty, R. Ragot, V. Pouthas, When time is up: CNV time course differentiates the roles of the hemispheres in the discrimination of short tone durations, Exp. Brain Res. 151 (3) (2003) 372–379.

[89] F. Macar, F. Vidal, The CNV peak: an index of decision making and temporal memory, Psychophysiology 40 (6) (2003) 950–954.

[90] P. Praamstra, D. Kourtis, H.F. Kwok, R. Oostenveld, Neurophysiology of implicit timing in serial choice reaction-time performance, J. Neurosci. 26 (20) (2006) 5448–5455.

[91] D.J. Serrien, R.B. Ivry, S.P. Swinnen, Dynamics of hemispheric specialization and integration in the context of motor control, Nat. Rev. Neurosci. 7 (2006) 160–166.

[92] D.V. Buonomano, J. Bramen, M. Khodadadifar, Influence of the interstimulus interval on temporal processing and learning: testing the state-dependent network model, Phil. Trans. R. Soc. Lond. B. Biol. Sci. 364 (2009) 1865–1873.

[93] R.M. Spencer, U. Karmarkar, R.B. Ivry, Evaluating dedicated and intrinsic models of temporal encoding by varying context, Philos. Trans. R. Soc. Lond. B. Biol. Sci. 364 (2009) 1853–1863.

The Neural Code for Number

Andreas Nieder

Animal Physiology, Institute of Neurobiology, University of Tuebingen,
Tuebingen, Germany

Summary

Basic numerical competence is rooted in biological primitives that can be explored in animals. Over the past years, the anatomical substrates and neuronal mechanisms of numerical cognition in primates have been unraveled down to the level of single neurons. Studies with behaviorally trained monkeys have identified a parieto-frontal network of individual neurons selectively tuned to the number of items and suggested mechanisms for their implementation. The properties of these neurons' numerosity tuning curves can explain fundamental psychophysical phenomena, such as the numerical distance and size effect. Functionally overlapping groups of parietal and prefrontal neurons represent not only numerable-discrete quantity (numerosity), but also innumerable-continuous quantity (extent), relations between quantities (proportions) and semantic associations between signs and abstract numerical categories, supporting the idea of a generalized magnitude system in the brain. These studies establish putative homologies between the monkey and human brain and demonstrate the suitability of nonhuman primates as model systems to explore the neurobiological roots of the brain's nonverbal quantification system, which constitutes the phylogenetic and ontogenetic foundation of all further, more elaborate numerical skills in humans.

Basic numerical competence does not depend on language; it is rooted in biological primitives that can already be found in animals. Animals possess impressive numerical capabilities and are able to nonverbally and approximately grasp the numerical properties of objects and events. Such a numerical estimation system for representing number as language-independent mental magnitudes (analog magnitude system) is thought to be a precursor on which verbal numerical representations build, and its neural foundations can be studied in animal models. This chapter reviews the progress that has been made in our understanding of the neuronal substrates and mechanisms of nonverbal numerical magnitude representations in primates.

Space, Time and Number in the Brain.
DOI: 10.1016/B978-0-12-385948-8.00008-6

© 2011 Elsevier Inc. All rights reserved.

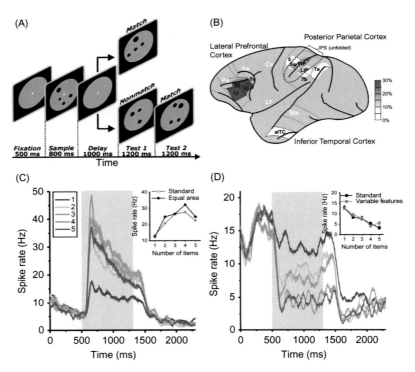

FIGURE 8.1 **Representation of visual cardinality in rhesus monkeys.** (A) Delayed match-to-sample task with visually presented numerosity as the stimulus dimension of interest. A trial started when the monkey grasped a lever and fixated at a central target. After 500 ms of pure fixation, the sample stimulus (800 ms) cued the monkey for a certain numerosity it had to memorize during a 1000-ms delay period. Then, the test1 stimulus was presented, which in 50% of cases was a match showing the same number of dots as cued during the sample period. In the other 50% of cases the test1 display was a non-match, which showed a different numerosity to the sample display. After a non-match test stimulus, a second test stimulus (test2) appeared that was always a match. To receive a fluid reward, monkeys were required to release the lever as soon as a match appeared. Trials were pseudo-randomized and balanced across all relevant features. Monkeys were required to maintain fixation throughout the sample and delay period. (B) Lateral view of a monkey brain showing the recording sites in LPFC, PPC and aITC. The proportion of numerosity-selective neurons in each area is color coded according to the color scale. The IPS is unfolded to show the different areas in the lateral and medial walls. Numbers on PFC indicate anatomical areas. (As, arcuate sulcus; Cs, central sulcus; LF, lateral fissure; LS, lunate sulcus; Ps, principal sulcus; Sts, Superior temporal sulcus). (C, D) Responses of single neurons that were recorded from the PFC (C) and the IPS (D). Both neurons show graded discharge during sample presentation (interval shaded in gray, 500–1300 ms) as a function of numerosities 1 to 5 (color-coded averaged discharge functions). The insets in the upper right corner show the tuning of both neurons and their responses to different control stimuli. The preferred numerosity was 4 for the PFC neuron (B), and 1 for the IPS neuron (C). Modified from [2].

NEURONS ENCODING NUMERICAL QUANTITY

Recordings in monkeys trained to discriminate numerosity demonstrated the capacity of single neurons to encode cardinality [1–3]. In the basic layout of the task, monkeys viewed a sequence of two displays separated by a memory delay and were required to judge whether the displays contained the same number of items (Fig. 8.1A). To ensure that the monkeys solved the task by judging number *per se* rather than simply memorizing sequences of visual patterns or exploiting low-level visual features that correlate with number, sensory cues (such as position, shape, overall area, circumference and density) were varied considerably and controlled for.

Numerosity-selective neurons were tuned to the number of items in a visual display, that is, they showed maximum activity to one of the presented quantities—a neuron's "preferred numerosity"—and a progressive drop off as the quantity became more remote from the preferred number [1,4]. Importantly, changes in the physical appearance of the displays had no effect on the activity of numerosity-selective neurons. A high proportion of numerosity detectors (Fig. 8.1B) was found in the lateral prefrontal cortex (PFC). In the posterior parietal cortex (PPC), numerosity-selective neurons were sparsely distributed in several areas, but relatively abundant in the fundus of the intraparietal sulcus (IPS), termed VIP [5]. There were few such cells in the anterior inferior temporal cortex (aITC) [2] (Fig. 8.1B).

Item numbers can be determined in two fundamentally different spatio-temporal presentation formats. When presented simultaneously as in multiple-item patterns, numerosity can be estimated at a single glance in a direct, perceptual-like way from a spatial arrangement. In contrast to a simultaneous presentation, the elements of a set can be presented one by one and, thus, need to be enumerated successively across time. Sequential enumeration is cognitively more demanding; it incorporates multiple encoding, memory and updating stages, and bears resemblance to mental addition. Sequential enumeration is particularly interesting in that it constitutes a nonverbal precursor of real counting; after all, verbal counting is a sequential enumeration process using number symbols (i.e. 1-2-3, etc.).

To address the neuronal representation of an abstract counting-like accumulation of sensory events and to compare it to the encoding of numerosity in simultaneous displays, Nieder *et al.* [3] recorded single-cell activity in the fundus of the IPS while monkeys performed a delayed match-to-sample task in which sample numerosity was specified either by single dots appearing one-by-one to indicate the number of items sequentially ("sequential protocol", Fig. 8.2A) or by multiple-dot patterns presented simultaneously ("simultaneous protocol", Fig. 8.1A). Temporal and spatial cues were counterbalanced across trials to ensure they could not be used by the animals to solve the task. In addition to the previously described neurons selective to numerosity in multiple-dot patterns, roughly 25% of the neurons in the fundus of the IPS also encoded sequentially presented numerical quantity (Fig. 8.2B). However, numerical quantity was represented by distinct populations of neurons during the ongoing spatial or temporal enumeration process (i.e. in the sample phase); cells encoding the number of sequential items were not tuned to numerosity in multiple-item displays, and *vice versa*. However, once the enumeration process was completed, and the monkeys had to store information, a third population of neurons coded numerosity both in the sequential and simultaneous protocol; about 20% of the cells were tuned to numerosity irrespective of whether is was cued simultaneously or in sequence. This argues for segregated processing of numerosity during the actual encoding stage in the parietal lobe, but also for a final convergence of the segregated information to form abstract quantity representations.

In another domain, cells in the superior parietal lobule (SPL) have been reported to keep track of the number of movements [6]. The authors trained monkeys to alternate between five arm movements of one type ("push" and "turn") and five of another. They found neurons in a somatosensory-responsive region (part of area 5) of the SPL that maintained the number of movements. Interestingly, transient and focal inactivation of area 5 with chemical agents significantly increased the error rate in the selection task [7]. This transient neural

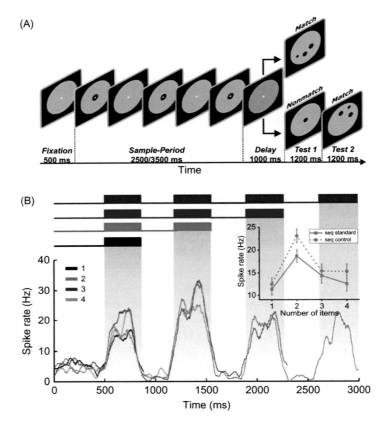

FIGURE 8.2 Coding of sequentially presented numerosity. (A) Sequential delayed match-to-numerosity task (here for numerosity 3). The sample numerosity was cued by sequentially presented items temporally separated by pauses containing no items. The temporal succession and duration of individual items were varied within and across quantities. (B) Responses of an example neuron in ventral intraparietal area (VIP) selective to the sequential quantity 2 (only one condition shown for clarity). Top panel illustrates the temporal succession of individual items (square pulses represent single items). The corresponding latency-corrected discharges for many repetitions of the protocol are plotted as averaged spike density functions. The first 500 ms represent the fixation period. Corresponding colors were used for the stimulation illustration and the plotting of the neural data. Gray shaded areas denote item presentation. The inset shows the tuning functions of the neuron to the standard and a control protocol (error bars represent S.E.M.) for four sequential dots. In both protocols, the neuron was tuned to numerosity 2. Modified from [3].

inactivation also caused omission errors that were not observed before the inactivation. A control task showed that the errors were not caused by motor deficits or impaired ability to select between two possible actions. These results indicate that area 5 is crucial for selecting actions on the basis of numerical information.

The PPC might be the first cortical stage that extracts visual and somatosensory numerical information because its neurons require shorter latencies to become numerosity selective than PFC neurons [2]. As PPC and PFC are functionally interconnected [8,9], that information might be conveyed directly or indirectly to the PFC where it is amplified and maintained to gain control over behavior.

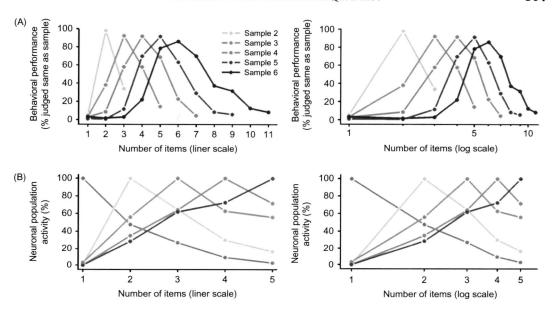

FIGURE 8.3 **Relation between monkey behavior and numerosity-selective neurons.** (A) Behavioral numerosity discrimination functions of two monkeys. The curves indicate whether they judged the first test stimulus as containing the same number of items as the sample display. The function peaks (and the color legend) indicate the sample numerosity from which each curve was derived. Behavioral filter functions are skewed on a linear scale (*left*), but symmetric on a logarithmic scale (*right*). (B) The averaged single-cell numerosity-tuning functions (from PFC) are also asymmetric on a linear scale, but symmetric after logarithmic transformation. Modified from [10].

Behavioral Significance of Numerosity-Selective Neurons

The activity of all numerosity-selective neurons, each tuned to a specific preferred numerosity, formed a bank of overlapping numerosity filters (Fig. 8.3B), mirroring the animals' behavioral performance (Fig. 8.3A). Interestingly, the neurons' sequentially arranged overlapping tuning curves preserved an inherent order of cardinalities. This is important because numerosities are not isolated categories, but exist in relation to one another (for example, 3 is greater than 2 and less than 4); they need to be sequentially ordered to allow meaningful quantity assignments.

The response properties of numerosity-selective cortical cells can explain basic psychophysical phenomena in monkeys, such as the numerical distance and size effect (Fig. 8.3). The *numerical distance effect* states that it is easier to discriminate quantities that are numerically remote from each other (say, 2 *vs* 6 is easier that 5 *vs* 6), while the *numerical size effect* captures the finding that pairs of numerosities of a constant numerical distance are easier to discriminate if the quantities are small (for example, 2 *vs* 3 is easier than 5 *vs* 6). The numerical distance effect results from the fact that the neural filter functions that are engaged in the discrimination of adjacent numerosities heavily overlap [10]. As a consequence, the signal-to-noise ratio of the neural signal detection process is low, and the monkeys make many errors. On the other hand, the filter functions of neurons that are tuned to remote numerosities barely overlap, which results in a high signal-to-noise ratio and, therefore, good performance in cases where the animal has to discriminate sets of a larger numerical distance. The behavioral consequences of the numerical size effect therefore accord to Weber's Law.

What scaling scheme describes the neurons' overlapping tuning curves that are ordered along a "number line" best (Fig. 8.3B)? Are neuronal numerical representations best described on a linear, or a nonlinear, possibly logarithmically compressed scale? The latter would be predicted if Fechner's Law holds. Fechner's Law states that the perceived magnitude (S) is a logarithmic function of stimulus intensity (I) multiplied by a modality and dimension specific constant (k). If the tuning functions for behavioral discrimination and single units are regarded as the monkeys' behavioral and neural numerical representations (Fig. 8.3), the crucial question then concerns which scaling scheme provides symmetric (i.e. Gaussian) probability density distributions. Both the performance and the single unit data for numerosity judgments are better described by a compressed, as opposed to a linear scale [10]. Therefore, single-neuron representations of numerical quantity in monkeys obey Fechner's Law.

The numerical size effect is directly related to the precision of the neuronal numerosity filters: the widths of the tuning curves (or neuronal numerical representations) increase linearly with preferred numerosities (i.e. on average, tuning precision deteriorates as the preferred quantity increases). Hence, more selective neural filters that do not overlap extensively are engaged if a monkey has to discriminate small numerosities (say, 1 and 2), which results in high signal-to-noise ratios and few errors in the discrimination. Conversely, if a monkey has to discriminate large numerosities (such as 4 and 5), the filter functions would overlap considerably. Therefore, the discrimination has a low signal-to-noise ratio, which leads to poor performance.

An important piece of evidence for the contribution of numerosity-selective neurons to behavioral performance came from the examination of error trials. When the monkeys made judgment errors, the neural activity for the preferred quantity was significantly reduced as compared to correct trials [1–4]. As a result of this (and the ordered representation of quantity), the activity to a given preferred numerosity on error trials was more similar to that elicited by adjacent non-preferred quantities on correct trials. In other words, if the neurons did not encode the numerosity properly, the monkeys were prone to mistakes.

Implementing Numerosity Detectors

How may numerosity-selective neurons tuned to preferred numerosities arise in the course of cortical processing? Purely sensory, non-numerical properties (such as wavelength and contrast in the visual system) are encoded already at the earliest processing stages of the sensory epithelia. Number, on the other hand, is a most abstract category devoid of specific sensory features; two cats and two calls have nothing in common, except that the size of their set is "two". How then may the cardinality of objects or events, the pure number of entities, be derived in terms of neuronal information processing?

Two main models have been proposed to explain the implementation of quantity information. The *mode-control model* by Meck and Church [11] works in series and suggests that each item is encoded by an impulse from a pacemaker, which is added to an accumulator (Fig. 8.4A). The magnitude in the accumulator at the end of the count is then read into memory, forming a representation of the number of a set. Thus, it is assumed that quantity is encoded by "summation coding", i.e. the monotonically increasing and decreasing response functions of the neurons (see also network model by Zorzi and Butterworth [12]).

Another model, the *neural filtering model* by Dehaene and Changeux [13] implements numerosity in parallel (Fig. 8.4B). First, each (visual) stimulus is coded as a local Gaussian

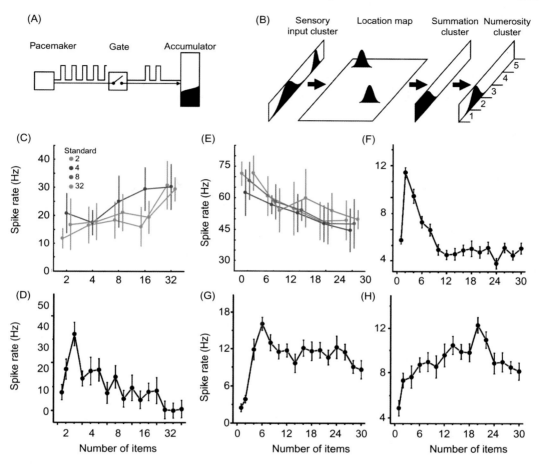

FIGURE 8.4 **Implementation of numerosity detectors.** (A) Mode-control model (after Meck and Church [11]). (B) Neural filtering model (after Dehaene and Changeux [13]). (C,D) Neurons in LIP discharge monotonically as a function of set size during an implicit numerosity task. Two single cells are depicted that show an increase (C) or decrease (D) of discharge rate, respectively, with increasing numerosity. Each neuron was tested with different standard (color code) and deviant numerosities (see text for explanation of the task) (from Roitman *et al.*[15]). (E–H) PFC neurons tuned to preferred numerosities in monkeys performing a delayed match-to-numerosity task. Preferred numerosity was 2 (E), 4 (F), 6 (G) and 20 (H). Modified from [4].

distribution of activation by topographically organized input clusters (simulating the retina). Next, items of different sizes are normalized to a size-independent code. At that stage, item size, which was initially coded by the number of active clusters on the retina (quantity code), is now encoded by the position of active clusters on a location map (position code). Clusters in the location map project to every unit of downstream "summation clusters", whose thresholds increase with increasing number and pool the total activity of the location map. The summation clusters finally project to "numerosity clusters". Numerosity clusters are characterized by central excitation and lateral inhibition so that each numerosity cluster responds only to a selected range of values of the total normalized activity, i.e. their preferred numerosity. Since the numerosity of a stimulus is encoded by peaked tuning functions with a preferred numerosity (causing maximum discharge) this mechanism is termed "labeled-line code". A similar architecture was proposed by Verguts and Fias [14] using a back-propagation network. Interestingly, summation units developed spontaneously in the second processing stage (the "hidden units") after tuned numerosity detectors were determined as output stage.

Even though numerosity representations derived with both model are noisy (approximate) and obey Weber's Law, the two models differ in important aspects. The mode-control model by Meck and Church [11] operates serially and assumes representation of cardinality on a linear scale, whereas in the neural filtering model by Dehaene and Changeux [13] numerosity is encoded in parallel and represented on a logarithmic scale (the same holds for the back-propagation model by Verguts and Fias [14]). Both models, however, have summation units implemented that accumulate number in a graded fashion prior to feeding into numerosity detectors at the output. As a putative physiological reflection of this computational stage in models of number processing, Roitman *et al.* [15] recorded neurons in the parietal lobe whose responses resembled the output of accumulator neurons with response functions that systematically increased or decreased with an increase of stimulus set size (Fig. 8.4C,D).

In this study [15], the activity of single neurons was recorded in the lateral intraparietal area (LIP) of monkeys performing a delayed saccade task. On each trial, monkeys maintained fixation on a central point while a saccade target was placed at a random location lateral of the fixation spot. When the fixation point was extinguished, the monkey shifted its gaze to the saccade target to receive a fluid reward. Prior to the monkey performing the saccade towards the target, a set of items (2, 4, 8, 16, or 32 dots) at the location of the recorded cell's receptive field informed the monkey about the amount of reward it would receive after a correct saccade. One of the five possible numerosities was selected as the standard, which was then presented in half of the trials. In such standard trials, the animal received a fixed amount of fluid as reward. In each of the remaining trials, one of the four deviant numerosities was shown, resulting in a slightly larger amount of fluid as reward. This encouraged the monkey to pay attention to the numerosities, even though they were not to be discriminated or otherwise used in the task.

Roitman and co-workers [15] found that the activity of most LIP neurons increased or decreased systematically with increasing number of elements during stimulus presentation (Fig. 8.4C,D) (irrespective of other stimulus features or cognitive demands). Thus, a population of neurons in LIP encoded the number of elements in a visual array in a roughly monotonic manner. The authors suggested that these two classes of number-selective neurons may be the physiological instantiation of the summation units and numerosity units proposed in neural network models of numerical representation; monotonic magnitude coding of LIP neurons may provide input to neurons in the PPC and PFC that compute cardinal numerical representations via tuning to preferred numerosities (Fig. 8.4E–H) [1–4].

In agreement with this hypothesis, monotonic neurons described in LIP would operate on an intermediate level of numerosity detection. The numerosity stimuli used by Roitman and coworkers [15] were carefully placed over the spatially confined response fields of LIP neurons and thus allowed the encoding of numerosity to be addressed within contiguous subsets of the visual. Final processing stages of abstract numerical information, however, are required to integrate across time, space and modality. Area VIP and the PFC are ideal candidate structures for a global representation of numerosity; both areas integrate multimodal input [16] and neurons in PFC in particular exhibit global cognitive processing

BOX 8.1

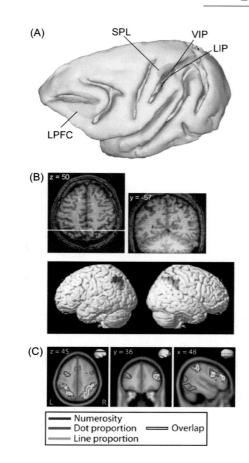

BOX 8.1 FIGURE 1 **Numerically responsive regions in the rhesus monkey and human brain, indicating homologies in neural substrates between both species.** (A) Dorso-lateral view of a rhesus macaque brain. The colored areas represent regions in which neurons that respond to numerosities have been identified via single-cell recordings. Areas include the lateral PFC (LPFC), the SPL, the ventral intraparietal area (VIP), which is located at the fundus of the intraparietal sulcus, and the LIP. (B) Regions in the human brain that responded to numerosity changes, as measured by BOLD-activation. Colored areas in the axial (top left) and coronal (top right) sections, as well as on the surface image indicate the IPS. From [18]. (C) Substantial overlap (outlined in white) of BOLD-activation in the human brain for numerosities, dot proportions and line proportions. Significant overlap was restricted to the bilateral parietal cortex surrounding the IPS, the precentral and prefrontal cortex. Modified from [19].

properties that are no longer spatially restricted [17]. Behavioral relevance is another aspect that could have a substantial effect on the coding scheme. All studies that required the monkeys to use cardinal numerical information explicitly to solve a task found a labeled-line code, irrespective of stimulus modality, presentation format and recording site [1,3,6], whereas numerosity was implicitly informative in the delayed saccade task [15] but discrimination was not required for the monkey to perform the task. Thus, the neuronal representation may change if quantity is encoded as an explicit category.

Tracing Numerosity Tuning in the Human Brain

If anatomical and functional similarities between the brains of nonhuman primates and humans do exist, equivalent areas in the brain should also be activated in humans when nonverbal cardinality is processed (see Box 8.1). Testing functional MRI (fMRI) adaptation with numerosities, Piazza *et al.* [18] found such a corresponding blood oxygenation level-dependent (BOLD) activation in the IPS of humans. The horizontal segment of the IPS significantly habituated to numerosity. Based on the recovery from BOLD-adaptation, Piazza *et al.* [18] could indirectly trace the average numerosity-tuning curve of the underlying neural population, which also showed a clear Weber-fraction signature. Using the same approach, Jacob and Nieder [19] later demonstrated a systematic recovery from BOLD-adaptation as a function of numerical distance both in the IPS and the PFC. Just as the single-neuron tuning curves in monkeys, these recovery functions were also significantly better described on a logarithmic than on a linear number scale.

CODING OF CONTINUOUS AND DISCRETE QUANTITY

To investigate how continuous quantity is encoded by single nerve cells and how it relates to numerosity representations, Tudusciuc and Nieder [20] trained two rhesus monkeys in a delayed match-to-sample task to discriminate different types of quantity randomly alternating within each session. In the "length protocol", the length of a line (out of four different lengths) needed to be discriminated (continuous-spatial quantity). In the "numerosity protocol" (Fig. 8.1A), the number of (one to four) items in multiple-dot displays (discrete-numerical quantity) was the relevant stimulus dimension. To ensure that the monkeys solved the task based on the relevant quantitative information, other co-varying features of the stimuli were again controlled, and the positions of the dots and lines were greatly varied.

After the monkeys solved more than 81% of the trials correctly for both the length and the numerosity protocols, single unit activity from the depth of the IPS was analyzed while the animals performed the task. About 20% of anatomically intermingled single neurons in the monkey IPS each encoded discrete-numerical (Fig. 8.5A), continuous-spatial (Fig. 8.5B), or both types of quantities (Fig. 8.5C), suggesting two partly overlapping populations of neurons within this area.

Can functionally overlapping groups of parietal neurons provide sufficient information for the monkey to make correct quantity judgments? To assess the discriminative power of small populations of neurons, Tudusciuc and Nieder [20] applied a population decoding technique [21] based on an artificial neuronal network [22]. The classifier was trained with neuronal responses (i.e. pre-processed spike trains) of a set of neurons recorded while the monkeys judged each of the eight quantity categories; at this stage, the classifier was informed about the stimulus configuration and learned the neuronal features which were best suited for identifying a given category. In the subsequent test phase, the classifier predicted the categories from novel neuronal responses of the same pool of neurons, i.e. from data it had not used for learning.

The quantitative results based on the statistical classifier demonstrated that the small population of quantity-selective neurons carried most of the categorical information; by exploiting the classical spike-rate measure which contributes to the monkeys' quantity discrimination performance, the classifier was able to accurately and robustly discriminate both continuous and discrete quantity classes. Interestingly, even the population of untuned neurons had a remarkable and significant quantity-coding ability, albeit to a lesser extent than the tuned neurons. This suggests that the classifier extracted, beyond the averaged spike rate, additional information from the temporal structure of the neuronal responses. Moreover, the comparison between the monkeys' neuronal and behavioral responses showed that the brain indeed utilizes this

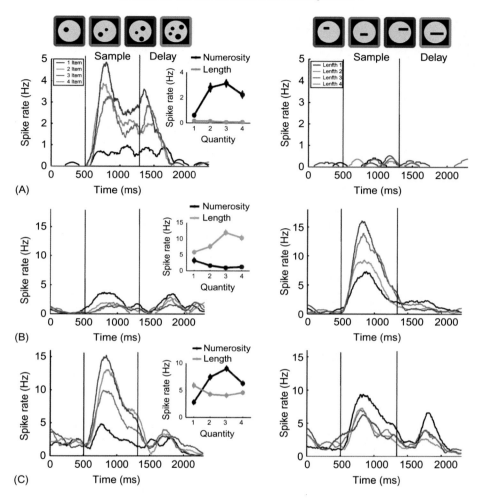

FIGURE 8.5 **Neuronal coding of continuous and discrete quantity.** (A–C) Three example neurons in the IPS exhibiting selectivity for quantity. Top panels in (A) illustrate the four different numerosities (*left*) and four different line lengths (*right*) used as stimuli. Left and right graphs illustrate the discharge rates (displayed as smoothed spike density histograms) of the same neuron in the numerosity and length protocol, respectively. The first 500 ms represent the fixation period. The area between the two black vertical bars represents the sample presentation, the following 1000 ms indicate the delay phase. Colors correspond to the quantity dimensions. The insets between two histograms depict the tuning functions of each of the three neurons to numerosity and length. (A) Neuron tuned to numerosity 3, but not to length. (B) Neuron tuned to the third longest line, but not to any tested numerosity. (C) Neuron encoding both discrete and continuous quantity. Modified from [20].

information for decision making; neuronal responses recorded whenever the monkeys failed to discriminate the quantity categories prevented the classifier from predicting the correct quantity category. Future studies need to clarify whether complex quantity judgments require an interplay with, or readout by, structures with more executive functions, such as the PFC [23].

CODING OF PROPORTIONS

Neurons in the prefrontal and posterior parietal cortices are selectively tuned to abstract quantity, and the cellular response characteristics can explain basic psychophysical phenomena in dealing with them. However, many vital decisions in animals require an estimation of the relation between two quantities, or proportion. Vallentin & Nieder [24] demonstrated that rhesus monkeys were able to grasp proportionality in a delayed match-to-sample test. They trained two rhesus monkeys to judge the length ratio (proportion) between two lines, a reference and a test line. The length ratios between the test and reference lines were 1:4, 2:4, 3:4 and 4:4 (Fig. 8.6). After demonstrating that the monkeys could discriminate spatial proportions, Vallentin and Nieder [24] investigated this capacity's neuronal underpinning and recorded from 526 randomly selected neurons of the PFC while the animals performed the proportion discrimination task. Both during the sample and delay presentation, 25% of the tested neurons were significantly tuned only to proportion, irrespective of the absolute lengths of the test and reference bars. Each of the selective neurons preferred one of the four tested proportions. Just as with numerosities or lines, a labeled-line code was found for the coding of proportions,

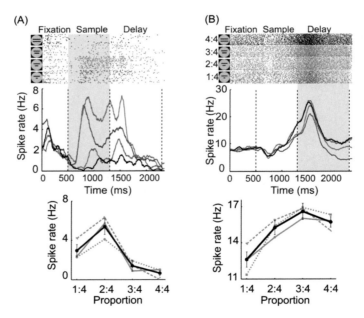

FIGURE 8.6 **Neuronal coding of proportions.** Single-cell responses of two example neurons during the fixation, sample and delay period are shown. Neurons were proportion-selective during the sample (A) or delay (B) period (marked in gray). In the top panel, the neuronal responses are plotted as dot-raster histograms (each dot represents an action potential, spike trains are sorted and color-coded according to the sample proportion illustrated by example stimuli on the left). Middle panels show spike density functions (activity to a given proportion averaged over all trials and smoothed by a 150-ms Gaussian kernel). The first 500ms represent the fixation period followed by an 800-ms sample and a 1000-ms delay phase (separated by vertical dotted lines). Bottom panels depict the tuning functions of the respective neurons for each of the three stimulus protocols derived from the periods of maximum proportion selectivity (error bars represent S.E.M.). Modified from [24].

with neurons exhibiting tuning curves and preferred proportions. The areas where such proportion-selective neurons were found coincided with PFC regions that also house numerosity-selective neurons. These data suggest that the perception of relational quantity is represented by the same frontal network and magnitude code as absolute quantity in the primate brain.

These single-cell data complement and refine recent functional imaging studies describing selectivity to quantity relations in a parieto-frontal network. Using an fMRI adaptation protocol to investigate automatic quantity processing, a recovery from repetition suppression was detected both for line and numerosity proportions in lateral PFC and PPC [25]. Because recovery from blood-oxygenation-level-dependent (BOLD)-adaptation was a function of ratio distance, populations of neurons in the human cortex also seem to be tuned to preferred proportions. Moreover, both numerosity and proportion seem to be processed by the same dedicated brain areas, as witnessed by a strong overlap of the distance effect for numerosity and proportions stimuli. Using the same methodology but presenting fractions in symbolic notation, Jacob and Nieder [26] could show that populations of neurons in human parietal cortex were tuned to preferred fractions and even generalize across the format of presentation. The distance effect was invariant to changes in notation from number to word fractions and strongest in the anterior IPS, a key region for the processing of whole numbers. The intraparietal cortex was also active in adults solving a fraction comparison problem [27]. These findings demonstrate that the primate brain uses the same analog magnitude code to represent both absolute and relative quantity. A fraction might be represented by its numerical value as a whole rather than by the numerical values of its numerator and denominator. Together with previous studies in the numerical domain, the current findings indicate close similarities between non-symbolic quantity processing in the human and monkey brain.

TOWARDS SYMBOLIC NUMBER REPRESENTATIONS

As shown previously, humans and animals share an evolutionarily old quantity representation system which allows the estimation of set sizes. Nonverbal numerical cognition, however, is limited to approximate quantity representations and rudimentary arithmetic operations. Language-endowed humans, on the other hand, invented number symbols (numerals and number words) during cultural evolution. These mental tools enable us to create precise quantity representations and perform exact calculation that is beyond the reach of any animal species.

Even though number symbols are of paramount importance in today's scientifically and technologically advanced culture, their invention dates back only a couple of thousand years [28]. Given the time scale of brain evolution, a *de novo* development of brain areas with distinct, culturally dependent number symbol functions is more than unlikely [29]. Rather, it is conceivable that brain structures that originally evolved for other purposes are built upon in the course of continuing evolutionary development [30]. According to the "redeployment hypothesis" [31] or "recycling hypothesis" [29,32], pre-existing cell assemblies are largely preserved, extended, and combined as networks become more complex.

In the number domain, existing neuronal components in PFC and IPS subserving nonverbal quantity representations could be used for the new purpose of number symbol encoding, without disrupting their participation in existing cognitive processes [33,34]. Guided by the faculty of language, children learn to use number symbols as mental tools during childhood. During this learning process, and as a prerequisite for the utilization of signs as numerical symbols, long-term associations between initially meaningless shapes (that later become numerals) and inherent semantic numerical categories must be established. This necessary, but by no means sufficient, step towards the utilization of number symbols in humans can also be mastered by different animal species [35,36].

To investigate the single-neuron mechanisms of semantic association, Diester and Nieder [37] mimicked such a semantic mapping process by training two monkeys to associate the *a priori* meaningless visual shapes of Arabic numerals (that became "signs", or more precisely, "indices" [38]) with the inherently meaningful numerosity of multiple-dot displays. After this long-term learning process was completed, a relatively large proportion of PFC neurons (24%) encoded plain numerical values, irrespective of whether they had been presented as a specific number of dots or as a visual sign. Such "association neurons" showed similar tuning during the course of the trial to both the direct numerosity in dot stimuli and the associated numerical values of signs. Interestingly, the tuning functions of association neurons showed a distance effect for both protocols, i.e. a drop-off of activity with increasing numerical distance from the preferred numerical value. This distance effect found in the sign protocol indicates that association neurons responded as a function of numerical value rather than visual shape *per se*. These findings argue for association neurons as a neuronal substrate for the semantic mapping processes between signs and categories.

In the same study [37], the activity of neurons in the fundus of the IPS was also recorded. In contrast to PFC, only 2% of all recorded IPS neurons associated signs with numerosities.

BOX 8.2

QUESTIONS FOR FUTURE RESEARCH

1. How do numerosity-selective neurons develop? Neurons that represent numerical information are abundant in PFC and PPC. Does the coding scheme change with experience of the subject? Long-term recording studies could answer these questions.

2. Are single-cell representations abstract or non-abstract? So far, numerosity-selective neurons have only been tested for single sensory modalities. Are single neurons responding modality-independent to preferred numerosities, i.e. are they supramodal?

3. How is the brain treating cardinal and ordinal aspects of numerical information? Numerical quantity and rank have been studied largely separately so far, and the relationship between mechanisms that underlie cardinality and serial order judgments remains elusive. However, if numerical capacities are two aspects of a common numerical faculty, should there not be similarities in neuronal processing?

4. What types of neural codes are implemented in the brain? Average firing rates nicely explain many fundamental psychophysical effects. But even in the absence of average rate information, statistical classifiers can extract behaviorally relevant information from single spike trains. What is the nature of this additional, temporal information in spike trains?

Moreover, the quality of neuronal association in the IPS was weak and occurred much later during the trial.

The conclusion drawn from these results is that, even though monkeys use the PFC and IPS for non-symbolic quantity representations, only the prefrontal part of this network is engaged in semantic shape–number associations. Interestingly, this pattern of brain areas seems to be preserved in children [39–41]. In contrast to adults, pre-school children lacking ample exposure to number symbols show elevated PFC activity when dealing with symbolic cardinalities. With age and proficiency, however, the activation seems to shift to parietal areas. The PFC could thus be ontogenetically and phylogenetically the first cortical area establishing semantic associations, which might be relocated to the parietal cortex in human adolescents in parallel with maturing language capabilities that endow our species with a sophisticated symbolic system [42].

For a list of questions that need to be addressed in future research, see Box 8.2.

References

[1] A. Nieder et al., Representation of the quantity of visual items in the primate prefrontal cortex, Science 297 (2002) 1708–1711.

[2] A. Nieder, E.K. Miller, A parieto-frontal network for visual numerical information in the monkey, Proc. Natl. Acad. Sci. U. S. A. 101 (2004) 7457–7462.

[3] A. Nieder et al., Temporal and spatial enumeration processes in the primate parietal cortex, Science 313 (2006) 1431–1435.

[4] A. Nieder, K. Merten, A labeled-line code for small and large numerosities in the monkey prefrontal cortex, J. Neurosci. 27 (2007) 5986–5993.

[5] CL Colby et al., Ventral intraparietal area of the macaque—anatomical location and visual response properties, J. Neurophysiol. 69 (1993) 902–914.

[6] H. Sawamura et al., Numerical representation for action in the parietal cortex of the monkey, Nature 415 (2002) 918–922.

[7] H. Sawamura et al., Deficits in action selection based on numerical information after inactivation of the posterior parietal cortex in monkeys, J. Neurophysiol. 104 (2010) 902–910.

[8] J. Quintana et al., Effects of cooling parietal cortex on prefrontal units in delay tasks, Brain Res. 503 (1989) 100–110.

[9] M.V. Chafee, P.S. Goldman-Rakic, Inactivation of parietal and prefrontal cortex reveals interdependence of neural activity during memory-guided saccades, J. Neurophysiol. 83 (2000) 1550–1566.

[10] A. Nieder, E.K. Miller, Coding of cognitive magnitude: Compressed scaling of numerical information in the primate prefrontal cortex, Neuron 37 (2003) 149–157.

[11] W.H. Meck, R.M. Church, A mode control model of counting and timing processes, J. Exp. Psychol.: An Behav. Proc. 9 (1983) 320–334.

[12] M. Zorzi, B. Butterworth, A computational model of number comparison, in: M. Hahn, S.C. Stoness, (Eds.), Proceedings of the Twenty First Annual Conference of the Cognitive Science Society, Erlbaum, (1999), pp. 778–783.

[13] S. Dehaene, J.P. Changeux, Development of elementary numerical abilities: A neural model, J. Cogn. Neurosci. 5 (1993) 390–407.

[14] T. Verguts, W. Fias, Representation of number in animals and humans: A neural model, J. Cogn. Neurosci. 16 (2004) 1493–1504.

[15] J.D. Roitman et al., Monotonic coding of numerosity in macaque lateral intraparietal area, PLoS Biol. 8 (2007) e208.

[16] J.R. Duhamel et al., Ventral intraparietal area of the macaque: congruent visual and somatic response properties, J. Neurophysiol. 79 (1998) 126–136.

[17] S. Everling et al., Filtering of neural signals by focused attention in the monkey prefrontal cortex, Nat. Neurosci. 5 (2002) 671–676.

[18] M. Piazza et al., Tuning curves for approximate numerosity in the human intraparietal sulcus, Neuron 44 (2004) 547–555.

[19] S.N. Jacob, A. Nieder, Tuning to non-symbolic proportions in the human frontoparietal cortex, Eur. J. Neurosci. 30 (2009) 1432–1442.

[20] O. Tudusciuc, A. Nieder, Neuronal population coding of continuous and discrete quantity in the primate posterior parietal cortex, Proc. Natl. Acad. Sci. U. S. A. 104 (2007) 14513–14518.

[21] M. Laubach, Wavelet-based processing of neuronal spike trains prior to discriminant analysis, J. Neurosci. Meth. 134 (2004) 159–168.

[22] T. Kohonen, Self-Organizing Maps, second ed., Springer-Verlag, Berlin, Germany, 1997.

[23] E.K. Miller, J.D. Cohen, An integrative theory of prefrontal cortex function, Annu. Rev. Neurosci. 24 (2001) 167–202.

[24] D. Vallentin, A. Nieder, Behavioural and prefrontal representation of spatial proportions in the monkey, Curr. Biol. 18 (2008) 1420–1425.

[25] S.N. Jacob, A. Nieder, Tuning to non-symbolic proportions in the human frontoparietal cortex, Eur. J. Neurosci. 30 (2009) 1432–1442.

[26] S.N. Jacob, A. Nieder, Notation-independent representation of fractions in the human parietal cortex, J. Neurosci. 29 (2009) 4652–4657.

[27] A. Ischebeck et al., The processing and representation of fractions within the brain: an fMRI investigation, Neuroimage 47 (2009) 403–413.

[28] G. Ifrah, The Universal History of Numbers : From Prehistory to the Invention of the Computer, Wiley, New York, 2000. 633 p.

[29] S. Dehaene, Evolution of Human Cortical Circuits for Reading and Arithmetic: The "Neuronal Recycling" Hypothesis, in: S Dehaene, et al.(Ed.), *From Monkey Brain to Human Brain*, MIT Press, pp. 133–157.

[30] S.J. Gould, Exaptation: A missing term in the science of form, Paleobiology 8 (1982) 4–15.

[31] M.L. Anderson, Evolution of cognitive function via redeployment of brain areas, Neuroscientist 13 (2007) 13–21.

[32] S. Dehaene, L. Cohen, Cultural recycling of cortical maps, Neuron 56 (2007) 384–398.

[33] M. Piazza et al., A magnitude code common to numerosities and number symbols in human intraparietal cortex, Neuron 53 (2007) 293–305.

[34] E. Eger et al., Deciphering cortical number coding from human brain activity patterns, Curr. Biol. 19 (2009) 1608–1615.

[35] S.T. Boysen, G.G. Berntson, Numerical competence in a chimpanzee (Pan troglodytes), J. Comp. Psychol. 103 (1989) 23–31.

[36] D.A. Washburn, D.M. Rumbaugh, Ordinal judgments of numerical symbols by macaques (Macaca mulatta), Psychol. Sci. 2 (1991) 190–193.

[37] I. Diester, A. Nieder, Semantic associations between signs and numerical categories in the prefrontal cortex, PLoS Biol. 5 (2007) e294.

[38] H. Wiese, Numbers, Language and the Human Mind, Cambridge University Press

[39] D. Ansari et al., Neural correlates of symbolic number processing in children and adults, Neuroreport 16 (2005) 1769–1773.

[40] S.M. Rivera et al., Developmental changes in mental arithmetic: evidence for increased functional specialization in the left inferior parietal cortex, Cereb. Cortex 15 (2005) 1779–1790.

[41] L. Kaufmann et al., Neural correlates of the number-size interference task in children, Neuroreport 17 (2006) 587–591.

[42] T. Deacon, The Symbolic Species: The Co-Evolution of Language and the Human Brain, Norton, London, 1997.

SHARED MECHANISMS FOR SPACE, TIME AND NUMBER?

Introduction, by Stanislas Dehaene

In the early 1990s, when I was studying parity judgments, I accidentally hit upon an unexpected finding. My research concerned how quickly human participants could decide whether a digit was odd or even. The central issue was whether they could do this digitally, like a computer, by simply looking at the last bit or the last digit, or whether they would be influenced by conceptual variables such as the magnitude of the number. Unexpectedly, the latter effect turned out to be massive. Independently of whether the digit was odd or even, number magnitude biased the subjects' responses in such a way that large numbers led to faster key presses on the right-hand side of space, and small numbers to faster key presses on the left-hand side of space. This Spatial Numerical Association of Response Codes or SNARC effect, as we called it, underscored the fact that number and space are intimately related concepts that cannot easily be disentangled, even if they are unrelated to the task at hand.

The SNARC effect and its variants quickly became a standard paradigm in numerical cognition. As of 2010, more than a hundred papers have been published on this topic, and several thousand human subjects have been tested with variants of the SNARC effect. The results reveal that cross-domain associations are much more varied than anyone ever expected: number is associated with space, but also with temporal duration, object size, grip size, saccade side, finger location... Furthermore, these interactions are often, but not always reciprocal, thus entwining space, time and number into a tangled knot of inter-related concepts.

In spite of these empirical advances, considerable controversy still surrounds the nature of the mechanisms that link space, time and number. Vincent Walsh introduced the influential ATOM theory (A Theory Of

Magnitude) or the concept that a single underlying magnitude representation underlies all three domains. This shared resources hypothesis is related to the earlier proposal, by Meck and Church, of a single accumulator mechanism capable of generating representations of both number and time. My own proposal, developed in close collaboration with Laurent Cohen and Philippe Pinel, departs from this view. I believe that distinct representations exist for the dimensions of space, time and number—and indeed, for many sub-levels of representation *within* these general domains, such as for ordinality *vs* cardinality, or duration *vs* absolute circadian time. I do not deny, however, that the cues for space, time and number may arise from partially shared accumulator systems, and that these representations are often intermingled within the same brain areas, linked by fast and automatic associations, and submitted to shared top-down processing operations such as attentional shifts. The metaphor of the "number line" summarizes this wealth of associations and inter-relations—yet it must be recognized that this is only a figure of speech and will ultimately have to be replaced by a detailed understanding of the underlying brain mechanisms.

The present section reviews some of the contemporary advances in this field, which go much beyond the classical SNARC effect. **Roi Cohen Kadosh** and **Limor Gertner** briefly examine the evidence from spatial synesthesia—the fact that some individuals vividly experience numerical or temporal concepts as occupying specific locations in space, to the extent that they can often draw sophisticated curvilinear or three-dimensional representations of their subjective number line. Based on recent experiments, they speculate as to the cerebral origins of these spectacular experiences, which might lie either in ventral visual cortex or, more likely perhaps, in the dorsal parietal route known to be involved in representing all three parameters of space, time and number.

David Burr, John Ross, Paola Binda, and **Concetta Morrone** bring a distinctly psychophysical paradigm to bear on this issue. They discovered a remarkable illusion: just before a subject makes a saccade, the perception of space and time is altered, such that these dimensions appear to be compressed to a subjective value smaller than objective reality. Very recently, they observed that number is similarly compressed. This finding, although not fully theorized, clearly shows that the three dimensions of space, time and number belong together and share intimate mechanisms of saccadic updating. This idea fits nicely with recent evidence that areas coding for saccadic eye movement are being activated during number processing and simple arithmetic (as discovered independently by André Knops, Ed Hubbard, Bertrand Thirion and myself, and by Tobias Loetscher and his colleagues). The brain mechanisms for updating our mental representations of the environment as we move our eyes, which play a crucial role in the stability of our perception, seem to be co-opted or "recycled" to support the higher conceptual representations underlying our sense of time and number.

The last two chapters in this section, by **Wim Fias, Jean-Philippe van Dijck** and **Wim Gevers**, and by **Yves Rossetti, Sophie Jacquin-Courtois, Masami Ishihara, Claudio Brozzoli** and **Fabrizio Doricchi** introduce complexities in this increasingly detailed picture of the interactions between space, time and number. Both chapters revisit the remarkable finding that "spatial" neglect in brain-lesioned patients can affect not only the bisection of physical lines, but also of numerical intervals, leading some patients to decide for instance, that 18, is in the middle of 10 and 19. Evidence from multiple patients now indicates that the spatial and numerical forms of neglect can be dissociated, and therefore do not imply a uniquely spatial format for the mental "number line". Furthermore, Wim Fias and his collaborators find that a purely ordinal representation of words in working memory, without magnitude coding, can by itself generate an analog of the SNARC effect. Finally both Wim Fias and Yves Rossetti emphasize the context-dependence of these spatial influences on time and number, which can be cancelled or even reversed by task instructions and task context. These findings stress the highly parallel, multifacetted and flexible associations that link the concepts of space, time and number. Incorporating these complex findings into a minimal model remains a daunting challenge for future theorists.

Synesthesia: Gluing Together Time, Number, and Space

*Roi Cohen Kadosh** and Limor Gertner[†]*

*Department of Experimental Psychology and Oxford Centre for Functional Magnetic Resonance Imaging of the Brain, University of Oxford, Oxford, UK
[†]Department of Psychology, and Zlotowski Center for Neuroscience, Ben-Gurion University of the Negev, Beer-Sheva, Israel

Recent research has suggested that the perception of time, number, and space is linked in humans and this association appears to be at the implicit level for most of the people. In contrast, in some people this association is triggered automatically, which results in an explicit and vivid experience of time and/or number in a predefined spatial location. This ability to "glue" time, number, and space together is called synesthesia, and we suggest here that it is a matter of quantitatively increased proficiencies in the synesthetic as compared to the non-synesthetic population to encode time, number, and space simultaneously. In this chapter, we describe the phenomenon of time and/or number, space (TNS) synesthesia, its possible neural mechanisms and its effect on everyday life functioning. Finally, we suggest that TNS synesthesia research can provide a better understanding of the link between time, number, and space processing in the general population.

Do you see numbers vividly in certain locations in space? For example, do you see the numbers 1 through 10 running from the right to the left and then continuing up right by 30°? Do you disagree with this description because you see numbers in another shape? Maybe instead of numbers you can see different units of time, such as hours, days of the week, months, or even years in a specific spatial location (Fig. 9.1)? If yes, you are probably one out of approximately five people who possess a distinct and explicit ability to combine time, number, and space [1,2], an ability that is implicit in the average population [3–5].

This phenomenon is termed synesthesia, a condition in which certain perceptual or conceptual stimuli (e.g., digits) trigger an additional concurrent experience (e.g., color, visuospatial experience) [6]. Recent studies have shown that synesthesia is a neurological

Space, Time and Number in the Brain.
DOI: 10.1016/B978-0-12-385948-8.00009-8

© 2011 Elsevier Inc. All rights reserved.

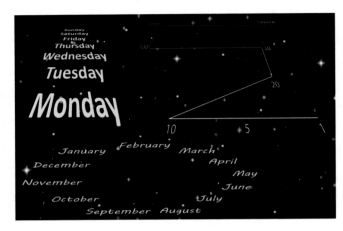

FIGURE 9.1   An example of 3D representations of time units (months, days of the week) and numbers in mental space, as depicted by different TNS synesthetes.

condition with a genetic basis that leads to an over-binding of different features [7]. Importantly, synesthesia is not restricted to TNS and can also be found for other psychological processes (e.g., seeing a grapheme, hearing sounds) that automatically trigger an additional experience (e.g., color, taste, smells, pain) in the absence of any direct stimulation for this experience [8–15]. For example, for some people who see digits in colors (termed digit–color synesthesia) an achromatic 7 will appear in a distinct color such as turquoise [16].

TNS synesthesia is not a newly reported phenomenon: researchers described this experience at the end of the 19th century (e.g., [17,18]). However, it has rarely been studied since then, as these earlier studies were based on introspection and together with the idiosyncrasy of synesthesia (but see [19–22], for challenging this latter point) led to little scientific interest. With the recent availability of more objective psychological methods together with rigorous neuroscientific techniques, synesthesia has seen a revival in the last 15 years and has been brought back into the realms of empirical science. Most synesthesia research, however, has focused on specific types of synesthesia, such as hearing–color synesthesia or grapheme–color synesthesia [10–13,15] and only recently have scientists begun to investigate TNS synesthesia (also sometimes referred to as: visuospatial synesthesia, sequence–space synesthesia, spatial forms, synesthetic spatial forms, time–space synesthesia, number–space synesthesia, number forms, number–form synesthesia, time lines, number lines [23]). These studies provide important insights into the way that time, number, and space are being represented by TNS synesthetes (e.g., [1,2,23–32]. Importantly, the differences and similarities between synesthetes and non-synesthetes have provided a better understanding of the underlying neurocognitive mechanisms for time, number, and space perception in the general population.

IS IT REALLY SYNESTHESIA?

Previous studies have considered synesthesia only when it involved connections between or within one of our five senses; sight, hearing, touch, smell and taste. Given that "a sense of space" is not counted typically among the five "physical" senses, one could ponder whether time, number, and space associations can be really considered as a type of synesthesia.

While recent estimates suggested that TNS synesthesia is far more likely to coincide with other varieties of synesthesia [2], the same spatial forms for numbers and time units were recognized in approximately 20% of the general population—quite a large proportion [1,2,9]. More specifically, recent studies have demonstrated the existence of TNS associations in non-synesthetic individuals (e.g., [8]). This similarity between TNS synesthetes and non-synesthetes is a matter of a degree on a single continuum, on which synesthetes represent the explicit, automatic, and consistent association between time, number, and space (for a neural evidence see [32]). In contrast, non-synesthetes represent the association between these dimensions in an implicit fashion, which is more influenced by task-induced strategies and their representation therefore seems more flexible (e.g., [2,25,26,28,29,31,33]). For example, there is a striking resemblance between the explicit representation of number and space in TNS synesthetes, and the implicit representation of number and space in non-synesthetes. Studies from different countries and educational systems have shown that between 62% and 66% of the TNS synesthetes report representing numbers with small numbers on the left and large numbers on the right side [2,24,34]. This prevalence is similar to the percentage of the non-synesthetes (65%) who represent numbers implicitly from left to right as the numbers increase, as indicated by the spatial–numerical association of response codes (SNARC) effect [35]. Yet, TNS synesthetes are singled out by their enhanced ability to consciously, consistently and automatically associate time and/or numbers with space [1,2,23–25,27–32,34,36].

The account for the allegedly contrasting evidence relies on the idea that both synesthetes and non-synesthetes share the same cognitive and neural mechanisms and the differences between them are down to different levels of conscious awareness and the intensity of the TNS association [8]. While non-synesthete individuals are unaware of their mental–spatial representations (and they are revealed only under certain experimental manipulations, such as posthypnotic suggestion [37]), TNS synesthetes are consciously and irrepressibly visualizing these representations each time they see, hear or think of them. Thus, it has been suggested that the synesthetic experience is not so much the result of a qualitatively different mechanism, but rather due to an extreme expression of a normal cognitive process (for further discussions see [8,23,24,38,39]). These quantitative differences between synesthetes and non-synesthetes are not unique in TNS synesthesia but have also been documented for other types of synesthesia [19,22,40–42]. This line of evidence thus renders synesthesia research an attractive research approach for the study of normal cognitive processes that are usually much less accessible in the non-synesthetes population.

THE EFFECT OF TNS SYNESTHESIA ON EVERYDAY COGNITIVE PROCESSES

How does TNS synesthesia affect everyday cognitive processes? Is it an advantage or a disadvantage to be a synesthete? Being able to answer these questions can provide us with insights in the functionality of the interaction between these dimensions in non-synesthetes. Recent studies indicate that there are benefits for the explicit representation of

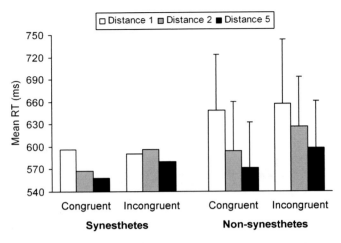

FIGURE 9.2   Mean reaction times (RTs) as a function of group, congruency and numerical distance. On the left, the performance of TNS synesthetes. A numerical distance effect has been observed only when the presentation on the computer screen was compatible with their synesthetic experience (congruent condition). Twelve non-synesthetes (on the right) show a numerical distance effect independent of the presentation of the numbers on the computer screen. Error bars are one standard error of the mean.

these dimensions by TNS synesthetes. It has been shown that people with time–space synesthesia have enhanced abilities in tasks that relate to time or space [1,23]. For example, it has been demonstrated that the performance of month–space synesthetes is better when the external stimuli are consistent with their month–space perception. Namely, synesthetes who visualize early months on the left and late months on the right were faster to make left-hand responses to the former and right-hand responses to the latter than vice versa, while synesthetes who represent early months on the right and late months on the left showed the opposite pattern [31]. Other studies have shown that there is a cost that is associated with TNS synesthesia and that TNS synesthetes tend to use less flexible strategies in a given task if it is not in line with their explicit representation. Similarly, number–space synesthetes exhibit slower processing times when asked to compare the quantity of two numbers when the numbers are incongruent to their explicit representation compared to congruent presentation of the numbers [2,25–27]. For example, Gertner et al. [25] compared the performance of three number–space synesthetes with non-synesthete controls on a standard number comparison task. As can be seen in Fig. 9.2, number–space synesthetes displayed a decrease in reaction time as the numerical distance between compared numbers increases (i.e. the numerical distance effect [43]) only when the numbers' positions on the screen were compatible with their relative position on the specific number-form. Namely, synesthete OT showed a distance effect when numbers were presented in a right-to-left orientation, which is congruent with his number-form. Synesthete SM displayed a distance effect only in her congruent condition, that is, when numbers were presented in a bottom-to-top orientation, and synesthete RS was generally much faster in left-to-right orientation trials, which is congruent with her number-form, and showed a distance effect only in this condition. In contrast, the non-synesthete controls showed the classic distance effect regardless of numbers orientation and/or position. These results suggest that the visuospatial uniquely defined number form interferes with the synesthete's ability to represent numbers in a flexible manner.

Similarly, while it seems that the synesthetes' general arithmetic abilities are not different from non-synesthetes, number–space synesthetes show rigidity that leads to underperformance when the most efficient way to solve an arithmetic problem requires a strategy that is not based on a visuospatial process [44] (e.g., small multiplication problems such as 3 × 3 which are based on rote retrieval, rather than visuospatial abilities, as in the case of subtraction problems [45]).

These studies show that having an explicit representation of time, number, and space can provide some benefits as the information is constantly available, but it can also lead to lower behavioral flexibility in solving a task effectively.

NEURAL PROCESSES OF TNS SYNESTHESIA

Which brain areas are involved in the case of TNS synesthesia? This question is not easy to answer. In contrast to the established specialized areas for colors, there are no selective regions involved in processing the ubiquitous spatial information. Moreover, the suggestion that TNS synesthetes and non-synesthetes might recruit the same mechanisms for the binding of time, number, and space makes the task of finding the exact neural distinction even more difficult [3,4,38,46–48]. Yet, there are two regions that present reasonable candidates for the manifestation of TNS synesthesia at the neural level: the striate cortex (V1 and V2) and the parietal cortex.

Striate Cortex

Neuroimaging studies on grapheme–color synesthesia showed that color processing areas (V4/V8) are also involved in the synesthetic experience of colors. Specifically, it was found that when presenting synesthetes with their inducer stimulus (word, grapheme or number), activation in the color-selective areas is observed [49–52]. However, most studies failed to find similar activation in the primary visual areas (V1 and V2) (for review see [10,11], but see [53]). For example, Hubbard and colleagues [49] found a correlation between behavioral performance and brain activation in grapheme–color synesthesia. In particular, participants who performed better on a behavioral crowding task also showed a larger activation in early retinotopic visual areas in response to spoken linguistic symbols (numbers and letters).

These findings of unusual activation of the striate and extrastriate cortex in grapheme–color synesthesia also suggests the involvement of these regions in TNS synesthesia, at least in cases when TNS synesthesia and grapheme–color coincide [2]. In turn, this might suggest a common neural origin.

Doricchi et al. [54] found behavioral differences in the bisection of mental and physical number lines. Based on previous imaging studies, they suggested that those two processes implicate different brain areas. Processing numerical information was consistently found to activate the intraparietal sulcus (IPS) bilaterally [47,55,56]. In contrast, physical line bisections were found to be dependent on the striate and extrastriate visual cortex [57].

We used this idea to introduce the following thought: if one assumes that spatial forms are equivalent to physical lines, in the sense that they share similar qualities of tangibility and vividness, then it would be reasonable to expect neural differences between synesthetes and non-synesthetes in the visual cortex. This idea deviates from a recent idea by Eagleman [24] who has suggested that areas in the temporal lobes that are involved in sequence processing might play a critical role in TNS synesthesia. In this scenario, the over-learned sequences, such as numbers, months, and days, that are represented in TNS synesthesia trigger an experience of objecthood. While this idea is plausible, it is still awaiting support for the idea that temporal lobe areas are involved in over-learned sequences in non-synesthetes and/or synesthetes.

Parietal Cortex

The literature on different types of magnitudes such as time, number, and space suggests that the neural circuits for these dimensions overlap in the parietal lobes [3,4,38,47], an idea that has been supported by non-invasive brain stimulation studies that impaired or enhanced time, number, and space perception in non-synesthetes (e.g., [58–66]). For example, Göbel and colleagues [64] found that transcranial magnetic stimulation (TMS) to the left and right angular gyrus (AG) impaired performance on a number comparison task by affecting the spatial number line.

In a recent study, Tang *et al.* [32] were the first to provide evidence supporting an involvement of the parietal lobe in TNS synesthesia. They found stronger brain activation in the left and right parietal lobes for number–space synesthetes as compared to controls when performing ordinal judgments.

Another study showed the necessity of the parietal lobe for TNS synesthesia. Spalding and Zangwill [67] reported on a patient who suffered from a lesion in left tempo-parietal regions caused by a gunshot. Several years later he still exhibited spatial problems, severe acalculia but no evidence of his TNS synesthesia. Apparently, prior to the incident he was experiencing forms of numbers, months, days of the week and letters of the alphabet, which disappeared following his injury. Thus, it seems that the parietal lobe is crucial for the representation of spatially ordered sequences such as time and numbers.

Taking all of this together, we suggest that striate cortex and/or the parietal cortex could provide us with a plausible platform for revealing differences in the neural circuits of TNS synesthetes and non-synesthetes.

It might very well be that, as in other types of synesthesia such as grapheme–color synesthesia [68], or mirror–touch synesthesia [69], two types (or even more) of synesthesia exist with different neural origins (e.g., striate cortex, parietal cortex). A better understanding of the neural bases might offer a lead toward its origin, including the developmental stages at which it might occur. Therefore, a careful investigation of the individual differences in the experience of TNS together with a better understanding of its neural mechanisms will provide a means for the delineation of these types of synesthesia and consequently a better knowledge of the neurocognitive mechanisms behind the implicit interaction of time, number, and space in non-synesthetes.

TNS SYNESTHESIA: SYMBOLIC OR NON-SYMBOLIC?

An open question currently is whether time and number in the case of TNS synesthesia are triggered by symbolic content (Arabic digits, dates) which is culturally mediated [70], or by their non-symbolic content (e.g., duration, numerosity), which has ontogenetic and phylogenetic origins [71]. We hypothesize that the synesthetic experience is triggered by the symbolic content of time/number. We reason that as in all the cases so far, the effects and the descriptions by the TNS synesthetes are based on symbolic stimuli. This idea emphasizes the impact of culture on shaping the synesthetic experience. It is interesting to note that many synesthetic experiences are induced by cultural tools, such as letters, numbers, time units, which develop later neurally, and are newer evolutionarily [72]. In addition, the current idea suggests that there is an interplay between semantic (in the case of digits or time) and non-semantic spatial information (in the case of space) that depends on egocentric and allocentric spatial representation [31,73].

Nevertheless, it might be that the neural substrate for TNS is based initially on the neural substrate that is dedicated to non-symbolic representations of time and number. Our idea is based on theories that see development of cognitive and perceptual abilities as a function of neuronal re-use. For example, the massive redeployment hypothesis [74], and the neuronal recycling hypothesis [75], suggest that neuronal re-use constitutes a fundamental evolutionary [74] or developmental [75] strategy for realizing cognitive functions. An earlier, and similar theory, called the Interactive Specialization approach has been put forward by Mark Johnson [76,77]). An interactive specialization-based theory would attribute synesthesia to a lack of neuronal specialization in the related lobes (e.g., parietal, occipital), which therefore results in the simultaneous processing of several magnitudes such as time/number/space [78].

CONCLUSIONS

We described here the case of explicit connections between time, number, and space, as shown by TNS synesthetes. Recent research has shown that while these explicit representations are beneficial for the general processing, they also lead to less flexibility and thus higher cognitive costs. At the neural level, it has been suggested that TNS synesthesia stems from amplification of the same brain areas that are involved in processing time, number, and space in non-synesthetes. Further research will be needed to trace the developmental trajectories, as well as the respective genetic and cultural influences of TNS synesthesia, which, in turn will provide a better understanding of the connection between time, number, and space in the general population.

Acknowledgments

We would like to thank Kathrin Cohen Kadosh, Ed Hubbard, and Wim Gevers for helpful comments. RCK is supported by the Wellcome Trust (WT88378).

References

[1] H. Mann, J. Korzenko, J.S.A. Carriere, M.J. Dixon, Time–space synesthesia—A cognitive advantage?, Conscious. Cogn. 18 (2009) 619–627.

[2] N. Sagiv, J. Simner, J. Collins, B. Butterworth, J. Ward, What is the relationship between synesthesia and visuo-spatial number forms?, Cognition 101 (2006) 114–128.

[3] D. Bueti, V. Walsh, The parietal cortex and the representation of time, space, number and other magnitudes, Philos. Trans. R. Soc. B: Biol. Sci. 364 (2009) 2369–2380.

[4] J.F. Cantlon, M.L. Platt, E.M. Brannon, Beyond the number domain, Trends Cogn. Sci. 13 (2009) 83–91.

[5] V. Walsh, A theory of magnitude: common cortical metrics of time, space and quantity, Trends Cogn. Sci. 7 (2003) 483–488.

[6] J. Simner, Defining synesthesia, Br. J. Psychol. (in press).

[7] J.E. Asher, J.A. Lamb, D. Brocklebank, J.B. Cazier, E. Maestrini, L. Addis, et al., A whole-genome scan and fine-mapping linkage study of auditory–visual synesthesia reveals evidence of linkage to chromosomes 2q24, 5q33, 6p12, and 12p12, Am. J. Hum. Genet. 84 (2009) 279–285.

[8] R. Cohen Kadosh, A. Henik, Can synesthesia research inform cognitive science?, Trends Cogn. Sci. 11 (2007) 177–184.

[9] R.C. Cytowic, D.M. Eagleman, Wednesday is Indigo Blue, Massachusetts Institute of Technology, Cambridge, 2009.

[10] M. Hochel, E.G. Milan, Synesthesia: the existing state of affairs, Cogn. Neuropsychol. 28 (2008) 93–117.

[11] E.M. Hubbard, V.S. Ramachandran, Neurocognitive mechanisms of synesthesia, Neuron 48 (2005) 509–520.

[12] A.N. Rich, J.B. Mattingley, Anomalous perception in synesthesia: a cognitive neuroscience perspective, Nat. Rev. Neurosci. 3 (2002) 43–52.

[13] L.C. Robertson, Binding, spatial attention and perceptual awareness, Nat. Rev. Neurosci. 4 (2003) 93–102.

[14] L.C. Robertson, N. Sagiv, (Eds.), Synesthesia: Perspectives from Cognitive Neuroscience, Oxford University Press, New York, 2004

[15] J. Ward, J.B. Mattingley, Synesthesia: an overview of contemporary findings and controversies, Cortex 42 (2006) 129–136.

[16] R. Cohen Kadosh, K. Cohen Kadosh, A. Henik, The neuronal correlate of bi-directional synesthesia: a combined ERP and fMRI study, J. Cogn. Neurosci. 19 (2007) 2050–2059.

[17] F. Galton, Visualised numerals, Nature 21 (1880) 494–495.

[18] F. Galton, Visualised numerals, Nature 21 (1880) 252–256.

[19] R. Cohen Kadosh, A. Henik, V. Walsh, Small is bright and big is dark in synesthesia, Curr. Biol. 17 (2007) R834–R835.

[20] A.N. Rich, J.L. Bradshaw, J.B. Mattingley, A systematic, large-scale study of synesthesia: implications for the role of early experience in lexical color associations, Cognition 98 (2005) 53–84.

[21] J. Simner, J. Ward, M. Lanz, A. Jansari, K. Noonan, L. Glover, et al., Non-random associations of graphemes to color in synesthetic and non-synesthetic populations, Cogn. Neuropsychol. 22 (2005) 1069–1085.

[22] J. Ward, B. Huckstep, E. Tsakanikos, Sound–color synesthesia: to what extent does it use cross-modal mechanisms common to us all?, Cortex 42 (2006) 264–280.

[23] J. Simner, Synesthetic visuo-spatial forms: viewing sequences in space, Cortex 45 (2009) 1138–1147.

[24] D.M. Eagleman, The objectification of overlearned sequences: a new view of spatial sequence synesthesia, Cortex 45 (2009) 1266–1277.

[25] L. Gertner, A. Henik, R. Cohen Kadosh, When 9 is not on the right: implications from number-form synesthesia, Conscious. Cogn. 18 (2009) 366–374.

[26] E.M. Hubbard, M. Ranzini, M. Piazza, S. Dehaene, What information is critical to elicit interference in number–form synesthesia?, Cortex 45 (2009) 1200–1216.

[27] M. Piazza, P. Pinel, S. Dehaene, Objective correlates of an unusual subjective experience: a single-case study of number–form synesthesia, Cogn. Neuropsychol. 23 (2006) 1162–1173.

[28] M.C. Price, Spatial forms and mental imagery, Cortex 45 (2009) 1229–1245.

[29] M.C. Price, R.A. Mentzoni, Where is January? The month-SNARC effect in sequence-form synesthetes, Cortex 44 (2008) 890–907.

[30] J. Simner, N. Mayo, M.J. Spiller, A foundation for savantism? Visuo-spatial synesthetes present with cognitive benefits, Cortex 45 (2009) 1246–1260.

[31] D. Smilek, A. Callejas, M.J. Dixon, P.M. Merikle, Ovals of time: time–space associations in synesthesia, Conscious. Cogn. 16 (2007) 507–519.

[32] J. Tang, J. Ward, B. Butterworth, Number forms in the brain, J. Cogn. Neurosci. 20 (2008) 1547–1556.

[33] M. Jarick, M.J. Dixon, M.T. Stewart, E.C. Maxwell, D. Smilek, A different outlook on time: visual and auditory month names elicit different mental vantage points for a time–space synaesthete, Cortex 45 (2009) 1217–1228.

[34] X. Seron, M. Pesenti, M.P. Noel, G. Deloche, J.A. Cornet, Images of numbers, or "When 98 is upper left and 6 sky blue", Cognition 44 (1992) 159–196.

[35] G. Wood, H.-C. Nuerk, K. Willmes, Crossed hands and the SNARC effect: a failure to replicate Dehaene, Bossini and Giraux (1993), Cortex 42 (2006) 1069–1079.

[36] E.M. Hubbard, What information is critical to elicit interference in number–form synesthesia?, Cortex 45 (2009) 1200–1216.

[37] R. Cohen Kadosh, A. Henik, A. Catena, V. Walsh, L.J. Fuentes, Induced cross-modal synesthetic experience without abnormal neuronal connections, Psychol. Sci. 20 (2009) 258–265.

[38] E.M. Hubbard, M. Piazza, P. Pinel, S. Dehaene, Interactions between number and space in parietal cortex, Nat. Rev. Neurosci. 6 (2005) 435–448.

[39] V.S. Ramachandran, E.M. Hubbard, Synesthesia - a window into perception, thought and language. J Conscious Stud. 8(2001) 3–34.

[40] G. Beeli, M. Esslen, L. Jancke, Frequency correlates in grapheme–color synesthesia, Psychol. Sci. 18 (2007) 788–792.

[41] R. Cohen Kadosh, A. Henik, V. Walsh, Synesthesia: learned or lost? Dev. Sci. 12 (2009) 484–491.

[42] D. Smilek, J.S.A. Carriere, M.J. Dixon, P.M. Merikle, Grapheme frequency and color luminance in grapheme–color synesthesia, Psychol. Sci. 18 (2007) 793–795.

[43] R.S. Moyer, T.K. Landauer, Time required for judgment of numerical inequality, Nature 215 (1967) 1519–1520.

[44] J. Ward, N. Sagiv, B. Butterworth, The impact of visuo-spatial number forms on simple arithmetic, Cortex 45 (2009) 1261–1265.

[45] S. Dehaene, N. Molko, L. Cohen, A.J. Wilson, Arithmetic and the brain, Curr. Opin. Neurobiol. 14 (2004) 218–224.

[46] N. Burgess, C.F. Doeller, C.M. Bird, Space for the brain in Cognitive Science, in: L. Tommasi, M.A. Peterson, L. Nadal, (Eds.), Cognitive Biology: Evolutionary and Developmental Perspectives on Mind, Brain, and Behavior, MIT Press, Cambridge, MA, 2009, pp. 61–82.

[47] R. Cohen Kadosh, J. Lammertyn, V. Izard, Are numbers special? An overview of chronometric, neuroimaging, developmental and comparative studies of magnitude representation, Prog. Neurobiol. 84 (2008) 132–147.

[48] P.A. Lewis, R.C. Miall, Distinct systems for automatic and cognitively controlled time measurement: evidence from neuroimaging, Curr. Opin. Neurobiol. 13 (2003) 250–255.

[49] E.M. Hubbard, A.C. Armanm, V.S. Ramachandran, G.M. Boynton, Individual differences among grapheme–color synesthetes: brain-behavior correlations, Neuron 45 (2005) 975–985.

[50] J.A. Nunn, L.J. Gregory, M. Brammer, S.C.R. Williams, D.M. Parslow, M.J. Morgan, et al., Functional magnetic resonance imaging of synesthesia: activation of V4/V8 by spoken words, Nat. Neurosci. 5 (2002) 371–375.

[51] R. Rouw, H.S. Scholte, Increased structural connectivity in grapheme–color synesthesia, Nat. Neurosci. 10 (2007) 792–797.

[52] J.M. Sperling, D. Prvulovic, D.E.J. Linden, W. Singer, A. Stirn, Neuronal correlates of graphemic color synesthesia: a fMRI study, Cortex 42 (2006) 295–303.

[53] A.N. Rich, M.A. Williams, A. Puce, A. Syngeniotis, M.A. Howard, F. McGlone, et al., Neural correlates of imagined and synesthetic colors, Neuropsychologia 44 (2006) 2918–2925.

[54] F. Doricchi, P. Guariglia, M. Gasparini, F. Tomaiuolo, Dissociation between physical and mental number line bisection in right hemisphere brain damage, Nat. Neurosci. 8 (2005) 1663–1665.

[55] R. Cohen Kadosh, V. Walsh, Numerical representation in the parietal lobes: abstract or not abstract?, Behav. Brain. Sci. 32 (2009) 313–373.

[56] S. Dehaene, M. Piazza, P. Pinel, L. Cohen, Three parietal circuits for number processing, Cogn. Neuropsychol. 20 (2003) 487–506.

[57] G.R. Fink, J.C. Marshall, N.J. Shah, P.H. Weiss, P.W. Halligan, M. Grosse-Ruyken, et al., Line bisection judgments implicate right parietal cortex and cerebellum as assessed by fMRI, Neurology 6 (2000) 1324–1331.

[58] I. Alexander, A. Cowey, V. Walsh, The right parietal cortex and time perception: back to Critchley and the Zeitraffer phenomenon, Cogn. Neuropsychol. 22 (2005) 306–315.

[59] R. Cohen Kadosh, K. Cohen Kadosh, T. Schuhmann, A. Kaas, R. Goebel, A. Henik, et al., Virtual dyscalculia induced by parietal-lobe TMS impairs automatic magnitude processing, Curr. Biol. 17 (2007) 689–693.

[60] R. Cohen Kadosh, N. Muggleton, J. Silvanto, V. Walsh, Double dissociation of format-dependent and number-specific neurons in human parietal cortex, Cereb. Cortex 20 (2010) 2166–2171.

[61] R. Cohen Kadosh, S. Soskic, T. Iuculano, R. Kanai, V. Walsh, Modulating neuronal activity produces specific and long lasting changes in numerical competence, Curr. Biol. 20(2010) 2016–2020.

[62] S.M. Goebel, M. Calabria, A. Farne, Y. Rossetti, Parietal rTMS distorts the mental number line: simulating 'spatial' neglect in healthy subjects, Neuropsychologia 44 (2006) 860–868.

[63] S.M. Goebel, M.F.S. Rushworth, V. Walsh, Inferior parietal rTMS affects performance in an addition task, Cortex 42 (2006) 771–776.

[64] S.M. Goebel, V. Walsh, M.F.S. Rushworth, The mental number line and the human angular gyrus, NeuroImage 14 (2001) 1278–1289.

[65] A. Knops, H.-C. Nuerk, R. Sparing, H. Foltys, K. Willmes, On the functional role of human parietal cortex in number processing: how gender mediates the impact of a 'virtual lesion' induced by rTMS, Neuropsychologia 44 (2006) 270–283.

[66] M. Sandrini, P.M. Rossini, C. Miniussi, The differential involvement of inferior parietal lobule in number comparison: a rTMS study, Neuropsychologia 14 (2004) 1278–1289.

[67] J.M.K. Spalding, O.L. Zangwill, Disturbance of number–form in a case of brain injury, J. Neurosurg. Neurosurg. Psychiatry 13 (1950) 24–29.

[68] M.J. Dixon, D. Smilek, P.M. Merikle, Not all synesthetes are created equal: projector versus associator synesthetes, Cogn. Affect. Behav. Neurosci. 4 (2004) 335–343.

[69] M.J. Banissy, J. Ward, Mirror-touch synesthesia is linked with empathy, Nat. Neurosci. 10 (2007) 815–816.

[70] D. Ansari, Effects of development and enculturation on number representation in the brain, Nat. Rev. Neurosci. 9 (2008) 278–291.

[71] E.M. Brannon, U. Suanda, K. Libertus, Increasing precision in temporal discriminations over development parallels the development of number discrimination, Dev. Sci. 10 (2007) 770–777.

[72] R. Cohen Kadosh, D.B. Terhune, Redefining synesthesia? Br. J. Psychol. (in press).

[73] N. Sagiv, J. Ward, Crossmodal interactions: lessons from synesthesia, in: S. Martinez-Conde, S.L. Macknik, L.M. Martinez, J.M. Alonso, P.U. Tse, (Eds.), Visual Perception Part 2, Volume 155: Fundamentals of Awareness, Multi-Sensory Integration and High-Order Perception (Progress in brain research series), Elsevier Science, London, 2006, pp. 263–275.

[74] M.L. Anderson, Evolution of cognitive function via redeployment of brain areas, The Neuroscientist 13 (2007) 13–21.

[75] S. Dehaene, L. Cohen, Cultural recycling of cortical maps, Neuron 56 (2007) 384–398.

[76] M.H. Johnson, Functional brain development in humans, Nat. Rev. Neurosci. 2 (2001) 475–483.

[77] M.H. Johnson, T. Grossman, K. Cohen Kadosh, Mapping functional brain development: building a social brain through interactive specialization, Dev. Psychol. 45 (2009) 151–159.

[78] R. Cohen Kadosh, L. Gertner, D.B. Terhume, Exceptional abilities in the spatial representation of numbers and time: Insights from synesthesia. The Neuroscientist (in press).

How is Number Associated with Space? The Role of Working Memory

Wim Fias,* Jean-Philippe van Dijck* and Wim Gevers†

*Department of Experimental Psychology, Ghent University, Belgium
†Unité de Recherches en Neurosciences Cognitives, Université Libre de Bruxelles, Belgium

Summary

A large body of evidence demonstrates that the processing of numbers and space are tightly related. Today, the dominant explanation for this interaction is the number line hypothesis. This hypothesis claims that the mental representation of numbers takes the form of a horizontally oriented line which is functionally homeomorphic to the way physical lines are represented. The aim of the present review is twofold. Firstly, we review recent evidence on number bisection bias in neglect and on the Spatial Numerical Association of Response Codes (SNARC) effect challenging the homeomorphic relationship between numerical and spatial processing. For the bisection bias, we present data that show a clear dissociation between number bisection and physical line bisection. Additionally, we present data on the SNARC effect showing that its origin is of a conceptual rather than visuospatial nature. Secondly, we present data that provide pointers towards a new theoretical framework which proposes that serial position in working memory may be an important determinant of the interactions between number and space.

It is generally accepted that the cognitive representation and processing of number and space are tightly linked. This is evident from introspective reports, for instance by mathematicians who describe their mathematical thinking as hinging on visual imagery. Also, math instruction and education rely strongly on visuospatial tools and strategies. Remarkably,

© 2011 Elsevier Inc. All rights reserved.

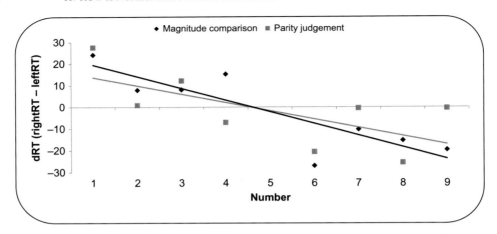

FIGURE 10.1   **SNARC-effect.** Depiction of the SNARC effect of both the parity judgment and magnitude comparison task, presenting the observed data and the regression lines, representing response time differences between right- and left-hand responses in function of the numerical magnitude. Positive values reflect faster left-hand than right-hand responses. The presented data reflect the effects of the baseline conditions described by van Dijck *et al.* [38].

the involvement of spatial processing in mathematical cognition is not restricted to complex mathematics but even applies to the basic and elementary representation of number.

Galton already described the introspective reports of people who experience vivid mental number line images in the 1880s (e.g., [1]). Later, Seron *et al.* [2] showed that these were more than incidental observations and confirmed that about 14% of a typical student population report mental number lines. Experiences of spatially defined mental number lines can be particularly strong and elaborated in synesthesia [3,4], a condition in which certain types of stimuli give rise to experiences in modalities that are normally not associated with such stimuli, for instance color sensations to number stimuli. Importantly, however, number–space interactions are not restricted to those who have the conscious experience of mental number lines. A number of empirical phenomena demonstrate that the involvement of space is a basic and essential aspect of number representation also in people who do not report having conscious experience of visuospatial number lines when they think about numbers.

In a seminal paper, Dehaene *et al.* [5] showed that, when subjects respond to numbers by pressing a left or a right response key, for instance in a parity judgment task, small numbers are responded to faster with the left hand than with the right hand, and large numbers receive faster right-hand than left-hand responses. This effect (see Fig. 10.1), indicating a Spatial Numerical Association of Response Codes (SNARC effect) has since then been replicated numerous times with paradigms using different stimulus and task configurations (for a review, see [6]).

Another phenomenon, reported for the first time by Zorzi *et al.* [7], is observed in many brain-damaged patients suffering from spatial hemineglect, most frequently after right hemisphere lesion. These patients fail to report, orient to, or verbally describe stimuli in the contralesional left hemispace (for a review, see [8]) as is, for instance, evident from tests like

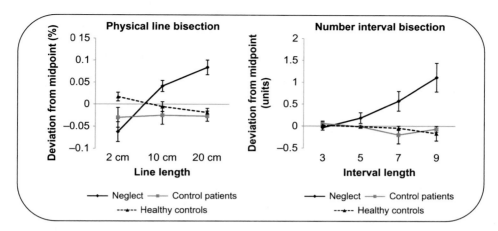

FIGURE 10.2   **Physical line and number interval bisection.** To test the hypothesis that the mental representation of numbers takes the form of a left to right oriented line, the relation between numbers and space has been investigated in right-brain-damaged neglect patients suffering from an attentional deficit for the left side of space. It was reasoned that when numbers were actually represented on such a representational format, their attentional deficit should give rise to a similar rightward bias when bisecting the mental number line as when indicating the midpoint of actual physical lines [7]. Here we present the results of a physical line and a number interval bisection task administered to neglect patients and two control groups [20], showing that neglect patients indeed shift the subjective midpoint of a numerical interval to the right (i.e. a positive deviation on the figure). This close resemblance in the performance of both tasks, led to the conclusion that the mental number line is more than a metaphor, and that its representational format is functionally isomorphic to that of physical lines (e.g., [7,13]).

physical line bisection where patients typically mark their perceived midpoint right from the veridical midpoint. When these patients are asked to name the number that is in the middle of a numerical interval (e.g., Which number is in the middle between 1 and 9?), they often produce a number that is larger than the true middle number, whereby the size of the bias is positively correlated to the size of the difference between the two numbers. Together with a cross-over effect (i.e. a tendency of a bias towards smaller numbers in small numerical intervals), the pattern of number bisection bias strongly resembles the bias observed when neglect patients bisect physical lines (see Fig. 10.2).

While the idea of a mental number line was originally conceived of as a metaphor (e.g., [9]), the strong similarity between number and physical line bisection has been taken as evidence in favor of a stronger version of the mental number line hypothesis that argues that the mental number line is not simply a metaphor but that the mental representation of numerical magnitude is considered to be homeomorphic to the representation of physical space (e.g., [10]), with a common mechanism of spatial attention operating on both numerical and physical space (e.g., [7,11]). The hypothesis of a homeomorphic mental number line has since become the dominant theoretical framework to account for various instances of number–space interactions (for a review, see for instance [12–14]).

In what follows, we will review recent evidence on number bisection bias in neglect and on the SNARC effect that challenges this interpretation. In doing so, we will provide pointers towards an alternative framework that proposes serial position in working memory as an important determinant of the interactions between number and space.

DISSOCIATING THE NUMBER INTERVAL BISECTION BIAS FROM THE LINE BISECTION BIAS

The parallelism between number interval bisection and physical line bisection in neglect offers a high degree of face validity to the mental number line hypothesis. Just like patients ignore the left side of physical space and, therefore, produce a rightward bias in line bisection, the patients are assumed to ignore the left side of the number line which then leads to a bisection towards the right side of the number line where the large numbers are located.

However, the idea of a functional isomorphism between bisection of physical and number space has been questioned. Doricchi *et al.* [15] (for a larger follow-up study, see [16]) observed a double dissociation between number interval bisection and physical line bisection. Those patients that established a strong bias in line bisection produced only a weak or no bias in number bisection and *vice versa*. This suggests that both tasks depend on at least partly dissociable mechanisms. Interestingly, Doricchi *et al.* observed the number interval bisection bias to occur only in those patients whose lesion comprised prefrontal cortex [15] and whose visuospatial and verbal working memory span was reduced [16]. This suggests that working memory span may play a crucial role in the number interval bisection task. However, by itself, a reduced span can explain generally inaccurate performance in the number interval bisection task, but is not sufficient to account for the systematic deviation towards the larger numbers.

Recently, van Dijck *et al.* [17] presented a single-case study in which a clear dissociation between number and line bisection was present within the same patient. Moreover, the performance of the patient was informative for how a working memory deficit can give rise to a systematic deviation towards larger numbers. This patient had an ischemic left hemisphere lesion mainly affecting temporo-parietal areas and extending into frontal cortex and accordingly exhibited a right-sided neglect for physical space (as tested with tasks like physical line bisection) as well as for representational space (as tested with the o'clock task [18] and the description of a memorized picture [19]). Surprisingly, the patient showed a number interval bisection bias towards the larger numbers, just like all other reports of number interval bisection bias after right hemisphere lesion and left-sided neglect. Thus, while physical line bisection was biased to the left because of her right neglect, number interval bisection bias remained directed towards the larger numbers. The possible explanation that this was due to a reversed mental number line (i.e. from right to left) was ruled out by the fact that the patient showed a normal SNARC effect (faster left- than right-hand responses to small numbers and *vice versa* for large numbers).

Interestingly, a close examination of the patient's working memory performance revealed a pattern that can explain the bisection bias. While her visuospatial memory span fell within the normal range, her verbal memory span was reduced to only three items, as measured with a forward letter span task. By means of a probe recognition task that measured the capacity of verbal working memory at different positions within the serial sequence to be remembered, it was found that the patient was specifically impaired in remembering items from the beginning of the working memory sequence (running against the primacy effect typically observed in working memory). Furthermore, with the use of a position recall task (where the patient had to reproduce the element at a specific position in the sequence), the nature of the errors was investigated. It was found that errors were primarily items that were positioned further in the sequence than the requested position. Clearly this position-specific impairment in verbal working memory provides a meaningful explanation for the patient's number bisection bias. After all, when the initial numbers of the to-be-bisected numerical sequences are not efficiently kept in mind and the bisection is performed on the remaining numbers, a shift towards the larger number is a logical consequence.

The involvement of verbal working memory in the bisection performance of this patient is further supported by the fact that the same directional bias that was observed in number interval bisection also occurred in a letter interval bisection (e.g., Which letter is in the middle between A and E?) and in a word bisection task (e.g., Which is the middle letter of the word 'voltage'?).

Although the experiments in this patient do not allow pinpointing the exact processes and representations involved in number interval bisection, they do allow concluding that number interval bisection bias can, despite its apparent similarity with physical line bisection, completely dissociate from it and even go in the opposite direction. It is true of course that generalizing from a single case study is not without problems, but the fact that position-specific working memory deficit can give rise to biased number interval bisection performance urges to seriously consider the involvement of working memory in future neuropsychological studies.

Of course, generalization of the interpretations from a single case study is not without problems. Therefore, van Dijck *et al.* [20] ran a group study evaluating whether number and physical line bisection depend on a shared spatial attention mechanism by exploring the extent to which both correlate. Right-hemisphere damaged neglect patients ($n = 9$), patients with right hemisphere lesion without neglect ($n = 5$) and healthy age-matched controls ($n = 12$) were included. All subjects were submitted to both the physical line bisection and the number interval bisection task. In addition, the SNARC effect was measured in both a parity judgment and a number comparison task. The results showed that only the neglect group showed a bisection bias in line and number interval bisection, as expected. All groups showed a SNARC effect in the parity judgment and in the number comparison tasks. The effects (bias for bisection tasks and the SNARC slopes for the parity judgment and the comparison tasks) were subjected to a principal component analysis. From the mental number line account, it is predicted that a single-factor component would be sufficient to capture the correlational structure between the space-related effects obtained in the different tasks. However, Principal Component Analysis (PCA) revealed that such solution is not the case. The results showed that a three-component solution provided the best fit of the data pattern. The first component was loaded by magnitude comparison and number interval bisection, the second component by parity judgment and number interval bisection and the third component only by physical line bisection.

This result clearly refutes the strong version of the mental number line hypothesis by showing that multiple factors are needed to capture the correlations between the tasks. However, given the fact that PCA is not well suited to determine the details of underlying mechanisms (especially when the number of subjects is relatively limited), further conclusions are not warranted. Nevertheless, both the single case and the group study demonstrate that a critical stance is needed towards the mental number line hypothesis as the sole explanatory mechanism of how number relates to space. In the following, we will focus on the SNARC effect and ask two questions. First, can the SNARC effect be dissociated from the mental number line explanation? Second, if it can be dissociated, then the question to the origin of the SNARC effect is open. Following the suggestions just described, the involvement of working memory in the SNARC effect will be explored.

DISSOCIATING SNARC FROM THE NUMBER LINE: CONCEPTUAL *VS* VISUOSPATIAL REPRESENTATIONS

People acquire knowledge about the world through sensory-motor experience. Hence, it is no wonder that high level cognition is grounded in sensorimotor experience [21] and that mental representations of this knowledge are at least to some extent analogous to the world they represent. Yet, it is also true that humans are a communicative species that use language to communicate thoughts and cognition with their conspecifics, the essential characteristic of language being that it summarizes information in structured and labeled categories. Hence, humans are also exposed to knowledge in a format that is abstracted away from direct physical reality. This makes it realistic to assume that information is not only represented in an analog way but also in a format that makes abstraction of instances of sensory-motor experience. This distinction is developed in the dual coding theory of Paivio [22] who claims that information is coded in an analog system and in a verbal–symbolic system. Along the same lines, but in the specific context of spatial representations, Kosslyn *et al.* [23,24] distinguished between categorical and coordinate spatial representations. The coordinate system codes for spatial position in a quantitatively precise way and the categorical system defines space in more qualitative and conceptually distinct classes (for instance, left *vs* right, or above *vs* below).

The mental number line hypothesis envisages only associations with the analog representational system: Numbers are positioned on a mental number line that is defined in the same metrics as physical space is mentally coded [7,12,25]. As such it can account for the number interval bisection bias in neglect and for the SNARC effect. Yet, recently it has been argued that the dimensional overlap between number and response location in the SNARC effect is not necessarily located at a visuospatial level but can also be situated at a categorical level, i.e. at a level of spatial representation that is not analogous to physical space but that is tightly linked to language. In this respect, Proctor *et al.* [26] developed the theoretical idea that the SNARC effect derives from a systematic association between the verbal concepts such as small and left, and large and right, based on the assumption that conceptual categorical dimensions (like left–right and small–large) have a specific polarity (e.g., left being negative and right positive; and similarly small being negative and large being positive). According to the polarity coding account it is the congruency between these polar codes that drives the SNARC effect. Similarly, but in a computationally explicit way, Gevers *et al.* [27] argued that the SNARC effect results from learned connections between a number's conceptual categorization as small or large and the conceptual category of the response (e.g., left or right).

A first empirical indication that the SNARC effect does not imply the existence of a mental number line was observed by Santens and Gevers [28]. Here, participants performed a regular magnitude comparison task with a fixed reference (i.e. 5), but instead of left–right responses, participants had to respond to a location that was close to or far from the initial finger position. On the mental number line, the numbers 4 and 6 are close to the number 5 whereas the numbers 1 and 9 are far from this reference number. Therefore, a direct mapping between the number line and the position of the response would result in faster 'close' than 'far' responses for the numbers 4 and 6 and faster 'far' than 'close' responses and the numbers 1 and 9. This was not observed. Small numbers (1 and 4) were fastest with the close response and large numbers (6 and 9) with the far response. This result is in line with a conceptual account that systematically associates small to close and large to far, following Proctor *et al.* [26].

Gevers *et al.* [29] followed up on this idea and designed an experimental paradigm that allowed the determination of the categorical *vs* visuospatial nature of the SNARC effect. The essential characteristic of this paradigm is that response buttons are variably (from trial to trial) labeled by response defining words (e.g., the label 'left' and the label 'right'). For instance, in a parity judgment task, subjects were asked to press the button wearing the label 'left' if the number was even, or to press the button labeled 'right' if the number was odd. In doing so, Gevers *et al.* could track whether the SNARC effect followed the visuospatial position of the hands emitting the response or the categorical concepts expressed by the labels. Both visuospatial and categorical coding could be observed when tested separately, but when both coding systems were directly pitted against one another, a pronounced dominance of the concepts expressed by the labels was observed, both in parity judgment and in number comparison. This observation provides direct evidence that numbers can interact with spatial representations at a conceptual level and that these interactions are the dominant ones for the SNARC. These results are difficult to reconcile with the homeomorphic mental number line hypothesis, because the conceptual nature of the underlying representation radically differs from the visuospatial coordinate system that is assumed to define the mental number line. At the same time, this implies that the idea of the involvement of a spatial attention mechanism in the SNARC effect is difficult to maintain.

THE SNARC EFFECT: A CRUCIAL ROLE FOR WORKING MEMORY

A number of research reports have shown that the associations between number and space are not absolute but depend on contextual aspects of the stimuli, the responses, and the task. This might suggest that the SNARC effect does not depend so much on long-term associations between numbers and space, as implied in the mental number line hypothesis, but rather on temporary representations.

First, the association between a specific number with left or right depends on the range in which that number occurs [5,30]. For instance, number 5 presented in the context of numbers ranging from 1 to 5 will receive faster right than left hand responses, but when that same number 5 occurs in the range 4 to 9, it will receive faster left- than right-hand responses. Similarly, when subjects are asked to envisage the numbers as being displayed on a clock face, the SNARC effect reverses, following the fact that now small numbers occur on the right side of the clock face and large numbers on the left side of the clock [31].

Second, the fact that the SNARC effect depends on response characteristics is shown by the fact that the left–right SNARC effect only occurs when responses have to be discriminated along the left–right dimension, suggesting that spatial coding needs to be part of the response or task set [32]. This was convincingly demonstrated by the experiments of Notebaert *et al.* [33] who showed that the SNARC effect can actually be reversed by creating new short-term memory associations between numbers and side of response. These associations were created by means of an inducer task where the letter X was presented either on the left or on the right side of fixation. Participants had to respond incompatibly to the location of the letter X (e.g., press left if it appears on the right side, press right if it appears on the left side). In this way, new associations are created between the position 'left' and the response 'right', and between the position 'right' and the response 'left' (see also [34]). The interest was to observe what these newly created associations would do with an intermixed SNARC task (e.g., centrally presented numbers that had to be judged on their orientation). The results showed that by creating these new short-term associations, the SNARC effect reversed. The effect of these short-term associations suggests an important role for working memory.

Third, and relatedly, it has been shown that Russian–Hebrew bilinguals show a normal SNARC effect when they had read a Russian text shortly before but a reversed SNARC effect when having read a Hebrew text before [35]. Similarly, Shaki and Gevers [36] showed that, in Israeli participants, the SNARC effect can reverse simply on the basis of the task instruction. Hebrew letters contain both ordinal (e.g., B comes after A in the alphabet) and magnitude meaning (e.g., the letter B is 2). When asked to judge the letters for their ordinal meaning, a SNARC effect was observed in line with their reading and writing direction (letters from the beginning of the alphabet—right response/letters far in the alphabetic sequence—left response). However, when asked to judge the letters on their magnitude meaning, a left-to-right SNARC effect was observed.

Observations such as these might indicate that numbers are not intrinsically related to space but that the relation is constructed during task execution, which might suggest a crucial role for working memory. This has been tested by evaluating the effect of working memory load on the SNARC effect. Herrerra *et al.* [37] and van Dijck *et al.* [38] showed that the SNARC effect in magnitude comparison disappears when visuospatial working memory is loaded (by Corsi block configurations). Van Dijck *et al.* additionally showed that, in parity judgment, it is verbal working memory load that abolished the SNARC effect. This indicates that the SNARC effect critically depends on the availability of working memory resources. Additionally, the results suggest that, depending on the task, verbal or visuospatial working memories are recruited.

Of course, just like a reduced working memory capacity is by itself not sufficient to explain the number interval bisection bias in neglect, the necessity of free working memory resources for the SNARC effect to occur does on itself say nothing about the nature of the underlying mechanism. Although such an association has never been reported, it might be plausible to assume that serial position in working memory is associated with left and right, with items in the initial positions being associated with left and items towards the end of the working memory sequence being associated with right.

To test this hypothesis, van Dijck and Fias [39] designed an experimental procedure that allowed the dissociation of the effects of position in a working memory sequence from position on a mental number line as a function of number magnitude. Subjects were presented with a randomly ordered series of numbers and were asked to remember these numbers to reproduce them later in the correct order. During the retention interval, left- and right-hand responses were measured by asking subjects to perform a parity judgment task and give a response only to those numbers that belonged to the remembered sequence. The results clearly showed that the position of the number in the working memory sequence was strongly associated with space: numbers from the beginning of the sequence were responded to faster with the left hand than with the right hand and *vice versa* for numbers towards the end of the sequence. Number magnitude, on the other hand, was not systematically associated with left or right responses.

If position in working memory relates to response preference, it should be possible to establish this position-based effect with whatever kind of information maintained in working memory. Hence, in the next experiment van Dijck and Fias [39] used fruit and vegetable names and asked subjects to perform a fruit/vegetable classification task during the retention interval. Again, a position-based effect on response preference was observed. Interestingly, the SNARC effect was also measured in the same subjects, using a traditional parity judgment tasks, i.e. without any working memory instructions. Crucially, the position-based effect with fruits and vegetables significantly correlated with the SNARC effect with numbers. This strongly suggests that the association between working memory position and space is what drives the SNARC effect, not the long-term numerical value.

These findings suggest that what happens is that, in order to achieve efficient task performance, participants store numbers in working memory as part of the task set and that, in doing so, they systematically order numbers as a function of their numerical magnitude, maybe as a helpful way of extending working memory capacity. From this explanation of the SNARC effect, a number of phenomena can be readily explained. First, it enables the explanation of the fact that the SNARC effect is obtained when number magnitude is completely irrelevant for the task [30]. It is not the task that has to be performed that is crucial, but if and how a number is systematically stored in working memory. Second, the range dependency of the SNARC effect [5,30] is a consequence of the fact that only numbers that belong to the task set are stored. Third, the fact that the SNARC effect also occurs for non-numerical stimuli with an intrinsic ordinal structure (letters of the alphabet [40], musical tones [41,42], arbitrary stimuli that have to be learned to be ordered [43–45]) is not surprising, given that not numerical value but systematic assignment to a serial position in working memory is important. Fourth, mapping small numbers to the beginning and large numbers to the end of the memorized task set sequence is the default mapping. However, task context can change this default mapping. This is the case for instance, when participants are asked to imagine numbers on a clock face (e.g., [31]). Similarly, the direction of the SNARC effect depends on reading habits (with a reversed SNARC effect in right-to-left reading cultures (with a reversed SNARC effect in right-to-left reading cultures [46]). It has been shown that the direction of the SNARC effect can rapidly change within the same participants, depending on whether they read a text from left-to-right or from right-to-left immediately before the measurement of the SNARC effect [35]. While this is hard to explain by a long-term oriented mental number line account, the positional working memory account easily explains this flexibility, although at this point it is not clear whether reading direction determines how the numbers belonging to the task set are positionally coded in working memory or, alternatively whether it is the position–space associations that are influenced by reading direction.

GENERAL DISCUSSION

The present review of our recent work challenges the dominant view that the mental representation of numerical magnitude takes the form of a mental number line which is homeomorphic with the representation of physical lines, and that there is a common spatial attention mechanism that operates both in physical space and in number space. We specifically considered the number interval bisection task in neglect and the SNARC effect, because these tasks have been considered prototypical exemplars of this homeomorphism.

Regarding the SNARC effect, our work generated results that are difficult to reconcile with the mental number line hypothesis. First, the spatial response code that is associated to numbers does not seem to be of a visuospatial nature, but is rather situated at the level of conceptual categories. Second, serial position in working memory is the primary determinant of associations with response codes, not numerical magnitude. The fact that the same serial position effects also occur for non-numerical stimuli implies that the spatial associations that are observed in the SNARC effect are not specific to number but are a side-effect of how serial position is coded in working memory and are related to spatial aspects of the response.

Also the single-case study and the patient group study revealed evidence that is not in line with what is expected from the mental number line hypothesis. Both studies converge with previously made observations that number interval bisection and physical line bisection can be dissociated (e.g., [15,16]). The single-case study actually showed physical bisection biases to the left whereas the number interval bisection bias remained towards the larger number.

Moreover, these patient studies are also suggestive of working memory being a crucial determinant of the bisection bias. The single-case study revealed that a position-specific deficit to initial items of the verbal working memory could explain the number interval bisection bias. The group study showed that the number interval bisection bias was not associated with line bisection, but with the SNARC effect. Because the SNARC effect is clearly determined by serial position in working memory and because the position-specific working memory impairment in the single-case study concur, we hypothesize that serial position drives the correlation between number bisection bias and the SNARC effect, thereby strengthening our hypothesis (derived from a single case) that also in number bisection the crucial variable is serial position.

In sum, the empirical work reviewed above questions the two key assumptions of the mental number line hypothesis: the homeomorphism between number and physical space and the common mechanism of spatial attention operating in both number and physical space. Instead, we propose that it is spatial associations that are defined in conceptual terms that are associated to number, and that it is not spatial attention operating on a mental number line, but a systematic coupling between number magnitude and ordinal position in working memory that constitutes the underlying mechanism. We realize that these are pointers towards an alternative framework but that we have not reached the stage of a fully elaborated functional explanation yet.

Clearly, the SNARC effect and the number bisection bias are not the sole phenomena that are indicators of interactions between number and space that have been taken as support for the mental number line hypothesis. First, Fischer *et al.* [11] showed that numbers can act as an endogenous cue in the Posner cueing paradigm, suggesting that numbers can induce shifts of spatial attention. Second, using fMRI, Knops *et al.* [47] showed that the pattern of neural activity in regions that are involved in planning saccades could distinguish between subtraction and addition, with subtraction being associated with leftward eye-movements and addition with rightward eye-movements. Although the causal involvement needs to be demonstrated, it might suggest a close link between spatial attention and mental calculation. Third, Ishihara *et al.* [48] showed that number-induced manual pointing to various horizontal spatial positions was facilitated when the location corresponded to the position on the mental number line, suggesting a close connection between numbers and visuomotor processes.

It might be that the mental number line is a valid hypothesis in these situations. At this point, however, we believe that any conclusions are premature in the absence of further testing. Given the fact that our work showed that the link between number and space is far more complex than we originally thought, a large body of work is needed to come to grips with this complexity.

In doing so, we might have to go beyond the boundaries that are typically drawn to demarcate research fields. For instance, how are spatial attention and working memory related? Hereby, recent work indicating an overlap in neural resources between attention and visuospatial working memory should be taken into account (e.g., [49]). A related question is whether spatial attention also plays a role in verbal working memory, as was recently suggested by Anderson *et al.* [50]. This, in turn, raises the old issue as to what extent visual and verbal working memory are interrelated. Are they organized in a modality-specific way as in the model of Baddeley and Hitch [51], or do they depend on modality-independent mechanisms [52,53]? Of course, also insights on how serial order processing in working memory is accomplished may turn out to be extremely relevant (e.g., [52,54,55]). It might be particularly useful to connect to the models that are designed in the context of serial order processing in working memory (see [56] for a review). Recently, Botvinick and Watanabe [57] explicitly made this connection by proposing a model on serial position in working memory that explicitly incorporated a mechanism that was based on number selective neural tuning (e.g., [58]).

Similarly, insight can be gained from the recently growing research line that tries to understand how instructions are implemented and executed (e.g., [59,60]). Because instructions are usually conveyed to the subject in verbal form, often referring to binary categorical labels as left or right (e.g., press left if even, press right if odd), one can ask the question whether this might be a causal factor for the dominance of the conceptual spatial representation in the SNARC effect. However, what happens when instructions are not delivered in terms of linguistic spatial categories (press left or press right)? The study of Ishihara *et al.* [48] might be indicative in this respect. Relatedly, one should think about the role of the specific task to be performed. For instance, why is it that parity judgment is affected by verbal working memory and magnitude comparison by visuospatial working memory [38]?

Another important avenue for further research is to better understand the nature and organization of knowledge representations about abstract concepts like space and number. Clearly, this knowledge is initially constructed from sensorimotor experience (for instance number occupying space or order going in a specific direction). But gradually these experiences are summarized in abstract concepts (like small *vs* large; left *vs* right; or individual numbers) and linked to language. A crucial question in the current context is to what extent these abstract concepts keep the characteristics of the representations involved in sensorimotor experience and are thus embodied (e.g., [61]) or, alternatively, become functionally separable from these concrete experiences (e.g., [62]), possibly mediated by language [63]. One can then ask refined questions as to what extent language-based conceptual knowledge *vs* knowledge more directly rooted in sensorimotor experience is invoked during number processing, probably depending on the nature of the task (e.g., [64] for a demonstration that exact addition relies on linguistic knowledge and approximate addition on visuospatial knowledge representations).

To conclude, having provided data that are incompatible with the mental number line hypothesis, our results may have raised more questions than it has provided answers. It was a fruitful approach to push the mental number line metaphor to the limits of the idea that number shares a type of representation that is homomorphic to physical space with spatial attention operating upon it. Yet, now the limits of this hypothesis are becoming clear and alternative hypotheses including conceptual knowledge and serial order in working memory need to be considered to come to a complete understanding of the complexity of number–space interactions. Referring to the location of the 24th Attention and Performance meeting, one could use the French expression "Reculer pour mieux sauter" to indicate what is ahead of us now.

BOX 10.1

THE ORIGIN OF NUMBER SPACE INTERACTIONS

Despite the compelling demonstrations of an intimate relation between the representations of space and numbers, two questions are still outstanding. Both pertain to the origin of the number–space interactions. The first question is a more general one: why is it that both domains are associated at a functional and neural level? The second is more specific and asks why there is a systematic directional preference in this association (why is a small number associated with left and a large number with right?).

At least three possible explanations have emerged in the literature (e.g., [65]). A first view holds that the functional overlap between numbers and space derives from experienced correlations between numbers and space (e.g., [5,66]). In our daily life, children often see numbers in typical and culturally consistent spatial configurations (e.g., on blackboards, in schoolbooks, on computer keyboards) and it is a well-established observation that such environmental and cultural factors are picked up and can have an influence on both behavioral and brain organization (e.g., [67]). Since these lay-outs of number are systematically organized in space (e.g., from left-to-right in Western cultures), this view naturally addresses both questions. Indeed, it has been shown that the direction of functional overlap between numbers and space critically depends on the direction of the reading system (which also determines the orientation in which number sequences are most commonly spatially depicted) of the tested subjects, whereby left-to-right readers associate small numbers with left and large numbers

BOX 10.1 (cont'd)

with right, and right-to-left readers in the opposite direction [35,46]. A recent study showed culturally dependent directions of number–space associations in preschoolers [68], suggesting that it is not reading direction *per se* but the culturally consistent organization of spatial lay-outs of ordinal information that are important.

A second view is that both domains are related to one another because of the shared vocabulary to talk about spatial and numerical entities (e.g., five is bigger than four, six is smaller than nine). It is assumed that, during development of their language skills, children pick up this equivalence, thereby determining and constraining the conceptual representation of both numbers and space (e.g., [69]). This view provides an answer to the first question but, without further assumptions, is largely silent regarding the nature of the specific directionality of the number space association. In line with this view, it has been recently demonstrated that the SNARC-effect is the expression of a congruency between verbal concepts rather than between numbers and a location in physical space [29,38]. A recent developmental study showed that such a conceptual relationship is already the dominant factor driving the SNARC-effect in third grade children, the youngest group tested [70].

A third and final view holds that the link between numbers and space is innate in the sense that it is the result of a process of recycling evolutionarily old, general-purpose mechanisms (like spatial processing) for more recent cognitive skills like number processing (e.g., [71]). For instance, Dehaene and colleagues [72] investigated the mental representation of numbers in an Amazonian tribe. Notwithstanding the fact that the members of this tribe lack a fully developed lexicon for numbers and formal (math) education, they spontaneously put numbers on a horizontal line when asked to map numbers to space (but see [73]). Other support for the native origin has been provided by de Hevia and Spelke [74] who demonstrated number–space interactions in nine-month-old infants, ruling out the idea that language acquisition and extensive experienced correlations between numbers and space are crucial for the emergence of a relation between both domains. So far, this account did not provide much evidence for the directional specificity issue.

In sum, it is clear that the origin of the relationship between numbers and space is multifaceted and cannot be reduced to one single mechanism. To the contrary, it seems that the functional overlap between both domains illustrates how environmental, cultural and linguistic experience can shape an innate biological tendency to link different domains of cognition. Our recent experiments (see main text) suggest that serial working memory position could be a crucial intermediate variable that determines how environment, culture and language effectuate the number space relationship. It is not unlikely that language and cultural experience structure the spatial organization of serial position in working memory and provide the systematicity in which ordinal information is mapped to positions in working memory. It is also reasonable to assume that number processing recruits and recycles the general-purpose resources provided by working memory because of its ordinal organization which it shares with the number system.

References

[1] F. Galton, Visualised numerals, Nature 21 (1880) 252–256.
[2] X. Seron et al., Images of numbers, or when 98 is upper left and 6 sky blue, Cognition 44 (1992) 159–196.
[3] R.C. Kadosh, A. Henik, Can synaesthesia research inform cognitive science?, Trends Cogn. Sci. 11 (2007) 177–184.
[4] W. Gevers et al., Bidirectionality in synesthesia evidence from a multiplication verification task, Exp. Psychol. 57 (2010) 178–184.
[5] S. Dehaene et al., The mental representation of parity and number magnitude, J. Exp. Psychol. Gen. 122 (1993) 371–396.
[6] W. Fias, M.H. Fischer, Spatial representation of number, in: J.I.D. Campbell, (Ed.), Handbook of Mathematical Cognition, Psychology Press, (2005), pp. 43–54.
[7] M. Zorzi et al., Brain damage—Neglect disrupts the mental number line, Nature 417 (2002) 138–139.
[8] P.W. Halligan et al., Spatial cognition: evidence from visual neglect, Trends Cogn. Sci. 7 (2003) 125–133.
[9] S. Dehaene, Precis of the number sense, Mind Lang. 16 (2001) 16–36.
[10] I. Stoianov et al., Visuospatial priming of the mental number line, Cognition 106 (2008) 770–779.
[11] M.H. Fischer et al., Perceiving numbers causes spatial shifts of attention, Nat. Neurosci. 6 (2003) 555–556.
[12] C. Umilta et al., The spatial representation of numbers: evidence from neglect and pseudoneglect, Exp. Brain Res. (2009) 561–569.
[13] E.M. Hubbard et al., Interactions between number and space in parietal cortex, Nat. Rev. Neurosci. 6 (2005) 435–448.
[14] G. Vallar, L. Girelli, Numerical representations: Abstract or supramodal? Some may be spatial, Behav. Brain Sci. 32 (2009) 354.
[15] F. Doricchi et al., Dissociation between physical and mental number line bisection in right hemisphere brain damage, Nat. Neurosci. 8 (2005) 1663–1665.
[16] F. Doricchi et al., Spatial orienting biases in the decimal numeral system, Curr. Biol. 19 (2009) 682–687.
[17] J.-P. van Dijck, et al., Non-Spatial Neglect for the Mental Number Line (under revision).
[18] D. Grossi et al., On the different roles of the cerebral hemispheres in mental-imagery—The o'clock test in 2 clinical cases, Brain Cogn. 10 (1989) 18–27.
[19] M. Denis et al., Visual perception and verbal descriptions as sources for generating mental representations: Evidence from representational neglect, Cogn. Neuropsychol. 19 (2002) 97–112.
[20] J.-P. van Dijck, et al., The internal structure of number space, in: J.-P. van Dijck (Ed.), The Cognitive Mechanisms of Spatial Numerical Associations, 2009. (Unpublished doctoral disertation).
[21] L.W. Barsalou, Perceptions of perceputal symbols , Behav. Brain Sci. 22 (1999) 637–660.
[22] A. Paivio, Mental Representations : A Dual Coding Approach, Oxford University Press
[23] S.M. Kosslyn, Evidence for 2 types of spatial relations—hemispheric specialization for categorical and coordinate relations, J. Exp. Psychol. Hum. Percept. Perform. 15 (1989) 723–735.
[24] S.M. Kosslyn, You can play 20 questions with nature and win: Categorical versus coordinate spatial relations as a case study, Neuropsychologia 44 (2006) 1519–1523.
[25] K. Priftis et al., Explicit versus implicit processing of representational space in neglect: Dissociations in accessing the mental number line, J. Cogn. Neurosci. 18 (2006) 680–688.
[26] R.W. Proctor, Y.S. Cho, Polarity correspondence: A general principle for performance of speeded binary classification tasks, Psychol. Bull. 132 (2006) 416–442.
[27] W. Gevers et al., Numbers and space: A computational model of the SNARC effect, J. Exp. Psychol. Hum. Percept. Perform. 32 (2006) 32–44.
[28] S. Santens, W. Gevers, The SNARC effect does not imply a mental number line, Cognition 108 (2008) 263–270.
[29] W. Gevers et al., Verbal–spatial and visuo-spatial coding of number–space interactions, J. Exp. Psychol. Gen. 139 (2010) 180–190.
[30] W. Fiasv et al., The importance of magnitude information in numerical processing: evidence from the SNARC effect, Math. Cogn. 2 (1996) 95–110.
[31] D. Bachtold et al., Stimulus–response compatibility in representational space, Neuropsychologia 36 (1998) 731–735.
[32] W. Gevers et al., Automatic response activation of implicit spatial information: Evidence from the SNARC effect, Acta Psychol. 122 (2006) 221–233.

[33] W. Notebaert et al., Shared spatial representations for numbers and space: the reversal of the SNARC and the Simon effects, J. Exp. Psychol. Hum. Percept. Perform. 32 (2006) 1197–1207.

[34] J.G. Marble, R.W. Proctor, Mixing location-relevant and location-irrelevant choice-reaction tasks: Influences of location mapping on the Simon effect, J. Exp. Psychol. Hum. Percept. Perform. 26 (2000) 1515–1533.

[35] S. Shaki, M.H. Fischer, Reading space into numbers—a cross-linguistic comparison of the SNARC effect, Cognition 108 (2008) 590–599.

[36] S. Shaki, W. Gevers, Cultural characteristics dissociate magnitude and ordinal information processing, J. Cross Cult. Psychol. (in press).

[37] A. Herrera et al., The role of working memory in the association between number magnitude and space, Acta Psychol. 128 (2008) 225–237.

[38] J.-P. van Dijck et al., Numbers are associated with different types of spatial information depending on the task, Cognition 113 (2009) 248–253.

[39] J.-P. Van Dijck, W. Fias, A working memory accout for spatial-numerical associations. Cognition 119(1) (2011) 114–119.

[40] W. Gevers et al., The mental representation of ordinal sequences is spatially organized, Cognition 87 (2003) B87–B95.

[41] P. Lidji et al., Spatial associations for musical stimuli: a piano in the head?, J. Exp. Psychol. Hum. Percept. Perform. 33 (2007) 1189–1207.

[42] E. Rusconi et al., Spatial representation of pitch height: the SMARC effect, Cognition 99 (2006) 113–129.

[43] P. Previtali et al., Placing order in space: the SNARC effect in serial learning, Exp. Brain Res. 201 (2010) 599–605.

[44] F. Van Opstal et al., The neural representation of extensively trained ordered sequences, Neuroimage 47 (2009) 367–375.

[45] S.F. Lourenco, Developmental origins and the extent of generalization in the representation of magnitude. in: 24th Attention and Performance Meeting, July 6–10, Paris, France, 2010.

[46] S. Zebian, Linkages between number, concepts, spatial thinking, and directionality of writing: the SNARC effect and the reverse SNARC effect in English and Arabic monoliterates, biliterates, and illiterate Arabic speakers, J. Cogn. Cult. 5 (2005) 165–190.

[47] A. Knops et al., Recruitment of an area involved in eye movements during mental arithmetic, Science 324 (2009) 1583–1585.

[48] M. Ishihara et al., Interaction between space and number representations during motor preparation in manual aiming, Neuropsychologia 44 (2006) 1009–1016.

[49] J. Lepsien, A.C. Nobre, Attentional modulation of object representations in working memory, Cereb. Cortex 17 (2007) 2072–2083.

[50] E.J. Anderson et al., Overlapping functional anatomy for working memory and visual search, Exp. Brain Res. 200 (2010) 91–107.

[51] A.D. Baddeley, G. Hitch, Working memory, in: G.H. Bower, (Ed.), The Psychology of Learning and Motivation, Academic Press, CA, 1974, pp. 47–90.

[52] S. Majerus et al., The commonality of neural networks for verbal and visual short-term memory, J. Cogn. Neurosci. 22 (2010) 2570–2593.

[53] L.E. Nystrom et al., Working memory for letters, shapes, and locations: fMRI evidence against stimulus-based regional organization in human prefrontal cortex, Neuroimage 11 (2000) 424–446.

[54] S. Majerus et al., The left intraparietal sulcus and verbal short-term memory: focus of attention or serial order?, Neuroimage 32 (2006) 880–891.

[55] C. Marshuetz et al., Order information in working memory: fMRI evidence for parietal and prefrontal mechanisms, J. Cogn. Neurosci. 12 (2000) 130–144.

[56] C. Marshuetz et al., Working memory for order and the parietal cortex: an event-related functional magnetic resonance imaging study, Neuroscience 139 (2006) 311–316.

[57] M. Botvinick, T. Watanabe, From numerosity to ordinal rank: a gain-field model of serial order representation in cortical working memory, J. Neurosci. 27 (2007) 8636–8642.

[58] A. Nieder et al., Representation of the Quantity of Visual Items in the Primate Prefrontal Cortex, Science 297 (2002) 1708–1711.

[59] M. Brass et al., Neural correlates of overcoming interference from instructed and implemented stimulus–response associations, J. Neurosci. 29 (2009) 1766–1772.

[60] F. Waszak et al., Cross-talk of instructed and applied arbitrary visuomotor mappings, Acta Psychol. 127 (2008) 30–35.

[61] G. Lakoff, M. Johnson, Philosophy in the Flesh: The Embodied Mind and its Challenge to Western Thought, Basic Books

[62] L. Boroditsky, M. Ramscar, The roles of body and mind in abstract thought, Psychol. Sci. 13 (2002) 185–189.

[63] L. Boroditsky, Linguistic Relativity, in: L. Nadel, (Ed.), Encyclopedia of Cognitive Science, MacMillan Press, pp. 917–921.

[64] S. Dehaene et al., Sources of mathematical thinking: behavioral and brain-imaging evidence, Science 284 (1999) 970–974.

[65] M. Srinivasan, S. Carey, The long and the short of it: on the nature and origin of functional overlap between representations of space and time, Cognition 116 (2010) 217–241.

[66] Q. Chen, T. Verguts, Beyond the mental number line: a neural network model of number–space interactions, Cogn. Psychol. 60 (2010) 218–240.

[67] T. Hedden et al., Cultural influences on neural substrates of attentional control, Psychol. Sci. 19 (2008) 12–17.

[68] M.-P. Noël, Spatial numerical associations in preschoolers, in: 24th Attention and Performance Meeting, July 6–10, Paris, France, 2010.

[69] D. Casasanto, L. Boroditsky, Time in the mind: using space to think about time, Cognition 106 (2008) 579–593.

[70] I. Imbo, J. De Brauwer, W. Fias, W. Gevers, The development of the SNARC-effect: evidence for early verbal–spatial coding (submitted).

[71] S. Dehaene, L. Cohen, Cultural recycling of cortical maps, Neuron 56 (2007) 384–398.

[72] S. Dehaene, Log or linear? Distinct intuitions of the number scale in western and amazonian indigene cultures, Science 320 (2008) 1217–1220.

[73] R. Núñez, No innate number line in the human brain. J. Cross Cult. Psychol. (in press).

[74] M.D. de Hevia, E.S. Spelke, Number–space mapping in human infants, Psychol. Sci. 21 (2010) 653–660.

Neglect "Around the Clock": Dissociating Number and Spatial Neglect in Right Brain Damage

Yves Rossetti*†, Sophie Jacquin-Courtois*†, Marilena Aiello‡§, Masami Ishihara¶, Claudio Brozzoli*, Fabrizio Doricchi‡§

*ImpAct (Integrative, Multisensory, Perception—Action Cognition Team), Centre de Recherche en Neurosciences de Lyon; Inserm U 2028; CNRS UMR 5292: Université de Lyon, Bron, France, †Mouvement et Handicap, Hôpital Henry Gabrielle, Hospices Civils de Lyon, St Genis Laval, France, ‡Dipartimento di Psicologia, Università degli Studi "La Sapienza", Roma, Italy, §Fondazione Santa Lucia IRCCS, Roma, Italy, ¶Department of Health Promotion Sciences, Tokyo Metropolitan University, Tokyo, Japan

Summary

Since the seminal observation of the SNARC effect by Dehaene, Bossini, and Giraux [(1993) *Journal of Experimental Psychology: General*, 122(3), 371–396] several studies have indicated the existence of an intrinsic-automatic spatial coding of number magnitudes. In the first part of this chapter we summarize recent work with healthy participants and expand on this original claim. Some of our evidence can be used to support a theory of spatial mapping of mental numbers onto mental space where smaller numbers are associated with the left and larger numbers with the right side of space. In the second part of the chapter we review investigations of spatial neglect and relate them to "small number neglect", which initially seemed to provide crucial support for a tight link between mechanisms of spatial attentional orienting and

© 2011 Elsevier Inc. All rights reserved.

the mental manipulation of number magnitudes [Zorzi *et al.* (2002). *Nature* 417, 138–139]. We will see that although left unilateral neglect after right-brain damage can occur in both visual and number space, recent behavioral dissociations, controlled studies and neuroanatomical correlations have consistently confirmed the functional dissociation of these two deficits and the absence of a causal effect of lateralized spatial–attentional impairments on numerical cognition. Finally, based on recent data gathered from experiments specifically designed to generate a mismatch in the "default" association of small numbers with the left side of space and large numbers with the right side of space, we argue that the pathological deviation toward larger numbers shown by right-brain-damaged patients in the bisection of number intervals may not arise from a basic spatial–attentional impairment. Taken together, these findings suggest that to assume a close phenomenological, functional and anatomical equivalence between orienting in visual space and orienting in representational number space could be partially misleading. It is concluded that careful reassessment of empirical evidence and consideration of the combined contributions of sensorimotor, conceptual, and working memory factors to mathematical cognition may provide a more coherent understanding of the adaptive interaction between spatial and mathematical thought.

In their seminal study, Dehaene, Bossini, and Giraux [1] described behavioral evidence for spatially oriented number lines in normal subjects. When asked to classify a single digit as being odd or even by pressing on one of two buttons, subjects reacted faster to smaller numbers with the left hand and more quickly to larger numbers with the right hand. Interestingly this effect could be reversed by crossing hands, showing that it is spatially based. Dehaene *et al.* [1] termed this effect the SNARC effect, standing for spatial numerical association of response codes. This effect reflects an automatic activation of number magnitude even when it is task-irrelevant (for reviews, see [2,3]). After briefly reviewing some of the work that enlarges on this phenomenon in the healthy brain, this chapter will examine the link between number and the spatial biases observed in spatial neglect. We will see that a number of studies agree about the co-occurrence of these two intriguing deficits in neglect, further evoking the existence of a default association between left–right and small–large. In addition, we will describe more recent studies that all confirm the absence of a causal link between the two deficits.

NUMBER–SPACE ASSOCIATION IN THE HEALTHY BRAIN

Three main questions have been addressed since Dehaene's pioneering study. First, the SNARC effect may depend on relative number magnitude and can be found with other ordinal dimensions (see beautiful data on this issue in Chapter 10 of this volume). Experiments examining this issue with a similar paradigm found that the ordinal information for both months and letters is spatially organized [4,5] (see also Chapter 10 of this volume). In addition, further investigations showed that this number–space link could be expanded to other dimensions such as time (e.g., see the introduction to this book by Stan Dehaene, Chapter 20 of this volume, and [6–9]).

The second main issue addressed in this field concerns the neuroanatomical correlates of the number–space association. Specifically, is this effect the result of shared resources or simply the result of anatomical vicinity? Brain imaging [2], lesion studies [10], and brain stimulation (e.g., [11]) experiments have addressed this intriguing question. Some of the results provided at the end of this chapter will address this issue.

Third, the origin of this left–right association to small–large numbers was investigated. In Western subjects, the left–right oriented number line seems to be like a default representation in that it can be altered if a different reference frame is introduced. Bächtold et al. [12] designed a very interesting number comparison experiment (involving deciding whether a target number is larger or smaller than the number 6) that could be performed in two ways. They elegantly showed that responses to digits 1–5 were faster with the left hand when the format reference, although only mental, was a ruler, while responses to the same digits were faster with the right hand when the mental reference was a clock face. A contrasting pattern of results was found for numbers larger than the reference number 6. This result suggested that the default left-to-right format of the mental number line is subject to contextual modifications.

In an elegantly simple experiment using a task derived from neglect examination, Fischer [13] reported data further supporting the fact that the left–right oriented number line seems to be the dominant default representation in European subjects. First, when subjects were asked to bisect long digit strings (e.g., 111…11 vs 999…99) with a pencil, they demonstrated a systematic pattern of results, i.e. small digits induced a left-bias in the bisection task whereas larger digits induced a right-bias. This effect was obtained [14] with lines made up of digit names expressed in letters (DEUX…DEUX vs NEUF…NEUF, which stand for TWO…TWO vs NINE…NINE in French) (Fig. 11.1A) and also applied even when the letter string was presented in mirror orientation (Fig. 11.1B). These experiments further support the hypothesis of an automatic association between numerical magnitude information and spatial response codes in the healthy brain. Interestingly, interactions between number and space are sensitive to cultural factors (see also Chapter 20 of this volume), as was indirectly suggested by Dehaene et al. [1]. Building on the effect of numbers on line bisection, we investigated manual bisection performed by French and Moroccan medical students with lines made up of Roman or Arabic letters representing small and large digits (Fig. 11.1C). The results obtained with French students on Roman letters replicated the findings of Calabria and Rossetti [14]. The French students did not show a significant effect on the Arabic version of the task. Even though the Moroccan students had been learning French since elementary school, had used it extensively at school, and their courses were conducted 100% in French (i.e. they can be considered as bilingual), their pattern of results was clearly different. When bisecting Arabic letter strings, they showed a bias towards the *right* for the *smaller* number, which suggests that their spatial–numerical association was different from that of the French students. In addition, they surprisingly showed no significant bias for the Roman letter stimuli.

Beyond its cultural and contextual aspects, the association between number and space appears to be quite robust. When it was compared to another obvious reference frame in which numbers are encoded using fingers [15,16], the spatial association was stronger than the finger association [17] (Fig. 11.2). In order to test this issue we used a corporeal modality, by investigating the attentional effects induced by numbers on the perception of touches delivered to fingers. When the right hand was in the palm-down position,

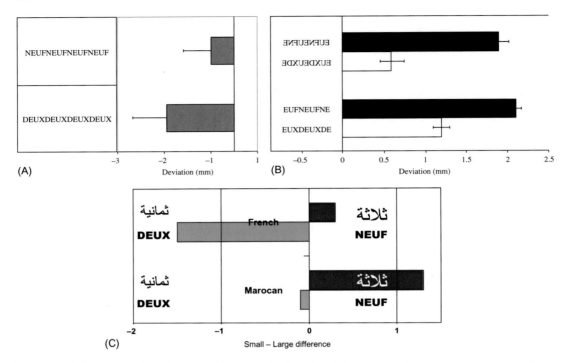

FIGURE 11.1   Number-line bisection. Building on Fischer *et al.* [13], bisection of lines consisting of letter strings was investigated. The string lines could be composed of letters making up the word "DEUX" or "NEUF" (Two and Nine in French, chosen for their resemblance). Bisections obtained for the higher number were biased to the right of the ones made for the smaller number and this held true whether the letter strings were oriented canonically (A) or in mirror image presentation (B), suggesting that direction of writing did not affect the numerical bias. In contrast, when bilingual Moroccan students were compared to non-bilingual French students on letter strings made up of Arabic characters [ثلاثة (thalatha) and ثمانية (thamania)], i.e. 3 and 8, again chosen to maximize resemblance) their bisections were biased towards the left for the larger number (C). This was not observed when Roman letter strings were used. This comparison emphasizes the importance of the role of reading direction for the native language as compared to current reading direction during the test. A and B adapted from [14].

subjects' detection of brief tactile stimuli applied to the little finger improved as a function of the preceding number magnitude. The opposite pattern of results was found when the same little finger was stimulated with the hand in the palm-up posture. In this condition, subjects' tactile performances actually decreased as the preceding number increased (see Fig. 11.2A, yellow panels). Results for the thumb mirrored those for the little finger (see Fig. 11.2A, blue panels). The spatial cueing effect arising in the external space coordinates was present irrespective of the emphasis in the instructions either concerning fingers (Fig. 11.2B: "you will feel a touch on either the thumb or the little finger") or side of space (Fig. 11.2C: "you will feel a touch on either the left or right side of your hand"). A similar modulation was indeed present in both manipulations. We thus found that the numerical cueing of touch does not follow a number–finger association, but a number–space association, akin to the mental number line. By using an embodied approach based on tactile perception, this study not only showed that number-based attentional cueing crosses sensory modalities but also demonstrated that number-based tactile priming is mapped early in life

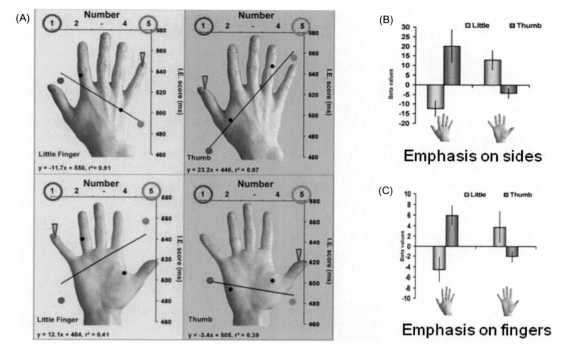

FIGURE 11.2 A conflict between space-based and finger-based representations of numbers. In this study, we investigated which spatial representation is dominant in the human brain: an embodied representation of numbers, arising from the finger-digit association common in Western European countries (thumb for digit 1 and little finger for digit 5) or a disembodied representation of numbers along the mental number line, in ascending order from left to right. (A) The tactile modality allowed us, through a simple postural manipulation of the hand (palm-up *vs* palm-down) to contrast the embodied and disembodied representations of numbers. A further manipulation was introduced to avoid any left–right arrangement in the response space, possible confounding of previous studies in the event they encouraged a space-based representation of numbers, and any motor bias in the response effector, that might favor a finger-based representation: subjects were asked to respond to tactile stimulation by pressing a centrally located pedal with one foot. Participants were thus requested to perform a simple tactile detection task by making speeded foot-pedal responses to a tactile stimulus delivered to either the thumb or the little finger of their right (preferred and counting) hands. When the right hand was in the palm-down position, subjects' detection of brief tactile stimuli applied to the little finger improved as a function of the preceding number magnitude. The larger the number, the better the performance in terms of an inverse efficiency (IE) score, jointly indexing accuracy, and response latency. The opposite pattern of results was found when the same little finger was stimulated with the hand in the palm-up posture. (B, C) Yellow bars: for stimuli applied to the little finger, a difference was apparent between the slopes of IE regression lines in the palm-down and palm-up positions (-4.55 *vs* $+3.70$, respectively; $P < 0.05$); blue bars: the opposite pattern for the stimuli applied on the thumb ($+5.94$ *vs* -2.04 for the palm-down and palm-up postures, respectively). Adapted from [17].

according to an extra-personal spatial representation, thus providing compelling support for the dominant role played by the spatial representation of numbers known as the "mental number line".

Now a crucial question surrounding the SNARC and its related effects is whether the left–right space association to small–large numbers supports the concept of a mental number line (Box 11.1; see also [18]). In most of the empirical data available, associations

BOX 11.1

EVIDENCE FOR CONTINUOUS MAPPING BETWEEN NUMBER AND SPACE

This experiment aimed at testing whether healthy individuals would automatically match number magnitude with spatial location in a continuous manner [19]. It had been previously shown that numbers can affect implicit parameters of motor control [64], but as for the SNARC paradigm, it remained difficult to ascribe the observed effects to a continuous mapping or to a simple categorization (see also [18]).

Participants were instructed to make a parity judgment to digits appearing on a touch screen. In each trial, they were asked to point at the odd numbers whilst ignoring the even numbers. Their motor task thus consisted of pointing to a given numeric

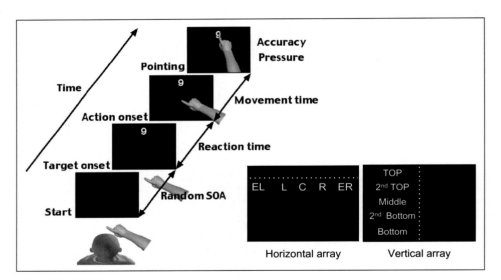

BOX 11.1 FIGURE 1   Method. A schematic representation of the experimental procedure. A numeric stimulus (either an odd number: 1, 3, 5, 7 or 9, or an even number: 2, 4, 6, or 8) was presented as the target at one of five horizontal locations [extreme left (EL), left (L), center (C), right (R), extreme right (ER)] on a touch screen. Participants (n = 12) were asked to point to the target by quickly moving their right index finger from the starting position to the target as soon as it appeared, but only when the target was an odd number (GO). They were asked to hold their finger on the starting position when the target was an even number (NO-GO). This instruction was used in order to ensure that the participants accessed semantic and not only topographic information from the number target. Reaction times were measured from the onset of the visual target until the release of the index finger from the starting position. The diagram shows an example of the target (No. 9) which appears at the "C" location. In a vertical pointing experiment (n = 10), procedures and stimuli in the experiment were identical to those used in horizontal number pointing except that the target was presented at one of five vertical locations (bottom, 2nd from the bottom, middle, 2nd from the top, top) on the screen.

BOX 11.1 *(cont'd)*

target (1, 3, 5, 7, or 9) as quickly and accurately as possible by moving their right index finger from the starting position. In the horizontal condition [19] the five target locations were organized along a horizontal array at the top of the touch panel. In the vertical condition [7] in each trial the target was presented at one of five vertical locations on the screen.

In the horizontal condition, analyses on pointing reaction times revealed a pure number magnitude effect with faster processing for smaller numbers (compared to larger numbers) at each of five individual target locations. The magnitude effect suggests that digits are represented on a unidimensional scale. A classical position effect was also obtained (see [65]). More interestingly, analyses revealed an interaction between number magnitude and position. In the horizontal condition, participants automatically and implicitly associated smaller numbers

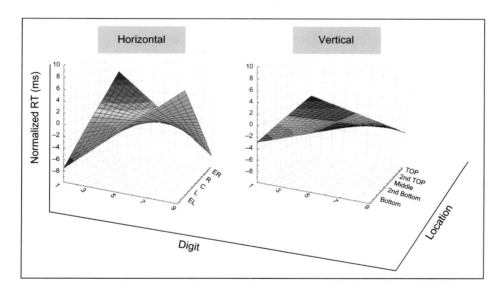

BOX 11.1 FIGURE 2 **Results.** The normalized reaction times representing "continuous" space–number mapping for the horizontal alignment of visual stimuli (left panel, derived from [19]) and for the vertical alignment of visual stimuli (right panel) [7]. Since the pointing action was executed in response to digits at different target locations, pointing reaction times include a variable motor preparation component needed for executing the pointing movement to each target (i.e. location effect). Additionally, pointing reaction times were modulated by number magnitudes (i.e. magnitude effect). To eliminate such influences from the reaction times and to look at a pure number-space congruent/incongruent effect without location and number magnitude influences, normalized reaction times were calculated. The curved surface was fitted to the resulted normalized reaction times by the least-squares method (see [19] for details). The space–number association for the vertical array of stimuli appeared to be weaker compared to the horizontal array. These findings demonstrate that in the vertical axis a facilitatory effect resulting from the number–space congruity is not as strong as for the horizontal array of stimuli.

BOX 11.1 *(cont'd)*

(i.e. numbers 1 and 3) with leftward locations and larger numbers (i.e. numbers 7 and 9) with rightward locations. In addition, the digit No. 5 induced the shortest processing time when it was presented in the central location (see [19]). These results suggest that horizontal space–number mapping is performed parametrically across the relative locations of the target in a given visual work space, which provides direct evidence for a continuous mapping between numbers and locations rather than for a simple left–right categorization.

In the vertical condition, a very similar simple magnitude effect was obtained. A marginally significant interaction between space and number was obtained with the vertical array. Normalized reaction time values obtained for digits 1 and 9 tended to be minimal when they were presented in the congruent location (i.e. Bottom and Top, respectively) and slightly increased when they were presented in the incongruent location (i.e. Top and Bottom, respectively). The comparison of normalized reaction times variation between horizontal and vertical arrays reveals that the space–number association is obviously much weaker for the vertical arrayed stimuli than for horizontal stimuli. This suggests that, at least in European subjects, the default and dominant spatial mapping used for number is a horizontal line on which numbers increase from left to right.

have been investigated in a categorical manner, i.e. by testing the association in a discrete way (left *vs* right, space, left *vs* right hand, small *vs* large numbers, …). In an attempt to investigate the existence of a *continuous* mapping of numbers and space, Ishihara *et al.* [7,19] tested for an implicit, default association of 5 digits (1, 3, 5, 7, 9) with five spatial locations. Number-targets were displayed on a touch-panel and subjects were asked to point at them when odd numbers were presented but to ignore even numbers. When the five spatial locations were arranged along a horizontal axis, subjects showed a strong interaction between digits and space, revealing a continuous mapping between number and space: RTs were relatively shorter for their implicitly mapped location, i.e. 1 on the left, 5 in the center, and 9 on the right. Interestingly, this interaction did not appear when the spatial locations were arranged vertically, unlike what has been suggested for Japanese subjects who are frequently exposed to vertical reading and writing [20]. This result provides a strong argument for an automatic, default mapping of digits onto a horizontal spatial array (see Box 11.1).

This section has concentrated on gathering arguments in support of an association between spatial and analogical numerical representations. The evidence reviewed suggests that there may be a default association between number and space that is compatible with the mental number line hypothesis. Several authors, however, challenged this view and provided alternative explanations for this phenomenological association (e.g., [18,21], and Chapter 10 in this volume). The following sections will address in more detail the supporting and challenging arguments to the space–number association hypothesis in the case of unilateral neglect.

NEGLECT IN VISUAL AND NUMBER SPACE

Right-brain-damaged patients affected by left unilateral neglect are characterized by a pathological attentional bias to the right side of space. This left-sided deficit encompasses eye and head deviations, visual, somatosensory and auditory sensory processing, action initiation and realization, and mental representations. It may affect the left side of space and/or the left side of individual objects [22]. When setting the midpoint in horizontal visual lines, patients typically shift the subjective line midpoint to the right of the objective one [23]. The combination of neglect and hemianopia makes this rightward bias more severe and can engender a significant and paradoxical leftward shift in the bisection of very short lines (the "cross-over" effect) [24,25].

In a seminal study published in 2002, Zorzi *et al.* [26] asked four right-brain-damaged (RBD) patients with left spatial neglect to mentally bisect, without calculating, 3-, 5-, 7- and 9-unit number intervals (i.e. saying what number is halfway between two orally presented numbers ; e.g., what is the midpoint between 21 and 29?). Compared with both a sample of four RBD patients without neglect and a sample of four healthy control participants, neglect patients showed a "rightward" shift towards greater numbers during the bisection of 5-, 7- and 9-unit number intervals (i.e. responses tended to be larger than the actual interval center). This shift increased as a function of interval length, as has been previously reported for physical line bisection. Three out of the four neglect patients also showed leftward "cross-over" in the bisection of short 3-unit number intervals (i.e. in this case, responses tended to be smaller than the actual interval center). These original findings seemingly provided crucial support for the idea that small numbers are automatically mapped on the left side of (representational) space and that this mapping is linked to brain mechanisms regulating the deployment of attention in space. This pioneering observation also suggested a superimposition of the networks underlying number representation and the orientation of spatial attention in the brain. This surprising aspect of neglect in the number space generated a whole new spate of research (for reviews, see [2,3,27,28]) on number representation in neglect patients [10,29–31] and neglect-like effects induced in healthy individuals (see Fig. 4 in [32]; [33]). Although this finding opened up a whole new line of enquiry into the study of the interaction between spatial and mathematical thought, the original investigation by Zorzi *et al.* [26] left a number of very relevant questions unanswered: (1) is the bisection bias in the mental number line correlated with a similar bias in the bisection of equivalent stimuli in visual space (i.e. horizontal lines)? (2) Is the bisection bias in number space positively correlated with neglect severity? (3) Is the bisection bias in number space caused by damage of the same cortical areas and subcortical white matter pathways whose damage provokes spatial neglect [34–36]? Since spatial neglect is a heterogenous syndrome, and since different visual, exploratory and representational/working memory features of the syndrome can impinge on different sectors of the right hemispheric parietal–frontal network regulating spatial attention [34–36], is the disruption of one of these anatomical–functional components responsible for the "rightward" shift in the bisection of number intervals ?

These points were specifically addressed in a study by Doricchi *et al.* [10]. Based on evidence showing important variations in performance on the line bisection test by neglect patients which suggests that left homonymous hemianopia accompanied by spatial neglect, increases both the rightward bias for the bisection of long horizontal lines and the leftward bias (i.e. "cross-over") for the bisection of very short lines, Doricchi and co-workers investigated bisection biases for visual and number space in a group of 11 RBD patients with neglect and in 5 RBD patients without neglect. Neglect patients population manifested a clear cut double dissociation. Some of the patients displayed very severe neglect on the bisection of visual lines and normal performance for the bisection of number intervals (i.e. comparable to that of controls). In contrast, other neglect patients showed the opposite trend, i.e. a strong rightward bias for the bisection of number intervals and performance on line bisection that fell within the range of the entire sample of patients included in the study. Correlational analyses confirmed the absence of any significant relationship between the rightward bias for the bisection of number intervals and measures of neglect severity. This was also true for the paradoxical leftward "cross-over" in the bisection of very short horizontal lines (i.e. 2 cm): in fact, this had no significant correlation with any equivalent effect in the bisection of the shortest number intervals (i.e. 3 units). The analysis of the anatomical correlates of the number interval bisection task revealed that the subcortical–cortical lesion of the prefrontal, rather than parietal, module of the network that underlies number processing in monkeys and humans was involved [37,38]. This finding led to the examination of patients' working memory. In the experimental sample, neglect patients who showed a "rightward shift" in the bisection of number intervals had the most severe spatial working memory impairments (i.e. Corsi span). Although the number of patients involved was relatively small, this latter finding suggested that the main pathological reason for the rightward bias in the bisection of number intervals lay in the patients' inability to construct or retain an active representation of the initial part of the number intervals on the mental number line.

Recently, a single-case study by van Dijck et al. [39] (for a full theoretical discussion and development of the role of working memory in number cognition see Chapter 10 of this volume) shed new light on this hypothesis. This work documents a striking behavioral dissociation by a left-brain-damaged patient suffering from right-sided neglect for extra-personal and representational space and left-sided neglect on the mental number line. A complete neuropsychological examination revealed that the apparent left-sided neglect in the bisection of number intervals was purely non-spatial in origin and was based on a poor memory for the initial items of verbal sequences presented visually at a fixed position in space. These findings clarify the possible role of working memory in the bisection of the mental number line, showing that effective position-based verbal working memory may be crucial for numerical tasks that are usually thought to involve purely spatial representations of numerical magnitudes.

Consistent double-dissociations between visual neglect and neglect in number space have been reported by other authors. For example, the two patients studied by Rossetti et al. [30] whose performance improved on the number interval bisection task after prism-adaptation showed no sign of neglect on the line bisection test. Loetscher and Brugger [40] and Loetscher et al. [41] demonstrated that patients with clearcut left spatial neglect on conventional line bisection or cancellation tasks display no lateral bias for the bisection of number intervals, on random number generation tasks or when asked to pick six lottery ticket numbers within the range 1–45.

The issue concerning the dissociation between lateral spatial biases in the bisection of visual lines and number intervals was recently re-assessed by Doricchi et al. [42] in an extended sample of 43 RBD patients (22 with and 21 without neglect) and 31 age-matched controls. This study explored whether the position of a number interval of a given length within a decade on the mental number line had any influence on the size and direction

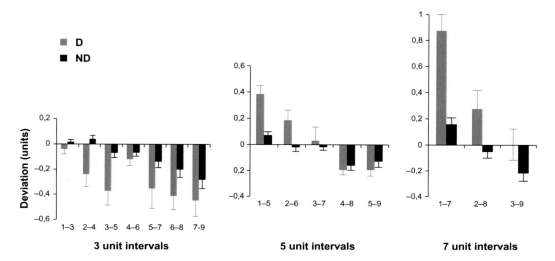

FIGURE 11.3 Bisection of number intervals as a function of their position within a decade. Bisection of 3-, 5- and 7-unit number intervals as a function of their position within a decade, in RBD and healthy elderly controls demonstrating significant rightward deviation (Deviating participants: D) and in RBD patients and healthy elderly controls showing no deviation (Non-Deviating participants: ND; modified from [42]). Positive values indicate rightward deviation and negative values leftward deviation from the objective midpoint (0 value on y-axis). For each interval, deviation is averaged from the bisection of intervals occupying the same position within the first three decades (e.g. deviation for the interval "1–7" corresponds to the average deviation across intervals "1–7", "11–17" and "21–27").

of the bisection error. As an example, the 7-unit interval "1–7" is positioned on the initial "left" part of the decade whereas the equivalent 7-unit interval "3–9" is positioned on the end "right" part of the decade: does this difference in interval position have an influence on bisection behavior? For large, 7-unit intervals a centripetal deviation toward the center of the decades was found in the bisection error: intervals were erroneously bisected further to the right the closer they were to the left starting point of a decade and further to the left the closer they were to the right endpoint of a decade (see Fig. 11.3). It is worth noticing that this effect was also present for intervals bridging different decades. A similar error trend was present with 5-unit intervals though here the centripetal error had shifted slightly towards the initial part of the decade. This tendency was even more pronounced with 3-unit intervals, where there was a null-error for intervals positioned on the left-side at the beginning of a decade, whereas the greater the proximity of the interval to the right-end of a decade the more the bisection error was shifted toward the left side of the interval. Interestingly, in a control study (second study in [42]) 31 healthy participants were asked to perform both the number intervals bisection task and a line bisection task, with 2-cm, 10-cm and 20-cm horizontal lines positioned in the left, central or right side of egocentric space. Whereas centripetal errors toward the center of decades were again found on the number task a centrifugal, rather than centripetal, error was observed for all line lengths on the line bisection task.

In addition to uncovering the effects of the recursive grouping of symbolic numerals within the tens on the non-symbolic spatial representation of magnitudes, this study provided confirmation of previous findings and new insights into the dissociation between neglect in visual and number space. In fact, no significant correlation was again found between neglect severity on line bisection or multiple item cancellation tasks and left side neglect in the bisection of number intervals. In contrast, neglect for number intervals correlated with poor immediate recall of sequences of spatial positions (Corsi span) and digits (Digit span). Most interestingly, the use of confidence intervals calculated over the entire sample of participants allowed us to classify participants as Deviating (D: 10 neglect, 5 non-neglect, 10 elderly healthy controls) or Non-Deviating (ND: 12 neglect, 16 non-neglect, 21 elderly healthy controls) on the bisection of number intervals. This showed that a number of healthy elderly participants (10) actually suffered from "neglect" in the bisection of the mental number line and, most of all, that the distribution of bisection errors as a function of interval position within a decade was different for D participants compared to ND participants (see Fig. 11.3). With 7- and 5-unit intervals, D showed enhanced rightward deviation in the bisection of number intervals located toward the "left" starting point of decades and made few or no errors with intervals located toward the right endpoint of decades. With 3-unit intervals the progressively increasing "leftward" bisection error for intervals located closer to the "right" end of the decade was greater for D than for ND participants. The study of anatomical correlates confirmed the role of prefrontal–frontal damage in number interval bisection and the well-known role of the inferior parietal lobe and the underlying parietal–frontal connections in neglect and line bisection [34–36,43,44].

The increasing rightward error displayed by D participants in the bisection of large 7-unit interval located to "left" side of decades offers another example of the apparent similarity between bisection behavior in visual and number space: in fact, it is well known that the pathological rightward shift in the bisection of long horizontal lines increases in patients with left spatial neglect as the egocentric position of lines moves leftward (i.e. toward the contralesional neglected space) [23]. However, repeated observation of no significant relationship between the extent of neglect and rightward shift in the bisection of number intervals clearly emphasizes the fact that phenomenological similarities in behavior can be misleading and do not necessarily imply functional or neuroanatomical equivalence. To further clarify this point, we reanalyzed line bisection and number interval bisection performance and, crucially, their correlation on a larger sample of RBD patients. This sample was obtained by merging the sample of 74 patients studied over several years by one of the authors of the present chapter (F. Doricchi) with a sample of 12 patients examined by Wim Fias and co-workers (unpublished data). No correlations between line and number interval bisection were found either in the entire sample (see Fig. 11.4C: Pearson's r = 0.09, $P = 0.36$) or in the subsamples of patients with (see Fig. 11.5C: Pearson's r = 0.1, $P = 0.52$) and without spatial neglect (see Fig. 11.6C: Pearson's r = 0.03, $P = 0.8$). To summarize, these findings clearly point towards the absence of a causal link between the pathological deviation of attention in visual space and the deviation toward higher numbers in the bisection of number intervals observed in RBD patients

Finally, it should be noted that Knops et al. [46] in a recent fMRI study using a multivariate approach for the analysis of the BOLD signal, showed that in the superior parietal lobes of the two hemispheres there are populations of neurons that are specifically activated by non-symbolic/symbolic subtraction and by the planning of leftward saccades and populations that are activated by non-symbolic/symbolic addition and by the planning of rightward saccades. Although the study suggests a link between saccadic programing and

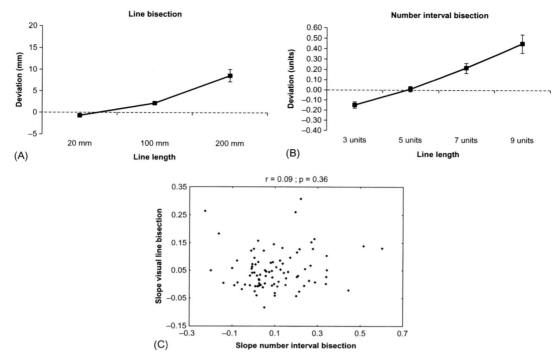

FIGURE 11.4 Line bisection and number interval bisection in right brain damage: patients with and without left spatial neglect (unpublished data by Doricchi and Fias). Bisection of visual horizontal lines and number intervals in a sample of 86 RBD patients (42 with left spatial neglect and 44 without neglect on the bisection of 200-mm lines. The cut off score, i.e. +6.5mm, is based on a sample of 206 RBD patients studied by Azouvi *et al.* [45]. (A) Bisection of horizontal visual lines (length: 20, 100 and 200mm). (B) Bisection of number intervals (size: 3-, 5-, 7- and 9-unit). In both (A) and (B) positive values indicate rightward deviation and negative values leftward deviation from the objective midpoint (0 value on y-axis); vertical bars indicate S.E. (C) Correlation between individual slopes describing the bisection deviation as a function of the length visual lines and the length of number intervals.

orienting in number-operational space, it leaves the issue of the hemispheric lateralization of the subtraction/addition neuron populations unresolved. Similarly, it would be very interesting to study whether left *vs* right brain damage can engender specific disruptions in addition *vs* subtraction abilities and associated, or dissociated, impairments in leftward *vs* rightward orienting.

A FURTHER TWIST TO NUMBER SPACE NEGLECT: BISECTING "AROUND THE CLOCK"

The clinical observation of number biases in patients with unilateral neglect is extremely easy and is done frequently. Following the studies of Zorzi *et al.* [26], Bächtold *et al.* [12], and Vuilleumier *et al.* [31], we had the opportunity to study a sub-population of selected neglect

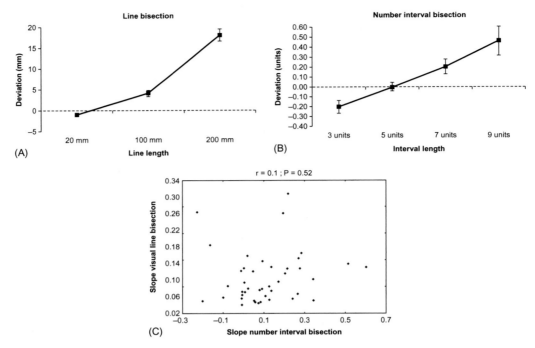

FIGURE 11.5 Line bisection and number interval bisection in right brain damage: patients with left spatial neglect (unpublished data by Doricchi and Fias). Bisection of horizontal visual lines and number intervals in the sample including 42 RBD patients with left spatial neglect. Panels (A), (B) and (C): same legend as Fig. 11.4.

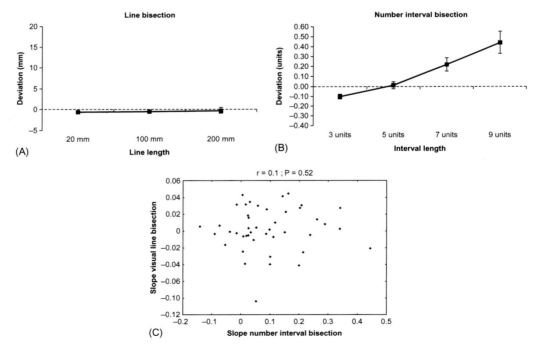

FIGURE 11.6 Line bisection and number interval bisection in right brain damage: patients without left spatial neglect (unpublished data by Doricchi and Fias). Bisection of horizontal visual lines and number intervals in the sample pertaining to 44 RBD patients without left spatial neglect. Panels (A), (B) and (C): same legend as Fig. 11.4.

patients who exhibited a peculiar behavior pattern when asked to perform the classical clock drawing task, where patients have to fill in the numbers on an empty clock face [47]. These patients all started with number 12, as most subjects do, but then used numbers ranging from 13 to 23 instead of the correct numbers ranging from 2 to 11 (see Fig. 11.7B–D). Even if it is common in France to refer to p.m. times as numbers greater than 12, numbers on all clock faces are always less than 13. We hypothesized that this pattern reflected a strong numerical bias towards larger numbers and systematically investigated five of these patients with a set of clock drawing tasks. Interestingly, only some of them exhibited spatial neglect on their clock drawings while the others placed them (the wrong numbers) at their appropriate virtual locations, suggesting a loose association between spatial and numerical deficits. Strikingly, when they were provided with an empty clock face containing a single numerical landmark (3, 6 or 9, at their canonical locations), their drawings included numbers higher than the landmark going up to 23 or 24 (Fig. 11.7E–G). Furthermore, some of them now revealed right spatial neglect: they frequently left an empty space between 12 and 3, or even more strikingly between 6 and 12. These tasks thus suggest that the patients were unable to activate numbers lower than the landmark. In the absence of a landmark, they thus used 12 as the default landmark and wrote larger numbers on the clock face. We conjectured that an impairment prevented patients from moving towards smaller numbers on their mental number line. As a matter of fact, the move from 12 to 1 during the normal drawing of a clock face requires a large jump towards smaller numbers on the mental number line; and when our patients ended their drawing with number 24, the jump to 1 was even greater. To investigate their ability to move towards smaller numbers, we asked them to draw clock faces counterclockwise (as in [48]). Surprisingly all patients were able to use correct numbers ranging from 12 to 1 when they performed counterclockwise. Starting with 12, all patients could count down to 1 and the spatial pattern of results described by Grossi was frequently observed, i.e. some patients placed numbers from 12 to 1 using only the left side of the clock face, while others used the entire clock space (Fig. 11.7H,I). This implies that their left-sided neglect was turned into a right-sided neglect on this particular test, showing a further dissociation between spatial and numerical performance. In addition, their ability to use the correct numbers proved that their previous pattern of results cannot be attributed to a general cognitive deficit. Improved competence on the counterclockwise versions would appear to indicate that these patients had preserved the capacity to move from the landmark to smaller numbers, but only if the size of the step was sufficiently small (i.e. 1 and not 11). Alternatively, it can be conjectured that moving spatially to the left from 12 was congruent with moving towards smaller numbers on the patients' mental number line, whereas in the first version of the task the requested jump from 12 to 1 was associated with a spatial movement to the right. In addition to these tasks, patients were also tested with empty clock faces including only the number 1 (Fig. 11.7J). Three of the patients made a very striking response: they started by adding 12 to the clock face, and then added a 3 next to the pre-existing 1 in order to transform it into 13 or 15, thus demonstrating the influence of the dominant landmark 12 even in its absence! This peculiar response can also be observed when more than one landmark is provided on the clock face, e.g., 12 and 1 (Fig. 11.7K), 12, 3, 6, and 9 (Fig. 11.7L) or even 12, 1, 2, and 3 (Fig. 7M).

The advantage of using the representation of a clock face to study number and space processing in brain damaged patients was originally demonstrated in an elegant study by

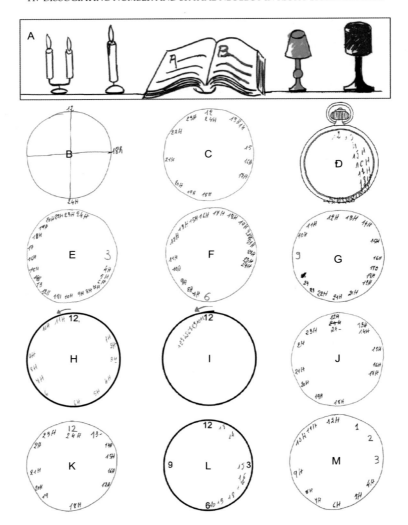

FIGURE 11.7 Clock drawings made by neglect patients. (A) Characteristic coloring made by a patient with left neglect. Not only is the left side of the original drawing omitted, but the left side of individual items is also missing. (B–D) A simple clock face test where numbers below 12 are omitted. (E–G) The clock face test performed with one pre-marked landmark number (3, 6, and 9). The patient systematically omits the numbers that are less than the landmark, giving rise to an apparent right neglect in the first two cases. (H,I) Counter-clockwise filling of the clock face showing that the number aspect of the task is improved whilst the spatial aspect may indicate right neglect. (J–M) Drawings with pre-marked landmarks that are either transformed or ignored by the patient. It is only when the three first numbers are indicated (M) that the patient can draw a correct clock face. From [47].

Vuilleumier *et al.* [31]. In the first experiment, RBD patients with and without contralesional neglect were required to press a key on the right when a target number was greater than a reference number (e.g., 5) and a left-hand one when the target was smaller. Results showed slower reaction times for the number "4" (the closest to the reference, on the neglected side) compared to other higher numbers. When the reference number was set at 7, the highest increase in reaction time was found for "6". These results showed that the time required to activate a number representation in neglect was systematically increased when the number was smaller than the reference value, whereas control subjects displayed a symmetrical increase on both sides of the reference. This result suggested that neglect patients are unable to activate smaller numbers on the left side of the mental number line. In an ensuing experiment, the authors also demonstrated that when asked to classify numbers as indicating hours earlier or later than six o'clock, neglect patients provided slower responses to numbers larger than "6", i.e. to numbers located on the left side of the clock face. Very interestingly, the study by Vuilleumier and co-workers suggests that comparing the performance of neglect patients in the bisection of number intervals with their performance in the "o'clock" task reveals whether the bias toward higher numbers in the bisection of number intervals is due to a pathological ipsilesional attention bias or whether it is due to a faulty representation of small magnitudes. In the first case, in fact, patients should display a congruent spatial bias in the two imagery tasks, i.e. bisection deviated toward higher numbers on the right side of number intervals and better performance with small time-hours located on the right side of the clock face. In contrast, a non-attentional deficit in the representation of small magnitudes should predict incongruent spatial biases on the two tasks, i.e. bisection deviated toward higher numbers on the right side of number intervals and better performance with high time-numbers on the left side of the clock face.

This line of reasoning constituted the rationale behind two complementary investigations that were independently run by Rossetti, Jacquin-Courtois and co-workers in Lyon and by Doricchi, Aiello and co-workers in Rome. These two studies are now merged into a single scientific communication [49,50]. It is worth noting that, unlike the investigation by Vuilleumier *et al.* [31], none of these studies adopted a SNARC-like paradigm requiring the explicit left *vs* right mapping of the (motor) response. As detailed below, these two studies provide convergent findings that are different from those that assess the coding of numbers on a clock face with a SNARC-like paradigm.

Just as it is possible to test number line bisection for letter strings *vs* mirror letter strings, it is possible to create a mismatch between the spatial and the mental number line reference frame in unilateral neglect. Jacquin-Courtois and Rossetti compared two mental number bisection tasks in a group of RBD patients with left spatial neglect (Fig. 11.8). In the clock version of the task, patients were seated in front of a large clock face made up of a circle and 12 numbers (diameter 145 mm, printed in the center of an A4 page). They were then asked to bisect pairs of numbers provided orally, in such a way that each pair corresponded to a horizontal or vertical line on the clock (e.g., 2 and 5, 7 and 23, 3 and 9, 4 and 8). As time numbers between 0 and 24 are currently used in France, we also included pairs with numbers higher than 12 (e.g., 15 to 21, 10 and 14). The crucial feature of the task was that bisections could be performed vertically on either the left or the right half of the clock face (e.g., 13 and 17 *vs* 19 and 23), and horizontally from left to right or right to left (e.g., 3 and 9 *vs* 9 to 15). In this task, the instructions given to the patient used an explicit reference to time around the clock, e.g., "what is midway between 1 o'clock and 5 o'clock?". The second bisection task, performed first, was similar to the classical number bisection task, and included all the same pairs of numbers to bisect, but it was performed without the clock face and in the classical way (e.g., what is midway between 3 and 9?). In both tasks,

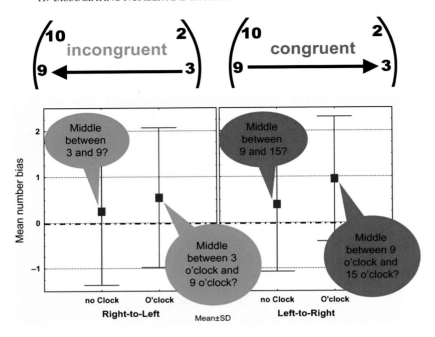

FIGURE 11.8   Number bisection around the clock. This experiment used two versions of the number bisection task. In addition to the classical version, an o'clock version was designed in which the task was performed in front of a large clock face and the question asked was, for example, "where is the middle between 3 o'clock and 9 o'clock". In each of these conditions two types of number pair that corresponded either to left-to-right or to right-to-left comparisons in the o'clock version were used. The left-to-right version is referred to as the congruent version, because both left-spatial neglect and small number neglect rightly predicted a bias towards larger numbers. In the right-to-left version, incongruent predictions resulted from the left spatial neglect and the small number neglect hypotheses: left neglect predicted that bisection responses should be biased to smaller numbers in the o'clock version whereas small number neglect should give rise to similar biases for the classical and the o'clock versions. The means (±SEM) for the neglect patient group displayed in this figure show that o'clock bisection responses were not biased towards smaller numbers. This clearly shows that spatial neglect cannot provide an explanation for the constant over-estimation of bisection responses.

emphasis was put on avoiding arithmetic calculations and preferably estimating the central number. Our main prediction was that if number bisections are processed on the basis of the spatial reference frame, patients' answers to right-to-left intervals should be biased toward smaller numbers in the clock version and biased towards larger numbers in the classical version. Two main results were obtained in this experiment. First, there was no significant difference between the horizontal bisections performed in the two versions of the task. In fact, the bias towards larger numbers was even slightly higher in the clock version, which was clearly incompatible with the spatial reference frame hypothesis (see Fig. 11.8). Second, the result obtained for vertical line bisection did not yield significant differences between the left side and the right side of the clock face. The main outcome of this study is that the spatial constraints imposed by the clock version of the number bisection task did not interfere in the expected way, i.e. there was no evidence of a spatial read-out of the numbers. This experiment, therefore, confirmed that the spatial bias and the numerical bias observed in spatial neglect cannot be assumed to depend on a single basic pathophysiological deficit.

In parallel, Doricchi, Aiello and co-workers considered that although neglect for the left side of number intervals is not systematically related to neglect for the left side of space, one can still assume that neglect in mental number space is only a special case of "imagery" neglect and that, as such, its occurrence can be independent of visual neglect (as in the case of clinical observations pioneered by Guariglia *et al.* [51]). This hypothesis suggested a systematic investigation of the relationship between neglect in mental number space and neglect for the left side of mental visual images. One consolidated instrument for the assessment of imagery neglect is the "o'clock" task devised by Grossi and co-workers [52]. In its original version, this task requires the mental comparison of the amplitude of two clock-hand angles indicating different times within the right or left half of the clock face. Typically, neglect patients have more difficulty comparing clock-hands' angles on the left side of the clock face. The correlation between neglect in the bisection of number intervals and imagery neglect in the "o'clock" task was assessed in 16 RBD patients with neglect and 21 RBD controls without neglect. Patients were administered a standardized battery for the assessment of spatial neglect, with the Number Interval Bisection task [26] and with the "o'clock task" [52]. The evaluation of correlations between the lateral bias in the bisection of number intervals, the severity of visual neglect and the severity of representational neglect in the "o'clock" task, revealed that the rightward shift towards higher numbers in the bisection of number intervals was significantly and exclusively correlated to better performance with higher times-numbers on the left side of the clock face (Pearson's $r = 0.4$, $P = 0.01$ for 7-unit number intervals, Pearson's $r = 0.34$, $P = 0.04$ for 9-unit intervals and Pearson's $r = 0.33$, $P = 0.04$ for the slope describing deviation as a function of number interval length). Put in other words, impaired spatial-imagery processing of small magnitudes was present when these were mapped on both the left and the right side of a mental visual image (i.e. as in the findings by Jacquin-Courtois and Rossetti reported in Fig. 11.8). The anatomical correlates of the two imagery tasks were defined using the Voxel Lesion Symptom Mapping approach [53]. This showed (Fig. 11.9) that the "rightward" error in the bisection of number intervals resulted from cortical–subcortical frontal–prefrontal damage (as previously documented with the classical lesion subtraction approach in [10,42]) whereas the rightward bias in the "o'clock" task was linked to lesion in the ventral temporal areas that code for the inherent left and right side of visual objects (i.e. "object-centered" coordinates) [36,54,55]. To summarize, this evidence allows for two important conclusions: (1) the right hemisphere supports the representation of small numerical magnitudes, regardless of their spatial mapping on the left or the right side of a mental layout; (2) unlike a clock face, number intervals on the mental number line, and possibly the mental number line itself, are not coded as objects with an inherent left and right side.

DISCUSSION AND CONCLUSIONS

The empirical evidence that we have reviewed in this chapter sketches a coherent outline of the available knowledge on the links between spatial and mathematical thought. On

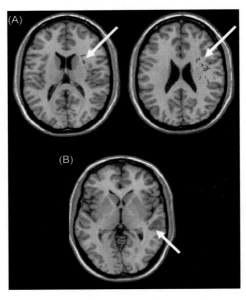

FIGURE 11.9   Anatomical correlates of the "Number Interval Bisection" and the "o'clock" tasks in right brain damage. Representative transverse slices show peaks of VLSM (Voxel Lesion Symptom Mapping) maps computed for (A) the slope describing rightward bisection deviation as a function of number interval length (Tailarach coordinates: top left: x = 28, y = 15, z = 16; top right: x = 30, y = 5, z = 24) ; (B) the rightward bias in the "o'clock" task (Talairach coordinates: x = 57, y = −24 , z = 0; modified from Aiello *et al.* [49]. Note that the cortical–subcortical ventral temporal lesion area correlated to rightward bias in the "o'clock" task corresponds to the area involved in the "object centered" coding of the left side of visual objects, described in the lesion study by Verdon *et al.* [36] and the perfusion imaging study by Medina *et al.* [54].

the one hand, a number of findings from healthy participants and the study of the effects of prism adaptation in brain damaged patients [30] seem to confirm that mathematical knowledge and sensorimotor mechanisms regulating action in space are lodged together and interact. On the other hand, evidence gathered from the study of RBD patients clearly provides no support for a causal link between deficits in the orienting of spatial attention (i.e. contralesional neglect) and phenomenologically similar deficits on tasks that assess the non-symbolic manipulation of numerical magnitudes (i.e. bisection of number intervals). Altogether these data offer a far more complex, and probably stimulating, scenario than what might be envisaged with a simple and point-to-point correspondence between brain mechanisms dedicated to the treatment of spatial attention and number magnitudes. This, on the one hand, does not mean that sensorimotor experience does not contribute to the acquisition and shaping of mathematical skills. Though, on the other hand, it clearly indicates that recycling [56] of sensorimotor networks for mathematical thought, is a complex process. This process can be enriched, in the maturing brain, by the parallel development of mechanisms that improve the voluntary planning and control of the allocation of attentional/motor resources and the development of working memory and language-based conceptual abilities. Based on this consideration, different interpretations of the dissociation between spatial–attentional and non-symbolic mathematical processing can be advanced. First, one can argue that dissociations arise because a specific task does not adequately tap the sensorimotor roots of mathematical processing: note, however, that in this case it is still assumed that, the sensorimotor component that the task fails to activate maintains its original functional properties and its full anatomical-functional integration within sensorimotor networks. Alternatively, it can be argued that dissociation between spatial and non-symbolic mathematical processing is observed because during the recycling process, the sensorimotor root of mathematical cognition ceases to be integrated into attentional–motor networks and is partially or totally blended into sensorimotor-independent networks subserving non-symbolic and/or symbolic mathematical operations.

Another point that needs careful consideration when we discuss the associations and dissociations between numerical and spatial coding that can be observed in the healthy brain is whether the influence of numerical cues on spatial processing is as strong as the reciprocal influence of spatial cues on number processing. As an example, in the paradigm devised by Fischer *et al.* [57] numerical cues presented at central fixation are spatially neutral: does this type of cue have the same effect as numerical cues presented at varying horizontal spatial positions as in the investigation by Ishihara *et al.* [19] or as in the case of line bisection [58] or number bisection tasks [59] in which number pairs are presented in a horizontal configuration with the smallest number on the spatially congruent left side or incongruent right side? This point is of relevance because spatial aspects of number representation can be sensitive to top-down control [60,61] and because the addition of an explicit spatial connotation to numerical cues may be more efficient at activating the default left-to-right organization of number magnitudes linked to reading habits and educational factors.

Although the evidence and hypotheses that we have sketched in this review do not allow for a coherent and complete understanding of number–space interaction, they offer insights into new exciting avenues of investigation. In the following paragraphs we will try to summarize a few questions that, in our opinion, should be assessed or re-assessed in future research

1. Is the spatial coding of number magnitudes linked to mechanisms regulating the automatic or the voluntary allocation of attentional resources? As an example, Fischer *et al.* [57] presented Arabic digits 1, 2 or 8, 9 at central fixation and reported observing an automatic facilitation in the detection of ensuing targets appearing to the left of fixation when these followed the presentation of small digits (1 and 2) and to the right of fixation when these followed the presentation of higher digits (8 and 9). This is usually considered as evidence for the automatic intrinsic link between number magnitude and reflexive shifts of attention. It is worth noting, however, that other authors using the same paradigm found weak facilitatory effects (i.e. around 2.5 ms, $P > 0.05$) [62] or no effect [63]. In contrast, other investigators have demonstrated that spatial–attentional facilitatory effects induced by numerical cues may crucially depend on the spatial–mental set that is voluntarily adopted by participants in the representation of numerical cues [60,61].

2. What role is played by the numerical–mental set maintained in working memory during the performance of tasks assessing the interaction between numbers and space? For example, in experiments that adopt the task devised by Fischer *et al.* [57], the use of magnitudes positioned at the extreme "left" or "right" side of a number decade (or a

fixed number range) may have favored the implicit dichotomic-conceptual recoding of cues as "left" ones (e.g., 1 and 2) or "right" ones (8 and 9), thus producing a SNARC-like effect. This "caveat" implies a number of very relevant empirical questions: Does the size of the sample of digits used as numerical cues have an influence on spatial–attentional facilitatory effects? Would facilitatory effects induced by digit-cues still be present when all the numbers in a decade are used cues? Would these effects show a continuous linear increment as a function of the progressively increasing positioning of numerical cues away from the center of a decade and towards the beginning or the end of the same decade?

To conclude, we would like to propose that current empirical evidence suggests that the assumption of a close phenomenological, functional and anatomical equivalence between orienting in number space and orienting in physical space may be untimely or, at least, partially misleading. A new look on the complex and combined contributions of sensorimotor, linguistic–conceptual, abstract–representational and working memory factors on the manipulation of number magnitudes (see also Chapter 10 in this volume) could perhaps provide a better and more coherent understanding of the adaptive and dynamic interaction between spatial and mathematical thought.

Acknowledgments

The authors wish to thank Drs Jacinta O'Shea, Alessandro Farnè, Gilles Rode, Mohamed Saoud and Wim Fias for stimulating discussions and Susana Franck, Ed Hubbard and Stanislas Deahene for editing a previous version of this chapter. Jean-Louis Borach contributed to some of the illustrations. This work was supported by Inserm and Hospices Civils de Lyon (YR and SJC) and by the Fondazione Santa Lucia IRCCS and Ministero Italiano della Universita' e della Ricerca Scientifica MIUR (FD).

References

[1] S. Dehaene, S. Bossini, P. Giraux, The mental representation of parity and number magnitude, J. Exp. Psychol. General 122 (3) (1993) 371–396.

[2] E.M. Hubbard, M. Piazza, P. Pinel, S. Dehaene, Interactions between number and space in parietal cortex, Nat. Rev. Neurosci. 6 (6) (2005) 435–448.

[3] G. Wood, K. Willmes, H.C. Nuerk, M.H. Fischer, On the cognitive link between space and number: a meta-analysis of the SNARC effect, Psychol. Sci. Q. 50 (2008) 489–525.

[4] W. Gevers, B. Reynvoet, W. Fias, The mental representation of ordinal sequences is spatially organized, Cognition 87 (2003) B87–B95.

[5] M. Zorzi, K. Priftis, F. Meneghello, R. Marenzi, C. Umiltà, The spatial representation of numerical and non-numerical sequences: evidence from neglect, Neuropsychologia 44 (7) (2006) 1061–1067.

[6] M. Ishihara, P.E. Keller, Y. Rossetti, W. Prinz, Horizontal spatial representations of time: evidence for the STEARC effect, Cortex 44 (2008) 454–461.

[7] M. Ishihara, Y. Rossetti, P.E. Keller, W. Prinz, Horizontal spatial representation of number and time: continuous number and categorical time lines, (2011 in press).

[8] V. Walsh, A theory of magnitude: common cortical metrics of time, space and quantity, Trends Cogn. Sci. 7 (11) (2003) 483–488.

[9] D. Bueti, V. Walsh, The parietal cortex and the representation of time, space, number and other magnitudes. Philos. Trans. R. Soc. Lond., B, Biol. Sci. 364 (2009) 1831–1840.

[10] F. Doricchi, P. Guariglia, M. Gasparini, F. Tomaiuolo, Dissociation between physical and mental number line bisection in right hemisphere brain damage, Nat. Neurosci. 8 (12) (2005) 1663–1665.

[11] S.M. Göbel, M. Calabria, A. Farne, Y. Rossetti, Parietal rTMS distorts the mental number line: simulating 'spatial' neglect in healthy subjects, Neuropsychologia 44 (2006) 860–868.

[12] D. Bächtold, M. Baumuller, P. Bruegger, Stimulus–response compatibility in representational space, Neuropsychologia 36 (1998) 731–735.

[13] M.H. Fischer, Number processing induces spatial performance biases, Neurology 57 (5) (2001) 822–826.

[14] M. Calabria, Y. Rossetti, Interference between number processing and line bisection: a methodology, Neuropsychologia 43 (5) (2005) 779–783.

[15] G. Wood, M.H. Fischer, Numbers, space, and action—from finger counting to the mental number line and beyond, Cortex 44 (4) (2008) 353–358.

[16] F. Domahs, K. Moeller, S. Huber, K. Willmes, H.C. Nuerk, Embodied numerosity: implicit hand-based representations influence symbolic number processing across cultures, Cognition 116 (2) (2010) 251–266.

[17] C. Brozzoli, M. Ishihara, S.M. Gobel, R. Salemme, Y. Rossetti, A. Farne, Touch perception reveals the dominance of spatial over digital representation of numbers, Proc. Natl. Acad. Sci. USA. 105 (2008) 5644–5648.

[18] S. Santens, W. Gevers, The SNARC effect does not imply a mental number line, Cognition 108 (2008) 263–270.

[19] M. Ishihara, S. Jacquin-Courtois, V. Flory, R. Salemme, K. Imanaka, Y. Rossetti, Interaction between space and number representations during motor preparation in manual aiming, Neuropsychologia 44 (2006) 1009–1016.

[20] Y. Ito, T. Hatta, Spatial structure of quantitative representation of numbers: evidence from the SNARC effect, Mem. Cognit. 32 (4) (2004) 662–673.

[21] M.H. Fischer, The future of SNARC could be stark… Cortex 42(8) (2006) 1066–1068.

[22] H. Ota, T. Fujii, M. Tabuchi, K. Sato, J. Saito, A. Yamadori, Different spatial processing for stimulus-centered and body-centered representations, Neurology 60 (11) (2003) 1846–1848.

[23] T. Schenkenberg, D.C. Bradford, E.T. Ajax, Line bisection and unilateral neglect in patients with neurologic impairment, Neurology 30 (5) (1980) 509–517.

[24] F. Doricchi, P. Guariglia, F. Figliozzi, M. Silvetti, G. Bruno, M. Gasparini, Causes of cross-over in unilateral neglect: between-group comparisons, within-patient dissociations and eye movements, Brain 128 (2005) 1386–1406.

[25] S. Ishiai, Y. Koyama, K. Seky, K. Hayashi, Y. Izumi, Approaches to subjective midpoint of horizontal lines in unilateral spatial neglect, Cortex 42 (2006) 685–691.

[26] M. Zorzi, K. Priftis, C. Umilta, Brain damage: neglect disrupts the mental number line, Nature 417 (2002) 138–139.

[27] C. Umiltà, K. Priftis, M. Zorzi, The spatial representation of numbers: evidence from neglect and pseudo-neglect, Exp. Brain Res. 192 (3) (2009) 561–569.

[28] S. Lacour, S. Jacquin, Y. Rossetti, Liens entre représentations spatiales et représentations numériques: apport de la négligence spatiale unilatérale et de la plasticité visuo-motrice. in: Y. Coello, S. Casalis, C. Moroni (Eds.), Vision, espace et cognition: fonctionnement normal et pathologique, Septentrion, 2004, pp. 61–72.

[29] K. Priftis, M. Zorzi, F. Meneghello, R. Marenzi, C. Umiltà, Explicit versus implicit processing of representational space in neglect: dissociations in accessing the mental number line, J. Cogn. Neurosci. 18 (4) (2006) 680–688.

[30] Y. Rossetti, S. Jacquin-Courtois, G. Rode, H. Ota, C. Michel, D. Boisson, Does action make the link between number and space representation? Visuo-manual adaptation improves number bisection in unilateral neglect, Psychol. Sci. 15 (6) (2004) 426–430.

[31] P. Vuilleumier, S. Ortigue, P. Brugger, The number space and neglect, Cortex 40 (2) (2004) 399–410.

[32] G. Rode, J. Luauté, T. Klos, S. Courtois-Jacquin, P. Revol, L. Pisella, et al., Bottom-up visuo-manual adaptation: consequences for spatial cognition, in: P. Haggard, Y. Rossetti, M. Kawato, (Eds.), Sensorimotor Foundations of Higher Cognition, Attention and Performance XXII, Oxford University Press.

[33] A.M. Loftus, M.E. Nicholls, J.B. Mattingley, J.L. Bradshaw, Left to right: representational biases for numbers and the effect of visuomotor adaptation, Cognition 107 (3) (2008) 1048–1058.

[34] P. Bartolomeo, M. Thiebaut de Schotten, F. Doricchi, Left unilateral neglect as a disconnection syndrome, Cereb. Cortex 45 (2007) 3127–3148.

[35] F. Doricchi, M.T. de Schotten, F. Tomaiuolo, P. Bartolomeo, White matter (dis) connections and gray matter (dys)functions in visual neglect: gaining insights into the brain networks of spatial awareness, Cortex 44 (8) (2008) 983–995.

[36] V. Verdon, S. Schwartz, K.O. Lovblad, C.A. Hauer, P. Vuilleumier, Neuroanatomy of hemispatial neglect and its functional components: a study using voxel-based lesion symptom mapping, Brain 133 (2010) 880–894.

[37] A. Nieder, E.K. Miller, A parieto-frontal network for visual numerical information in the monkey, Proc. Natl. Acad. Sci. USA. 101 (19) (2004) 7457–7462.

[38] S. Dehaene, N. Molko, L. Cohen, A.J. Wilson, Arithmetic and the brain, Curr. Opin. Neurobiol. 14 (2004) 218–224.

[39] J.P. van Dijck, W. Gevers, C. Lafosse, F. Doricchi, W. Fias, Non-spatial neglect for the mental number line, Neuropsychologia (under review).

[40] T. Loetscher, P. Brügger, Random number generation in neglect patients reveals enhanced response stereotypy, but no neglect in number space, Neuropsychologia 47 (1) (2009) 276–279.

[41] T. Loetscher, M.E. Nocholls, N.J. Towse, J.L. Bradshaw, P. Brügger, Lucky numbers: spatial neglect affects physical, but not representational, choices in a Lotto task, Cortex 46 (5) (2010) 685–690.

[42] F. Doricchi, S. Merola, M. Aiello, P. Guariglia, M. Bruschini, W. Gevers, et al., Spatial orienting biases in the decimal numeral system, Curr. Biol. 19 (8) (2009) 682–687.

[43] J. Binder, R. Marshall, R. Lazar, J. Benjamin, J.P. Mohr, Distinct syndromes of hemineglect, Arch. Neurol. 49 (1992) 1187–1194.

[44] G.R. Fink, J.C. Marshall, N.J. Shah, P.H. Weiss, P.W. Halligan, M. Grosse-Ruyken, et al., Line bisection judgments implicate right parietal cortex and cerebellum as assessed by fMRI, Neurology 54 (2000) 1324–1331.

[45] P. Azouvi, C. Samuel, A. Louis-Dreyfus, T. Bernati, P. Bartolomeo, J-M. Beis, et al., Sensitivity of clinical and behavioral tests of spatial neglect after right hemisphere stroke, J. Neurol. Neurosurg. Psychiatry 73 (2002) 160–166.

[46] A. Knops, B. Thirion, E.M. Hubbard, V. Michel, S. Dehaene, Recruitment of an area involved in eye movements during mental arithmetic, Science 324 (5934) (2009) 1583–1585.

[47] Y. Rossetti, S. Jacquin-Courtois, P. Revol, S. Lacour, G. Rode, Jamais avant midi: biais spatial et numérique dans le dessin d'horloge des héminégligents, in: Oral Communication at the Annual Meeting of the Société de Neuropsychologie de Langue Française, Paris, December 3d 2004.

[48] D. Grossi, G. Di Cesare, L. Trojano, Left on the right or viceversa: a case of "alternating" constructional allochiria, Cortex 40 (3) (2004) 511–518.

[49] M. Aiello, S. Courtois-Jacquin, S. Merola, T. Ottaviani, D. Bueti, F. Tomaiuolo, et al., No inherent left and right side in human mental number line, (2011, in prep.).

[50] M. Aiello, S. Courtois-Jacquin, S. Merola, T. Ottaviani, D. Bueti, F. Tomaiuolo, et al., Right brain damage: bias towards higher numbers in the bisection of number intervals is spatially and attentionally independent (poster presented at the second meeting of the European Societies of Neuropsychology—ESN—Amsterdam 22–24 September 2010).

[51] C. Guariglia, A. Padovani, P. Pantano, L. Pizzamiglio, Unilateral neglect restricted to visual imagery, Nature 364 (6434) (1993) 235–237.

[52] D. Grossi, A. Modafferi, L. Pelosi, L. Trojano, On the different roles of the cerebral hemispheres in mental imagery – the clock test in two clinical cases, Brain Cogn. 10 (1) (1989) 18–27.

[53] E. Bates, S.M. Wilson, A.P. Saygin, F. Dick, M.I. Sereno, R.T. Knight, et al., Voxel-based lesion-symptom mapping, Nat. Neurosci. 6 (2003) 448–450.

[54] J. Medina, V. Kannan, M.A. Pawlak, J.T. Kleinman, M. Newhart, C. Davis, et al., Neural substrates of visuospatial processing in distinct reference frames: evidence from unilateral spatial neglect, J. Cogn. Neurosci. 21 (2009) 2073–2084.

[55] G. Committeri, G. Galati, A.L. Paradis, L. Pizzamiglio, A. Berthoz, D. LeBihan, Reference frames for spatial cognition: different brain areas are involved in viewer-, object-, and landmark-centered judgments about object location, J. Cogn. Neurosci. 16 (9) (2004) 1517–1535.

[56] S. Dehaene, L. Cohen, Cultural recycling of cortical maps, Neuron 56 (2) (2007) 384–398.

[57] M. Fischer, A. D. Castel, M.D. Dodd J. Pratt, Perceiving number causes spatial shifts of attention. Nat Neurosci. 6(2003) 555–556).

[58] D. de Hevia, L. Girelli, G. Vallar, Numbers and space: a cognitive illusion? Exp. Brain Res. 168 (1–2) (2006) 254–264.

[59] M.R. Longo, S.F. Lourenco, Spatial attention and the mental number line: evidence for characteristic biases and compression, Neuropsychologia 45 (2007) 1400–1407.

[60] G. Galfano, E. Rusconi, C. Umilta, Number magnitude orients attention, but not against one's will, Psychon. Bull. Rev. 13 (5) (2006) 869–874.

[61] J. Ristic, A. Wright, A. Kingstone, The number line effect reflects top-down control, Psychon. Bull. Rev. 13 (5) (2006) 862–868.

[62] M. Ranzini, S. Dehaene, M. Piazza, E.M. Hubbard, Neural mechanisms of attentional shifts due to irrelevant spatial and numerical cues, Neuropsychologia 47 (12) (2009) 2615–2624.

[63] M. Jarick, M.J. Dixon, E.C. Maxwell, M.E.R. Nicholls, D. Smilek, The ups and downs (and lefts and rights) of synaesthetic number forms: validation from spatial cueing and SNARC-type tasks, Cortex 45 (10) (2009) 1190–1199.

[64] M. Andres, M. Davare, M. Pesenti, E. Olivier, X. Seron, Number magnitude and grip aperture interaction, Neuroreport 15 (2004) 2773–2777.

[65] M. Ishihara, K. Imanaka, Motor preparation of manual aiming at a visual target manipulated in size, luminance contrast, and location, Perception 36 (2007) 1375–1390.

Saccades Compress Space, Time, and Number*

David C. Burr†‡, John Ross‡, Paola Binda†¶,
M.Concetta Morrone**††*

*Department of Psychology, Università Degli Studi di Firenze,
Firenze, Italy; †Institute of Neuroscience,
CNR—Pisa, Pisa, Italy; ‡School of Psychology, University of Western
Australia, Western Australia, Australia; ¶Italian Institute of Technology—
Robotics, Brain and Cognitive Sciences Department, Genova, Italy;
**Department of Physiological Sciences, Università di Pisa,
Pisa, Italy; ††Scientific Institute Stella Maris, Pisa, Italy

Summary

It has been suggested that space, time, and number are represented on a common subjective scale. Saccadic eye movements provide a fascinating test. Saccades compress the *perceived magnitude* of spatial separations and temporal intervals to about half their true value. Do they also compress number? They do, and compression follows a very similar time-course for all three attributes, maximal at saccadic onset, falling back to veridicality within a window of about 50 ms. These results reinforce the suggestion of a common perceptual metric, probably mediated by the intraparietal cortex; they further suggest that before every saccade, the common metric for all three is reset, possibly to pave the way for a fresh analysis of the post-saccadic state of affairs.

*Reprinted from Trends in Cognitive Sciences, Vol 14, David C. Burr, John Ross, Paola Binda, M. Concetta Morrone, Saccades compress space, time and number, pg 528–533, 2010, with permission from Elsevier.

SPACE, TIME, AND NUMBER AS VISUAL PRIMITIVES

Space, time, and number are three central descriptors of visual events. By knowing where, when, and how many, we have an approximate representation of a scene. We still do not know who or what, we lack detail, but we have a crude and preliminary sketch sufficient to orient ourselves and to navigate through the environment. Over the past decade, many studies have suggested that these primitives share common processing paths in the primate visual system. In this essay we interpret the available behavioral, neuropsychological and neurophysiological data as evidence for the existence of a common metric for space, time, and number. This hypothesis predicts that changes in the metric of the three perceptual attributes should co-vary. We show that during a saccadic eye movement—a critical moment for the visual system—space, time, and number are all affected in a comparable way: the metric of all three is compressed.

A COMMON METRIC FOR MAGNITUDE

S. S. Stevens [1], distrusting the assumption that *just noticeable differences (JNDs)* were subjectively equal [2], introduced the psychophysical method of magnitude estimation, which requires subjects to match the ratio of two sensory magnitudes (such as loudness) to the ratio of two numbers. The ease with which subjects can make the match, and Stevens's success in amassing a mountain of evidence for a power law linking sensory to physical magnitudes, suggested the existence of a common metric (for a review, see [2]). The exponents of the power law can be greater than unity (expansive, like pain), less than unity (compressive, like loudness) or equal to one (linear). Interestingly, both space and time have exponents near unity, suggesting that both are perceived in the same way as number, up to a scaling factor. More recently, Walsh [3] explicitly proposed that a single magnitude system, resident in the parietal cortex, is responsible for the approximate computation of quantity, be it number, space, or time—or perhaps anything else.

A VISUAL SENSE OF NUMBER

Adult humans in literate and numerate societies have almost all learnt to count, which enables them to estimate number accurately, if slowly and laboriously. However, when deprived of the ability or opportunity to count, we—along with many nonhuman species— can still give a rapid estimate of the number of items in a set, though with much reduced accuracy. As first observed by the economist Jevons [4] error increases with set size in accordance with Weber's law [5,6], as it does for brightness, length, speed, shape and time [7], suggesting that, like them, subjective number (numerosity) is a perceptual attribute. Burr and Ross [8] pointed out that if number is a primary stimulus attribute it should be susceptible to adaptation, and showed that it is: prior adaptation to a more numerous visual stimulus causes a subsequent test stimulus to appear startlingly less numerous (see supplementary material to [8]): stimulus elements in the test stimulus seem to have disappeared after high adaptation and to have appeared out of nowhere after low adaptation.

Many have assumed that the estimation of the numerosity of a dot cloud has little to do with other numeric tasks, and may even derive from other visual attributes, such as texture density [9]. However, a series of experiments [10] has shown clearly that numerosity is estimated directly, not derived from texture density, or anything else; and importantly, the precision with which children can estimate the numerosity of a dot cloud predicts future mathematical ability [11].

INTERACTIONS BETWEEN SPACE, TIME, AND NUMBER

Space and number are intrinsically linked [12–14]. Hadamard [15], who interviewed many mathematicians of his day, reported that many "see" their solutions first and verify them later. Even more impressively, "mental abacus" users—who do mental arithmetic by moving the beads on an imagined abacus—are able to use their visual system to perform exact computations, reinforcing the role of spatial representation and showing that language is not necessary for the representation of exact number [16].

Sir Frances Galton [17] hypothesized that numerosities are perceived spatially, along a mental line, and that the perceptual machinery dealing with spatial extent is exploited to manipulate numerical quantities. Sometimes people can describe their own internal number line; surprisingly, this varies widely across individuals and in most cases it is not straight, or even regular. The notion of a "number line" has received support from a series of studies on the SNARC effect (Spatial Numerical Association of Response Codes), in which smaller numbers elicit faster responses in the left space and larger numbers in right space, as if the mental number line were mapped onto a spatial representation going from left to right [18]. This link of number to space could help explain why nonhuman species with highly developed visual systems can recognize numbers and perform some elementary arithmetic operations like ordering, adding, subtracting and halving (e.g., [19]). Interestingly, amblyopia, a visual condition closely associated with poor spatial resolution and spatial distortions, also affects numerosity judgments outside the subitizing range [20].

Experimental evidence has linked number to time as well as to space. Trained animals (rats or pigeons) discriminate duration and numerosity equally well, and administration of methamphetamine produces equal distortions in both tasks [21]. In double-task experiments, counting interferes with duration judgments and *vice versa* [22]; and a link between time and space has been repeatedly suggested in recent years. Spatial neglect is associated with an overestimate of duration [23], and event time seems to be spatially local [24,25].

The intraparietal sulcus (IPS) and the prefrontal cortex (PFC) of the primate are both involved in encoding of space, time, and number. Neurons tuned to number have been identified in nonhuman primates in parietal areas including the Ventral Intra-Parietal area (VIP) and the Lateral Intra-Parietal (LIP), as well as in a lateral pre-frontal region [26–28]. All these cortical structures have spatially selective receptive fields and are implicated in many important spatial tasks, such as attention and planning of saccades and reaching movements [29]. These areas are also involved in encoding time and number. Many cells respond to the number of items in their receptive fields in a graded manner [27], some preferring small numbers of items, others large numbers. This graded coding of numerosity could be the first step towards creating the selectivity to specific numbers, observed within the fundus of the IPS and in PFC [26]. Many LIP neurons are also modulated by judgments of sub-second intervals [30], indicating that these areas, implicated in numerosity and space processing, also encode temporal intervals. Many human fMRI studies indicate that posterior parietal areas are crucial both for the perception of time [31,32] and number

---

BOX 12.1

PREDICTIVE REMAPPING OF VISUAL NEURONS DURING SACCADES

Visual neurons encode space in retinotopic coordinates, meaning that the region where they respond to stimuli (receptive field) is fixed on the retina, and hence moves with the eyes. A stimulus displayed at a given position in external space drives different populations of cells before and after an eye movement. How do we maintain a stable representation of the visual world across saccades?

In a landmark paper, Duhamel, Colby and Goldberg [39] reported that receptive fields of many neurons in the LIP change drastically at the time of saccades, shifting in the direction of the saccade, *before* the eyes have moved. They respond to a given position in the external space both before and (for a brief period of time) after the eye movement, potentially bridging retinotopic maps across saccades [57]. fMRI experiments support the existence of the phenomenon in the human brain as well [58,59]. This "predictive remapping" has been observed in several areas of monkey cortex, including the frontal eye fields [60] and extra-striate visual areas [61,62]; but the parietal cortex—particularly LIP—is the area where the predictive behavior is most pervasive, seen in 40–50% of cells [39]. There

is evidence that the remapping is mediated by a non-visual corollary discharge, probably originating in the superior colliculus, and acting on the prefrontal cortex [57]. The corollary discharge signal may reach parietal and extra-striate areas by top-down modulation from the prefrontal cortex.

Most researchers believe that the behavior of these cells is responsible both for perceptual stability and for the transient distortions of visual perception observed at the time of saccades. Predictive remapping produces a transient alteration of spatial codes, and has been linked to the perisaccadic shift or compression of perceived position [40,48,52,63]. As LIP neurons have been shown to encode information about stimulus timing [30] and number [27], they could also be implicated in the peri-saccadic compression of time [48,49] and numerosity [51]. Recent evidence suggests that neurons in superior colliculus and frontal eye fields encode time with an amplitude magnitude code [64]. It is not yet known whether this encoding strategy is affected by the peri-saccadic update, but this would seem to be very likely.

---

[33]—although the PFC, subcortical nuclei (basal ganglia) and the cerebellum are also clearly involved in time perceptioin [34,35]. Lesions to areas located in the proximity of the intraparietal sulcus are associated with numerical deficits in patients [18,36], and repetitive TMS affects both the SNARC effect [37] and temporal judgments [38].

The intraparietal region, and area LIP in particular, is perhaps best known for its role in "remapping" spatial information during saccadic eye movements [39]. Just before each saccade, the receptive fields of many neurons shift in the direction of the saccade. Although the exact role of this anticipatory shift is still not clear (see Box 12.1), most assume that it is related to maintaining stability across saccades. As Fig. 12.1 illustrates schematically, areas where perisaccadic remapping has been observed and areas where numerosity and

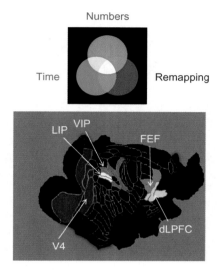

FIGURE 12.1 **Time, numbers and perisaccadic remapping in the brain.** Flattened cortical surface of a monkey right hemisphere; borders define cortical areas identified in the partitioning scheme by Lewis and Van Essen [65] (the anatomical image with the area-borders was downloaded from the Sums database http://sumsdb.wustl.edu/sums/index.jsp and visualized with Caret http://brainvis.wustl.edu/wiki/index.php/Caret). Areas where the studies in Table 12.1 identified neurons modulated by numerosity were colored in red, those modulated by temporal duration in green, and areas where perisaccadic remapping were reported in blue. The co-occurrence of two or more of these characteristics is indicated by the summation of the corresponding colors (see legend). Please note that this figure is intended only as a schematic representation, and the reader is referred to the original papers for the exact localization of the recording sites. Also it is clearly not an exhaustive account, but shows only those areas that have been studied for these attributes to date. dLPFC, dorso-lateral PFC (which includes Brodmann areas 45 and 46).

TABLE 12.1

	Study	Areas
Time	Leon and Shadlen 2003 [30]	LIP
	Genovesio *et al.* 2005 [66]	46-8-9-6
Numbers	Sawamura *et al.* 2002 [28]	5-2
	Nieder and Miller 2004 [26]	dLPFC-PPC
	Roitman *et al.* 2007 [27]	LIP
Remapping	Duhamel *et al.* 1992 [39]	LIP
	Tolias *et al.* 2001 [62]	V4
	Nakamura and Colby 2002 [61]	V2-V3-V3A
	Umeno and Goldberg 1997 [67]	FEF

temporal information are encoded overlap considerably—the three attributes are represented within fronto-parietal networks, which intersect at the level of key areas such as LIP (see also Table 12.1). Imaging work suggests a similar picture with humans, although the complexity of the terminology used to identify human cortical areas makes the task of localizing functional circuits and their overlap particularly difficult. Note that Fig. 12.1 is not intended as an exhaustive meta-analysis, but a schematic indication of the areas that have been studied to date: as more areas are studied in greater detail, the extent of overlap may well greatly increase.

EFFECTS OF SACCADES ON SPACE, TIME, AND NUMBER

Although several investigators have postulated links between space, time, and number, the evidence for them is often circumstantial and somewhat weak. Much relies on the coincidence of neural areas (e.g. intraparietal cortex), and on small advantages in reaction times, that can often be put down to "congruency effects". That reaction times are faster to small numbers on the left and larger on the right does not necessarily imply a hard-wired connection. For example, many of us who have spent far too much time producing graphs like Fig. 12.3B associate hot colors with large responses and cold colors with small. If we showed faster reaction times for large–red and small–blue, we would not necessarily believe that color and number were linked. To search for stronger links between the three attributes, we investigated the effect of saccadic eye-movements on space, time, and number. If spatial, temporal and numeral representations share a neural substrate in the posterior parietal cortex, and if visual responses on these areas are strongly affected by saccadic eye movements (Box 12.1), then saccades should interfere in similar ways with the perception of all three perceptual attributes: space, time, and number.

Saccades have dramatic but selective effects on visual processing (see, for example, [40]). Some stimuli (modulated in luminance at low frequencies) flashed before or during saccades are strongly suppressed, while others (chromatic, or high-frequency luminance stimuli) are not [41]. The effects begin before the eyes begin to move (and are therefore not caused by smearing) and do not occur when the saccades are simulated by fast-motion of the scene [42]. The apparent position of visual stimuli flashed briefly about the time of a saccade is also misplaced [43–45], usually in the direction of the impending saccade. But the effects are in fact more complicated: saccades do not cause only a simple shift in perceived position, but a *compression* of visual space [46,47]. As Fig. 12.2A shows, bars flashed briefly long before or after saccade are seen veridically, in their correct physical positions. Near the time of the saccade, however, there are huge mislocalization errors, and the direction of the errors is always towards the saccadic target: stimuli flashed to the left of the saccadic target (for a rightward saccade) are seen displaced rightwards, while stimuli flashed beyond it are displaced leftwards, in all cases towards the saccadic target. Stimuli flashed between -10 and $+20°$—some $30°$ of visual space—are all seen near the saccadic target at saccadic onset. This compression, which cannot result from the simple addition of a single "efference copy" vector to the retinal eccentricity signal, is very real, causing multiple bars straddling the saccadic target to collapse down to a single bar [46,47], so much is the distance between them underestimated.

Saccades cause not only a shift and compression of space, but also similar effects in the perception of event time, both shifts and compression [48,49]. Figure 12.2B illustrates the compression. A pair of bars flashed 100 ms apart is seen veridically when displayed well before or after saccadic onset, but near saccadic onset the apparent interval between them is strongly compressed, to about half its true value. The compression follows a very similar time-course to that for spatial compression. We have pointed out that the compression of

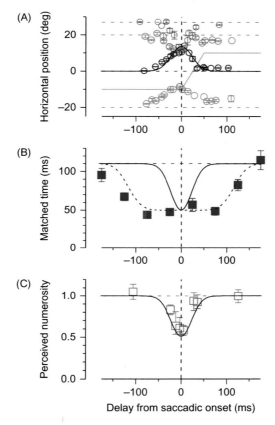

FIGURE 12.2 **Peri-saccadic distortion of space, time, and number.** Perceptual distortions for stimuli presented briefly at about the time of a large (20°) saccadic eye movement (continuous gray line in panel A). In all plots saccadic onset is indicated by a vertical dotted line. (A) Perceived spatial location of a bar flashed at four different locations (hollow circles, separate colors) as a function of the time of its presentation relative to the saccade onset. For each presentation, subjects reported perceived bar location relative to a memorized ruler. Localization during fixation is shown with dotted lines. Modified with permission from [46]. (B) Perceived temporal separation of two bars flashed with an interval of 100 ms; the abscissa shows the average time of the bars relative to saccadic onset. Subjects reported (in forced choice) which of two pairs of bars (one peri-saccadic, one post-saccadic) was separated by a longer temporal interval. The data were fitted by a cumulative Gaussian psychometric function, whose mean estimates the perceived duration of the peri-saccadic interval (ordinate of the figure). From these data, we calculated the predicted time-course of the temporal compression signal (continuous curve), by deconvolving the spline-fit of the data (dashed line) with the temporal separation of the two markers of the experiment (100 ms) increased by the duration of the dynamics (130 ms). Note that the predicted time-course is much more tightly tuned than the data, because the data were collected with a broad temporal stimulus (100 ms long) that necessarily blurs the effects over time. The dashed horizontal line reports perceived duration in steady fixation conditions. Modified with permission from [49]. (C) Estimated relative numerosity for a set of 30 random dots flashed perisaccadically, normalized by the steady fixation estimate (dashed horizontal line) [51]. This experiment was like the one with time, except that subjects judged which of two dot-stimuli was more numerous: one with fixed numerosity, presented well before the saccade, the other with variable numerosity presented peri-saccadically. For each time bin (relative to saccadic onset), and also for fixation, we calculated a psychometric function, yielding a PSE. The plot reports the ratio of number of dots in the probe when presented during fixation to that presented during saccades. The black continuous curves in A, B & C are Gaussians functions with the same mean and standard deviation that best fit all data.

space–time, around the time of rapid shifts of information, has strong analogies with special relativity [50].

Space and time are compressed just before and during saccades. What happens to the numerosity of visual elements? To address this question, we asked subjects to compare the number of elements in a random test array flashed at the time of a saccade to that of a reference stimulus presented well before the saccade [51]. Figure 12.2C illustrates how apparent numerosity varied with time relative to the saccade. Well before or after the saccade, numerosity estimation is veridical, but near saccadic onset there is a large and systematic underestimation of number—perceived numerosity is nearly halved. The time-course of the compression follows closely those of space and of time. As with saccadic compression, neither space, nor time or number is affected by simulating the saccade with a fast mirror motion [46,48,51].

Rarely in biology do independent and unrelated measurements follow so closely the same dynamics. Discarding the unlikely possibility of pure chance, the similar time-courses point to the existence of common mechanisms—probably resident in parietal cortex (Fig. 12.1)—which modulate the metrics of space, time, and number. We presume that the compression of all three attributes results from neural processes that occur at the time of saccades to preserve visual stability. When the eyes move, the visual representation of the world must be remapped into new coordinates, and this remapping commences before the eyes actually move, with a rapid and complex deformation of visual receptive fields, most commonly observed in the intraparietal cortex.

The shifting of receptive fields is best understood by considering simultaneously both the spatial and temporal events [52,53]. Figure 12.3A is a cartoon drawn from a recording of an LIP neuron to stimulation to the "future receptive field" (the part of space that will become the receptive field after the saccade) before, during and after the saccade [54]. The responses are aligned to the saccade, and sorted by stimulus presentation time. The first spikes to all stimuli occur at about the same time, implying that pre- and post-saccadic stimulation to this part of space (corresponding to different retinal positions) cause very similar spike trains. A higher-order cell monitoring the response has no way of distinguishing whether a particular spike results from early pre-saccadic stimulation to the "future receptive field" or later post-saccadic stimulation of the "classic receptive field". The region in space–time that elicits identical responses, all arriving at the same time, defines the transient receptive field of the cell, in space and in time, illustrated schematically in Fig. 12.3B. In retinal coordinates, it is oriented in space–time in the direction of the retinal motion caused by the saccade, and therefore cancels its effect (a similar argument for motion was proposed in [55]). The spatio-temporal structure of the receptive field at the time of saccades shows how tightly space and time are linked. It is not immediately obvious how this will also lead to a compression of number, other than that the same neural mechanisms that encode space and time also encode number, and those with a graded response to number also have receptive fields clearly circumscribed in space.

Spatial location, duration and numerosity form an approximate representation of a stimulus set; as such, the three attributes may well be expected to undergo similar distortions, ensuring that they always co-vary. At this stage it is unclear whether it is the representation of these attributes that is changed, or the mechanism that decodes them: either could cause compression. Concurrent deformation of space, time, and number has the advantage of maintaining ratios, invariant with the area of the stimuli on the retinal

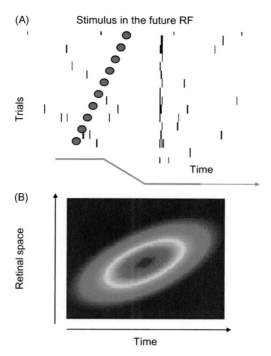

FIGURE 12.3 **Transient spatio-temporal receptive field during remapping.** (A) Cartoon drawn from data of Wang *et al.* [54] showing spike responses of a typical LIP cell (short bars) to stimulation in the "future receptive field" (that becomes the classical receptive field after the eye movement). The responses are all aligned to the saccade, and sorted by stimulus presentation time. The systematic delays in the responses cause all spikes to occur at a similar time, and therefore indistinguishable. (B) Schematic spatiotemporal receptive field of the neuron, defining the region of confusion in space–time with the same spiking pattern (hot colors indicating stronger responses). The spatio-temporal receptive field is oriented in space–time along the same direction of the retinal motion, and thereby annuls it.

surface, and its cortical representation (which changes considerably with each eye movement), facilitating transfer of information from one fixation to the next. Perhaps, during the rapid perisaccadic updating process, the brain cannot manage the usual large information bandwidth, so it reduces the informational load (keeping important ratios constant), by compression.

CONCLUSIONS

The results we consider here support the idea of close connections between space, time, and number, perhaps because all three representations are mapped onto a common magnitude line, as assumed by Stevens [2] and proposed by Walsh [3]. The compression could be a direct result of the rapid receptive field shifts accompanying (and preceding) saccades, for the quasi-relativistic reasons suggested by Morrone, Ross and Burr [50]. On each saccade, visual representations need to be updated to maintain stability as the retinal image is pitched about by movements of the eyes. Spatial updating cannot be a trivial process, and presumably places heavy demands on the available visual resources. This may cause the system to compress the spatial, temporal and numeric information, reducing informational load, and hence demand on processing resources. With all three compressed, the relationship between space, time, and number would be preserved to allow trans-saccadic information to be rescaled to the post-saccadic retinal image, paving the way for a fresh analysis of the visual scene from the post-saccadic perspective [56].

GLOSSARY

Saccades

rapid ballistic eye movements made on average three times a second to direct gaze towards objects of interest.

Power Law

a "law" proposed by S.S. Stevens, according to which perceived magnitudes increase proportionally to physical magnitudes raised to a power. The exponents can be greater than unity (expansive), less than unity (compressive) or equal to one (linear). Much data collected with Stevens's method of "magnitude estimation" supports his "law".

Weber "Law"

refers to a range of experimental findings showing that responses to smaller numerosities are faster and/or more accurate in the left space, and larger numerosities are advantaged in right space.

Receptive Field

a structured region of a sensory surface (such as retina or skin) where an appropriate (or "adequate") stimulus (such as a flash of light) causes a sensory cell to respond. Visual receptive fields can also be defined in external space.

Acknowledgments

This research was supported by the Italian Ministry of Universities and Research, the Australian Research Council, and by EC projects "MEMORY" (FP6-NEST) and "STANIB" (FP7-ERC).

References

[1] S.S. Stevens, E.C. Poulton, The estimation of loudness by unpracticed observers, J. Exp. Psychol. 51 (1956) 71–78.

[2] S.S. Stevens, On the psychophysical law, Psychol. Rev. 64 (1957) 153–181.

[3] V. Walsh, A theory of magnitude: common cortical metrics of time, space and quantity, Trends Cogn. Sci. 7 (2003) 483–488.

[4] W.S. Jevons, The power of numerical discrimination, Nature 3 (1871) 363–372.

[5] J. Ross, Visual discrimination of number without counting, Perception 32 (2003) 867–870.

[6] J. Whalen et al., Nonverbal counting in humans: the psychophysics of number representation, Psychol. Sci. 10 (1999) 130–137.

[7] G.T. Fechner et al., Elemente der psychophysik, Breitkopf und Härtel, Leipzig, 1860. (reprinted by Thoemmes Press (Bristol) 1999)

[8] D. Burr, J. Ross, A visual sense of number, Curr. Biol. 18 (2008) 425–428.

[9] F.H. Durgin, Texture density adaptation and visual number revisited, Curr. Biol. 18 (2008) R855–R856.

[10] J. Ross, D.C. Burr, Vision senses number directly, J. Vis. 10 (2010) 11–18.

[11] J. Halberda et al., Individual differences in non-verbal number acuity correlate with maths achievement, Nature 455 (2008). 665–668.

[12] S. Dehaene et al., Abstract representations of numbers in the animal and human brain, Trends Neurosci. 21 (1998) 355–361.

[13] B. Butterworth, The mathematical brain, Macmillan, London, 1999.

[14] S. Dehaene, The Number Sense: How the Mind Creates Mathematics, Penguin, London, 1997.

[15] J.S. Hadamard, An Essay on the Psychology of Invention in the Mathematical Field, Dover Publications, New York, 1954.

[16] M.C. Frank, Symposium: Is number visual? Is vision numerical? Investigating the relationship between visual representations and the property of magnitude, J. Vis. 9 (2009) 11.

[17] F. Galton, Visualised numerals, Nature 21 (1880) 494–495.

[18] S. Dehaene et al., The mental representation of parity and numerical magnitude, J. Exp. Psychol. Gen. 122 (1993) 371–396.

[19] E.M. Brannon, H.S. Terrace, Ordering of the numerosities 1 to 9 by monkeys, Science 282 (1998) 746–749.

[20] V. Sharma et al., Undercounting features and missing features: evidence for a high-level deficit in strabismic amblyopia, Nat. Neurosci. 3 (2000) 496–501.

[21] W.H. Meck, R.M. Church, A mode control model of counting and timing processes, J. Exp. Psychol. Anim. Behav. Process. 9 (1983) 320–334.

[22] S.W. Brown, Attentional resources in timing: interference effects in concurrent temporal and nontemporal working memory tasks, Percept. Psychophys. 59 (1997) 1118–1140.

[23] G. Basso et al., Time perception in a neglected space, Neuroreport 7 (1996) 2111–2114.

[24] D. Burr et al., Neural mechanisms for timing visual events are spatially selective in real-world coordinates, Nat. Neurosci. 10 (2007) 423–425.

[25] A. Johnston et al., Spatially localized distortions of event time, Curr. Biol. 16 (2006) 472–479.

[26] A. Nieder, E.K. Miller, A parieto-frontal network for visual numerical information in the monkey, Proc. Natl. Acad. Sci. U.S.A. 101 (2004) 7457–7462.

[27] J.D. Roitman et al., Monotonic coding of numerosity in macaque lateral intraparietal area, PLoS Biol. 5 (2007) e208.

[28] H. Sawamura et al., Numerical representation for action in the parietal cortex of the monkey, Nature 415 (2002) 918–922.

[29] R.A. Andersen, C.A. Buneo, Intentional maps in posterior parietal cortex, Annu. Rev. Neurosci. 25 (2002) 189–220.

[30] M.I. Leon, M.N. Shadlen, Representation of time by neurons in the posterior parietal cortex of the macaque, Neuron 38 (2003) 317–327.

[31] J.T. Coull et al., Functional anatomy of the attentional modulation of time estimation, Science 303 (2004) 1506–1508.

[32] D. Bueti et al., Encoding of temporal probabilities in the human brain, J. Neurosci. 30 (2010) 4343–4352.

[33] S. Dehaene et al., Three parietal circuits for number processing, Cogn. Neuropsychol. 20 (2003) 487–506.

[34] R.B. Ivry, R.M. Spencer, The neural representation of time, Curr. Opin. Neurobiol. 14 (2004) 225–232.

[35] P.A. Lewis, R.C. Miall, Remembering the time: A continuous clock, Trends Cogn. Sci. 10 (2006) 401–406.

[36] N. Molko et al., Functional and structural alterations of the intraparietal sulcus in a developmental dyscalculia of genetic origin, Neuron 40 (2003) 847–858.

[37] M. Oliveri et al., Overestimation of numerical distances in the left side of space, Neurology 63 (2004) 2139–2141.

[38] D. Bueti et al., Sensory and association cortex in time perception, J. Cogn. Neurosci. 20 (2008) 1054–1062.

[39] J.R. Duhamel et al., The updating of the representation of visual space in parietal cortex by intended eye movements, Science 255 (1992) 90–92.

[40] J. Ross et al., Changes in visual perception at the time of saccades, Trends Neurosci. 24 (2001) 113–121.

[41] D.C. Burr et al., Selective suppression of the magnocellular visual pathway during saccadic eye movements, Nature 371 (1994) 511–513.

[42] M.R. Diamond et al., Extraretinal control of saccadic suppression, J. Neurosci. 20 (2000) 3449–3455.

[43] L. Matin, D.G. Pearce, Visual perception of direction for stimuli flashed during voluntary saccadic eye movements, Science 148 (1965) 1485–1488.

[44] S. Mateeff, Saccadic eye movements and localization of visual stimuli, Percept. Psychophys. 24 (1978) 215–224.

[45] J. Schlag, M. Schlag-Rey, Illusory localization of stimuli flashed in the dark before saccades, Vision Res. 35 (1995) 2347–2357.

[46] M.C. Morrone et al., Apparent position of visual targets during real and simulated saccadic eye movements, J. Neurosci. 17 (1997) 7941–7953.

[47] J. Ross et al., Compression of visual space before saccades, Nature 386 (1997) 598–601.

[48] P. Binda et al., Spatiotemporal distortions of visual perception at the time of saccades, J. Neurosci. 29 (2009) 13147–13157.

[49] M.C. Morrone et al., Saccadic eye movements cause compression of time as well as space, Nat. Neurosci. 8 (2005) 950–954.

[50] M.C. Morrone et al., Keeping vision stable: rapid updating of spatiotopic receptive fields may cause relativistic-like effects, in: R. Nijhawan, B. Khurana, (Eds.), Space and Time in Perception and Action, Cambridge University Press, pp. 52–62.

[51] P. Binda, M.C. Morrone, J. Ross, D.C. Burr, Underestimation of perceived number at the time of saccades, Vision Res. 51 (2000) 34–42.

[52] D.C. Burr, M.C. Morrone, Vision: keeping the world still when the eyes move, Curr. Biol. 20 (2010) R442–444.

[53] C.D. Burr, M.C. Morrone, Spatiotopic coding and remapping in humans. Phil. Trans. Roy. Soc. 366 (2011) 504–515.

[54] X. Wang, et al., Perisaccadic elongation of receptive fields in the lateral intraparietal area (lip). in: Society for Neuroscience, Program No. 855.816/FF822 2008 Neuroscience Meeting Planner. Online.

[55] C.D. Burr, J. Ross, Visual processing of motion, Trends Neurosci. 9 (1986).

[56] J. Ross, A. Ma-Wyatt, Saccades actively maintain perceptual continuity, Nat. Neurosci. 7 (2004) 65–69.

[57] R.H. Wurtz, Neuronal mechanisms of visual stability, Vision Res. 48 (2008) 2070–2089.

[58] E.P. Merriam et al., Spatial updating in human parietal cortex, Neuron 39 (2003) 361–373.

[59] E.P. Merriam et al., Remapping in human visual cortex, J. Neurophysiol. 97 (2007) 1738–1755.

[60] M.A. Sommer, R.H. Wurtz, Influence of the thalamus on spatial visual processing in frontal cortex, Nature 444 (2006) 374–377.

[61] K. Nakamura, C.L. Colby, Updating of the visual representation in monkey striate and extrastriate cortex during saccades, Proc. Natl. Acad. Sci. U.S.A. 99 (2002) 4026–4031.

[62] A.S. Tolias et al., Eye movements modulate visual receptive fields of v4 neurons, Neuron 29 (2001) 757–767.

[63] F.H. Hamker et al., The peri-saccadic perception of objects and space, PLoS Comput. Biol. 4 (2008) e31.

[64] J.P. Mayo, M.A. Sommer, Encoding of brief time interval judgments in single neurons, J. Vis. (2010). (VSS 2010 conference proceedings).

[65] J.W. Lewis, D.C. Van Essen, Mapping of architectonic subdivisions in the macaque monkey, with emphasis on parieto-occipital cortex, J. Comp. Neurol. 428 (2000) 79–111.

[66] A. Genovesio et al., Prefrontal cortex activity related to abstract response strategies, Neuron 47 (2005) 307–320.

[67] M.M. Umeno, M.E. Goldberg, Spatial processing in the monkey frontal eye field. I predictive visual responses. J. Neurophysiol. 78 (1997) 1373–1383.

ORIGINS OF PROTO-MATHEMATICAL INTUITIONS

Introduction, by Stanislas Dehaene

Whenever they suddenly discover the solution to a difficult problem, mathematicians often claim that they relied on their "intuition". But what is an intuition? Several elements can contribute toward its definition: an intuition is fast, effortless, insightful, non-conscious and closed to introspection. In my book *The Number Sense* and elsewhere, I proposed that the most basic of our human intuitions relate to what Elizabeth Spelke calls "core knowledge"—the disparate set of knowledge that we inherit from our evolutionary past and which is present early on in infancy. According to this hypothesis, intuitions of geometry and arithmetic draw upon a store of fundamental knowledge accumulated over millions of years of evolution in a physical world which, at the scale we live in, is spatially, temporally and numerically structured. However, with education, our intuitions can be trained to reach far beyond this elementary core. Indeed, with practice, mathematicians can gain intuitive knowledge about high-level concepts such as complex numbers, infinite spaces or group theory. Yet the ultimate foundation of these mathematical constructions probably lies in a narrow set of principles, grounded in generations of interactions with a structured environment and the corresponding internalization through natural selection, of elementary mechanisms of spatial, temporal and numerical computation in the brain.

Within this context, two questions are essential. First, from a phylogenetic perspective, can we experimentally evaluate which species possess spatial, temporal and numerical representations, and begin to understand the evolutionary pathways that gave rise to them? Second, from an ontogenetic perspective, what are the developmental and, ultimately, the molecular and genetic mechanisms that allow intuitive representations of space, time and number to emerge in human children and even infants?

The scope of the issues I have just enumerated is so vast that the chapters in this section address them only partially. In a first chapter, eminent specialists of animal cognition **Daniel Haun, Fiona Jordan, Giorgio Vallortigara** and **Nicky Clayton** review whether and how non-human animals, including primates, birds and even fish, gain knowledge of space, time and number. Animal models provide these researchers with the opportunity to ask several unique questions. In chicks and fish, studies of newborn animals as well as controlled rearing studies (where animals spend their youth in a restricted environment) establish the fact that the sense of space and of number can develop in spite of the near-absence of interaction with a structured environment. Even newly hatched chicks can discriminate number and may even exhibit a preference for a left-to-right mapping of number onto space! Furthermore, studies of non-human primates afford tentative inferences about the specific evolutionary endowment of the human species. Finally, studies of more distant animals such as crows and jays demand that we revise our concepts about what were once thought to be uniquely human abilities for planning, memory, and mental time travel.

In a second chapter, **Elizabeth Brannon** and **Dustin Merritt,** using systematic behavioral studies of humans and macaques, flesh out the evolutionary origins of the human number system. As emphasized in the title of one of their previous papers, the capacities for "basic math in monkeys and college students" turn out to be remarkably related. The semantic distance and congruity effects that characterize number comparison behavior are very similar and suggest virtually identical coding and decision making mechanisms. Even the rudiments of the concept of zero turn out to be intuitive for macaque monkeys, inasmuch as they can apprehend the notion of an empty set and order it appropriately in respect to other sets of objects. Approximate addition and subtraction with concrete sets are also easily within the monkey's grasp, again with psychophysics quite similar to that of humans. All in all, this research strongly suggests that an approximate arithmetic system is part of the human evolutionary heritage and dates back at least 25 million years to when the human and macaque lineage diverged.

Finally, **Stella Lourenco** and **Matthew Longo** demonstrate that the correspondence between space, time and number also belongs to the core knowledge inherited by human infants. They describe clever experiments which prove that infants generalize the larger/smaller relation across dimensions of numerosity, temporal duration, and physical size. This finding fits well with the fact that children are quick to learn that the words "large" and "small" apply to all of these dimensions. It also meshes with Piaget's earlier findings concerning the child's tendency to confuse these dimensions when making explicit decisions. According to Lourenco and Longo, our human evolutionary heritage includes a general magnitude system that applies not only to space, time and number, but may also extend to pitch and other linear dimensions.

With such clear behavioral and ethological data in hand, numerical cognition research is gearing up to ask new major questions: How is the infant brain wired to support its early competences? Can we identify which genes are involved, and through which developmental pathways they interact to promote the ultimate emergence of neural structures biased to encode the concepts of space, time and number? In spite of recent advances in brain-imaging which, for example, made possible Véronique Izard's recent discovery of distinct ventral and dorsal responses to object identity and number in the baby brain, the biological origins of our Kantian *a priori* intuitions remain a vast *terra incognita* ripe for further research.

Origins of Spatial, Temporal, and Numerical Cognition: Insights from Comparative Psychology*

Daniel B.M. Haun[*†‡], Fiona M. Jordan[†], Giorgio Vallortigara[§], Nicky S. Clayton[¶]*

[*]Max Planck Institute for Evolutionary Anthropology, Leipzig, Germany; [†]Max Planck Institute for Psycholinguistics, Nijmegen, The Netherlands; [‡]University of Portsmouth, Department of Psychology, Portsmouth, UK; [§]Centre for Mind/Brain Sciences, University of Trento, Rovereto, Italy; [¶]Department of Experimental Psychology, University of Cambridge, Cambridge, UK

Summary

Contemporary comparative cognition has a large repertoire of animal models and methods, with concurrent theoretical advances that are providing initial answers to critical questions about human cognition. What cognitive traits are uniquely human? What are the species-typical inherited predispositions of the human mind? What is the human mind capable of without certain types of specific experiences with the surrounding environment? Here we review recent findings from the domains of space, time, and number cognition. These findings are produced using different comparative methodologies relying on different animal species, namely different birds and the nonhuman great apes. The study of these species not only reveals the range of cognitive abilities across vertebrates, but forwards our understanding of human cognition in crucial ways.

*Reprinted from Trends in Cognitive Sciences, Vol 14, Daniel B.M. Haun, Fiona M. Jordan, Giorgio Vallortigara, Nicky S. Clayton, Origins of spatial, temporal and numerical cognition: Insights from comparative psychology, pg 552–560, 2010, with permission from Elsevier.

RESEARCHING HUMAN COGNITION THROUGH THE STUDY OF OTHER SPECIES

"He who understands baboon would do more towards Metaphysics than Locke" **Charles Darwin, 1838, Notebook M84e**

In this short note, 21 years before publication of the *Origin of Species*, Charles Darwin recognized the value of studying animal cognition for human psychology. Implicit here is the idea that cognitive processes are biological adaptations with evolutionary histories, and therefore cognition is tractable to between-species mapping of similarities and differences in cognitive abilities. The last two decades have seen a steady growth in the number of species studied and the types of methodological approaches used in the growing field of comparative cognition [1,2]. Concurrently, this work has become highly interdisciplinary between biology, psychology, neuroscience, genetics, linguistics, and anthropology. Here we review lines of evidence in which the study of other animal species have informed our understanding of the structure and evolution of three core domains of human cognition: space, number, and time. We demonstrate how different methodologies in comparative cognition not only reveal the range of cognitive abilities within the animal kingdom, but forward our understanding of human cognition in crucial ways, allowing us to address seemingly intractable questions such as (1) are some cognitive capacities in place at birth? (2) what is the evolutionary endowment of human cognition? and (3) which cognitive abilities are uniquely human?

ARE SOME COGNITIVE CAPACITIES IN PLACE AT BIRTH?

In the past, rigorous controlled-rearing experiments with nonhuman animals have allowed scientists to establish which mechanisms are present at birth and the impact of specific experiences on shaping some basic perceptual-motor capacities [3]. One example is given in the classic "visual cliff" studies showing that the ability to judge depth through motion parallax is in place at birth in a variety of animal species [4]. This pioneering work, however, did not venture into more complex cognitive capacities, such as the cognition of space, number, or time. Recently, however, it has been proposed that complex human cognitive achievements such as mathematics and geometry, which are uniquely human in their full linguistic and symbolic realization, rest nevertheless on a set of core knowledge systems that humans share with other animals [5]. Because of their limited behavioral repertoire, the study of cognitive capacities in human infants is limited, as it is in the young of altricial (slow-developing) species in general. It is for this reason that investigating species that are precocial with regard to their pattern of motor and sensory development makes possible sophisticated behavioral analyses of early ages, scoping the influence of specific experiences on inborn cognition.

Precocial Animal Models

Being a precocial species, the domestic chick (*Gallus gallus*) has been a very successful animal model system for tackling some classical issues in developmental psychology such as the origins of both social cognition (e.g., biological motion [6], causal agency [7]) and physical cognition (e.g., object permanence [8]). The heuristic value of research with chicks for human developmental studies has been particularly apparent in the area of early social predispositions. Visually inexperienced chicks at their first exposure to point-light animation sequences exhibit a spontaneous preference to approach biological motion patterns [9]. These findings stimulated a substantial body of research concerning perception of biological motion in human newborns (e.g., [10,11]) that revealed astonishingly similar predispositions.

Chicks have also been recently used to investigate the origins of space and number cognition. Neurobiological evidence suggests basic homology in the avian and mammalian brain for a key neural structure involved in space cognition (hippocampal formation) and possibly for associative areas involved in number cognition as well (mesopallium) [12].

For example, much interest has been devoted to the issue of how humans and animals regain their sense of direction when they become disoriented. There appears to be impressive sensitivity to surface layout geometry in guiding spatial reorientation [13,14]. For example, when an animal observes the hiding of a target in one corner of a rectangular enclosure, and is then inertially disoriented, it subsequently shows selective searching at the two geometrically correct corners of the enclosure, avoiding the corners with incorrect metric (short/long) and sense (left/right) properties in the arrangement of surfaces [13,14].

Competing theories have been formulated as to how animals and humans reorient themselves in these circumstances, which include Fodorian modular encapsulated computations of the shape of the extended surfaces layout [15], combination of environmental cues weighted according to their experienced reliability [16], image-matching processes operating on panoramic 2D projections of current and remembered environments [17]. Several empirical studies have been carried out in both vertebrates [18–20] and invertebrates [21] in an attempt to decide about the relative merits of the different theories. One approach has been to investigate whether the system for reorientation does possess some of the hallmarks of a Fodorian module, such as specific genetic bases [22], specific neural mechanisms [23,24] and whether it develops in the absence of relevant experience of navigating in a geometrically structured layout. The last issue is of course important even irrespective of a Fodorian approach, and can be successfully addressed using controlled-rearing studies.

In rectangular enclosures, geometric information is fully available because of the presence of metrically distinct surfaces connected at right angles and two principal axes of symmetry. In circular enclosures, in contrast, this geometric information is removed and there is an infinite number of principal axes. In C-shaped enclosures no right angles or differences in wall length are available but the first principal axis is still usable to encode shape. Chicks reared soon after hatching in home-cages with these different geometric shapes proved to be equally capable of learning and performing navigational tasks based on geometric information [18,25]. This suggests that effective use of geometric information for spatial reorientation in principle does not require experience in environments with right angles and metrically distinct surfaces. Recently, further evidence that at least some aspects of spatial representations are present at birth arose from single-cell recording studies, showing that when rat pups explore an open environment outside the nest for the first time, head-direction cells show adult-like properties from the beginning; place and grid cells are also present from the beginning but their selectivity refines gradually [26,27].

It could be argued that the pattern of development of precocial species may be peculiar, and not generalizable to humans (note, however, that rats are an altricial species as well).

Nonetheless, these findings provide evidence that, in principle, a capacity can develop fully in the absence of a *specific* experiential contribution. Some differences between altricial and precocial species may turn out to be the by-product of maturation of other mechanisms rather than the outcome of specific learning. For instance, the ability to mentally complete partly occluded objects (amodal completion) is apparent in chicks soon after hatching [28], which could be taken as evidence for mechanisms that do not require experience, whereas in human infants this ability is only present from about four months of age [29]. Recently, however, it has been shown that when stroboscopic motion is used instead of continuous motion (the former being processed early in development by sub-cortical structures), human neonates of only a few hours of life show evidence of amodal completion similar to that of chicks [30]. Thus, in altricial species, maturation of other brain areas seems to be necessary in order to exhibit in behavior the mental competences which are predisposed at birth. Similarly, the results obtained in chicks [31] suggest that basic features of natural geometry are largely in place at birth—though of course in humans language and other types of non-geometric experience may influence the development of uniquely human forms of spatial knowledge [32].

Even though specific experiences may be not crucial in encoding surface geometry, it could be that they are important in the combined use of geometric and non-geometric information (e.g., features like the color of a wall) for reorientation. Some results with an altricial species of fish (*Archocentrus nigrofasciatus*) seem to suggest that when geometric and non-geometric information are set in conflict, rearing experience could affect the relative dominance of featural (landmark) and geometric information [33]. The same effect was not observed in chicks [18], suggesting that experiences might play different roles in the relative reliance of use of geometric and non-geometric information in altricial and precocial species, though this will require confirmation through more species comparisons.

Numerical cognition in chicks is also apparent early in development and parallels closely that observed in human infants. For example, in small identical object arrays, infants represent the total continuous extent of the visual array rather than its numerosity [34] or, according to some authors, both continuous extent and numerosity [35]. However, objects with contrasting sets of properties provoke infants to respond to the number of objects rather than to their continuous extent [36]. Similarly, newborn chicks have been tested for their sensitivity to number *vs* continuous extent of artificial objects that they had been reared with soon after hatching [37]. When the objects were similar, chicks chose the set of objects of larger numerosity, irrespective of the number of objects they had been reared with. However, when chicks were reared with objects that differed in their aspect (color, size, and shape) and then tested with completely novel objects (but controlled for continuous extent), they chose to associate with a set of objects comprising the same number of elements they had been reared with during imprinting. Early availability of small numerosity discrimination by chicks suggests that these abilities are in place at birth [38]. Even basic arithmetic seems available in very young chicks [39], which are capable of computing exact addition and subtraction on small numbers of social partners, with no previous experience of appearance and disappearance of such objects (Fig. 13.1). Finally, a disposition to map the numerical number line from left to right, possibly as a result of left visual hemifield (right hemisphere) dominance [40], has been reported [37]. Hence the disposition to map number and space is apparent very early in development in these precocial species.

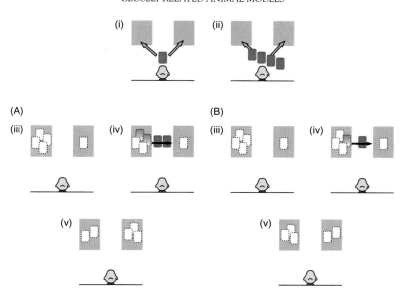

FIGURE 13.1 Newly hatched domestic chicks were imprinted on five identical objects and then one ball was hidden behind one screen (i) and four balls were hidden—one by one—behind the other screen (ii). The sequence of events and the directions were randomized between trials. At the end of the first displacement event, therefore, either four or one ball(s) were hidden behind each screen (iii). At this point, in condition (A) two balls moved—one by one—from the screen hiding four to the one hiding a single ball (iv). At test (v) chicks approached the larger number of imprinting balls, even though it was not behind the screen where the larger number of balls had initially disappeared. In condition (B), only one ball moved from the screen hiding four to the one hiding a single ball (iv). At test (v) chicks rejoined the larger number of imprinting balls, which was not behind the screen where the final hiding of balls had been observed.

WHAT IS THE EVOLUTIONARY ENDOWMENT OF HUMAN COGNITION?

Inherited cognitive capacities and preferences are not necessarily present at birth, but may emerge only later in ontogeny. Children might be inherently prepared to acquire an ability or preference over time [41]. We here refer to the question of whether any variance found in a late-blooming human cognitive capacity is due to species-typical genetic variance [42]. For example, capacities for relational thought [43], false belief reasoning [44] and the ability to think about the past and imagine the future [45] do not fully develop before roughly four years of age. While these sophisticated capacities are not present at birth, there is no *a priori* reason to exclude the possibility that heritable factors construct childrens' abilities in these late-blooming cognitive domains. Since they develop later in life, neither data from human infants nor precocial species will shed light on the nature of these inherited predispositions.

CLOSELY RELATED ANIMAL MODELS

Taxonomically informed cross-species comparisons within our immediate primate family, the great apes, offer a way to investigate the evolutionary history of late-blooming human

BOX 13.1

PHYLOGENETIC COMPARATIVE METHODS

Controlling for Evolutionary Relatedness

Analysing diversity in cognitive ability across species requires methods that control for the hierarchical relatedness of organisms through the branching process of descent [88]. Standard statistical tests on non-independent species data will overestimate the degrees of freedom available and increase the risk of Type I error. Evolutionary biologists have, therefore, developed a range of computational methods to (a) build trees (phylogenies) that describe species relationships, and (b) track the evolution of traits on those phylogenies [89,90] PCMs). Trees are usually inferred from gene sequence data, but morphological [91] and behavioral [92] data can also be used. Given a phylogenetic hypothesis about historical relatedness and the variable distribution of a trait at the tree "tips", we can use statistical approaches to infer the nature and likelihood of the underlying evolutionary processes.

Reconstructing Ancestral States

The present can reveal the past: PCMs can be used to reconstruct the ancestral state of a trait (behavioral, cognitive, morphological, even cultural) for the nodes (common ancestors) in a phylogeny that describes the history of a group of species. This "virtual

archaeology" process allows us to establish the directionality of trait change, to test models of evolution, and to incorporate independent information, such as fossil data, in hypothesis-testing. Methods use the data at the tips of the trees, a tree or set of trees, and some optimality approach or model of evolution. Different methods offer a range of approaches, from basic to highly sophisticated, and are implemented in a range of software packages [93].

Other Questions and Applications

Both practically and principally, many evolutionary questions can only be addressed in a phylogenetic framework [94,95]: the inference of ancestral states, calculating rates of evolution, assessing the degree of phylogenetic signal in the data, and examining the mode of evolutionary change (e.g., punctual *vs* gradual). Standard regression models can be used to analyze adaptive change and correlated evolution but only after similarity due to shared ancestry is accounted for. For comparative psychology, these methods offer great potential, as they can also be used to study intra-species variation. Within humans, ethnolinguistic groups are population entities for cultural and linguistic evolution [96,97], and phylogenetic methods have also been used to study chimpanzee cultural diversity [98].

cognitive skills. For this purpose, "heritable" cognitive characteristics should be seen as part of the evolutionary endowment of the species, that is, inherited from a last common ancestor (LCA) through descent with modification of a set of reliably reoccurring developmental resources [42]. In evolutionary biology, cross-species comparisons and historical reconstruction employ a set of statistical techniques called phylogenetic comparative methods (PCM). Amongst other possibilities (see Box 13.1) these methods allow us to reconstruct probable ancestral states of shared, but variable, cognitive traits [46–50] (Fig. 13.2).

(A) Categorical data, parsimony model, branch lengths arbitrary

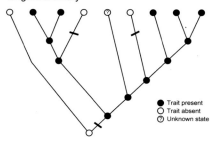

FIGURE 13.2 Ancestral states can be inferred with the combination of species data and a phylogenetic tree. The particular PCM that is used makes a difference to inferences about convergent and homologous evolution, shown in the first two trees. The same set of data and species relationships are shown. Black dots represent presence of a cognitive ability, white is absence, ? is unknown. (A) An intuitive "eyeballing" approach similar to parsimony reconstruction minimizes the number of evolutionary changes [47]. The trait is gained once and lost twice (changes = black bars), and the species can be inferred to share the trait as a result of descent (homology). (B) The same data and phylogeny, this time using a likelihood model where rates of gain and loss are different and change is proportional to branch length. Ancestral nodes show very different reconstructions (and uncertainty) compared to (A). In this case, the trait may be as a result of convergent evolution in the two bracketed groups. (C) Continuous data reconstructions for a morphological trait, e.g., limb length. A large number of equally probable solutions are summarized by the distributions. Narrow curves represent certainty, while flatter curves show there is ambiguity. The gray node is compared to fossil evidence; the fossil falls within the reconstruction distribution.

(B) Categorical data, likelihood model, branch lengths proportional

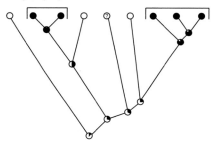

(C) Continuous data, likelihood model

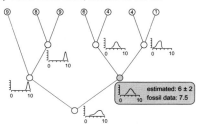

The power of phylogenetic inference depends on sample size (the number of species) and the completeness of the tested family of species. For humans, a complete set of species with a single common ancestor that, in turn, is not ancestral to any other species is the great ape clade: orangutans (*Pongo pygmaeus*), gorillas (*Gorilla gorilla*), bonobos (*Pan paniscus*), chimpanzees (*Pan troglodytes*) and humans (*Homo sapiens*) (Fig. 13.3). Widespread samples of distantly related species, as they are often used in comparative analysis [47], are not always desirable—including, for example, just one of the 15 lesser apes (*Gibbon* species [51]) will increase the sample by 1 but disproportionately violate completeness requirements (5/5 great apes *vs* 6/20 apes). Sample validity is also important. Since testing many highly endangered species is a major investment in resources, time, and effort, compromises are necessary. Recent studies have attempted to increase sample validity by testing fewer species but

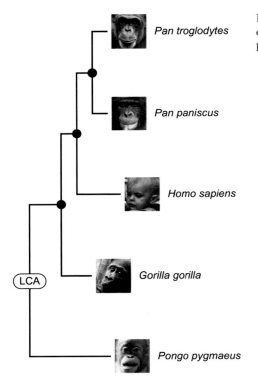

FIGURE 13.3   Consensus phylogeny of the great apes based on results from the 10k Tree Project [100]. Branch lengths are proportional to the amount of genetic change.

increasing the number of individuals [52] or by sampling small numbers from multiple populations [48]. In this section we review studies that use matched methods for comparing cognition across all great apes (for reviews of cognition of space, time, and number in individual primate species, see [53]).

A recent study showed that all five great ape species share the ability to track the invisible displacement of hidden objects in space, but at varying levels of proficiency [54]. This kind of variation allows us to apply phylogenetic comparative methods to infer the performance levels of the LCA of all great apes: the ability to track invisible displacements above chance level appears to be part of the evolutionary inheritance in all extant great apes. All great apes were also highly successful at tracking object displacements during visible rotations of a surface platform. When the rotation was invisible, i.e. participants had to rely on feature cues of either the cups or the surface to infer the hidden movement, only human children above five years of age, but not younger children and no other great apes, succeeded [55]. Thus, while object tracking during rotation is a shared great ape ability, the ability to infer invisible rotations based on feature cues of either objects or the supporting surface appears to be, at least amongst great apes, particularly pronounced in humans. Another cognitive domain in which humans have been claimed to be especially skilled is the domain of spatial relational reasoning [43,56]. All five great ape species are highly skilled when judging relations based on simple spatial rules such as alignment and proximity. However, only children above four years of age, bonobos, and chimpanzees display some mastery of reasoning by more abstract spatial–relational similarity, such as two objects being the right-most object in their respective arrays [48]. Mapped against their phylogenetic relationships, great ape skills in the proximity-reasoning task appear to change gradually through evolutionary history, but there appears to be a greater increase in the preference for abstract relations between the LCA of gorillas, chimpanzees and humans than in other branches on the tree. Given more data across a greater range of species, we shall be able to statistically determine where there are unusual "punctuational" events in the evolution of cognitive capacities and preferences [57] (Fig. 13.2A).

Tests that compare cognitive abilities across several species may suffer from the problem of unfair comparisons. Differences in ability could be dismissed by claims that experiments are simply not well-adapted to suit all species equally [58]. These problems can in part be alleviated by carefully designed studies that assess performance in a test condition relative to an established control condition which all species have passed [59]. In addition, researchers can compare relative performance in the preferences amongst multiple solutions to the same task across species [49]. For example, all but one species (bonobos were indifferent) demonstrated a clear preference for a place-based over a feature-based memory strategy [49] in an object displacement task. Based on a phylogenetic interpretation, we can infer a preference for space cues over feature cues in the LCA. Here it is important to note that "inherited" does not imply "inflexible": great apes are, irrespective of their shared preference, able to apply feature cues successfully under different task constraints [60]. Furthermore, the preference is likely reversed in human children between one and three years of age [49]. Similarly all great apes displayed common preferences when processing spatial relations. All great ape species, including four-year-old human children, displayed a preference for processing spatial relations using allocentric environmental cues over view-dependent egocentric cues [50]. Similar to the preference for place over feature, this preference for allocentric processing can then be inferred as part of our heritage as great apes. Inherited does not imply invariant, however: this allocentric preference not only changes across ontogeny but also depends on the cultural context in which children grow up [50].

A similar phylogenetic perspective can be taken for other domains such as cognition of number or time. Basic performance characteristics in quantity discrimination tasks are shared across animal taxa [61] including great apes [52,62]. All tested great apes can select the larger of two quantities by approximation, both when presented simultaneously and in sequence, even when the quantities are large and the numerical distance between them is small [62]. Similar performance levels have been reported for human children from roughly six years of age onwards [63], indicating a common heritage of the proximate number system [64]. Other numerical skills such as the ability to order sets of quantities (ordinal skills) [65] may evolve in tandem with quantity discrimination (cardinal skills), or they may have independent evolutionary histories: applying PCMs to a carefully selected array of species would provide insight into the interdependence of these cognitive features (see Box 13.1). Similar questions may be asked in the cognitive domain of time. Although very little great ape research exists, it has been shown that while monkeys (rhesus macaques) failed to remember the "when" component of an event, chimpanzees, bonobos (and arguably, orangutans) remembered when an event took place [66]. Further tests with gorillas and orangutans will be needed to confirm these results and thus allow investigation of the evolutionary history of time-related cognitive abilities.

WHICH COGNITIVE ABILITIES ARE UNIQUELY HUMAN?

Not all cognitive traits that are shared between species are the outcome of common evolutionary history; similarities in cognitive abilities and biases may emerge independently in distantly related species (Fig. 13.2B). These cases of *convergent evolution* place human cognitive skills in their evolutionary context within the animal kingdom: distantly related animal models can tell us whether complex cognitive abilities arose only once, thus producing outcomes that are shared only by descendants of a common ancestor (homologous traits), or whether these outcomes emerge independently through convergent evolution in distantly related taxa that have similar problems to solve. Cases of convergent evolution also allow us to identify similar evolutionary pressures, thus enabling the discovery of the proximate mechanisms that produce complex equifinal outcomes in two or more lineages [67]. PCMs can arbitrate if convergent or homologous evolution is more likely for particular traits (Fig. 13.2B), and coevolutionary methods can test hypotheses about the relevant selective pressures acting on cognitive evolution [68].

DISTANTLY RELATED ANIMAL MODELS

Mental time travel enables an individual to travel back in the mind's eye to recall previous events (episodic memory) and to travel forwards in the mind's eye to imagine future needs (episodic prospection). Many have assumed that this ability is unique to humans [45,69], particularly when episodic memory and future planning are defined in terms of the conscious experience of recollecting past events and imagining or pre-experiencing future events.

However, this is a highly controversial topic (most recently [70,71]). The absence of any agreed behavioral markers of conscious experience [72] presents an insurmountable barrier to demonstrating such cognitive skills in animal models; for how could we ever know if a nonhuman animal has a sense of self that it can project to another time [70,71]? Over the past 12 years, however, a suite of studies on birds and mammals, challenge the assumption that mental time travel is unique to humans by focusing on strictly observable behavioral criteria. Tulving's original definition of episodic memory in nonhuman animals identified episodic recall as the retrieval of information about three things: *where* a unique event took place, *what* occurred during the episode, and *when* the episode happened [73]. The advantage of this definition is that the simultaneous retrieval and integration of such tripartite information may be demonstrated behaviorally in animals. Later, the term "episodic-like memory" was coined to refer to this ability [74]. While at least some great ape species could be shown to pass tests of what-when-where memory [66] other primates which are more distantly related to humans failed to remember the "when" component of past episodes [75]. This pattern might be taken to indicate a recent change in homologous evolution within the primate family. However the finding that some species of food-caching birds pass the same criteria additionally suggests an interesting case of convergent evolutionary history [74,76].

There are good functional reasons for believing that food-caching birds would need to rely on specific past experiences about what happened where and when. Food-caching birds hide perishable caches as well as non-perishable ones so there would be much selective advantage in them remembering what they had cached, where, and when. A series of controlled experiments have demonstrated that western scrub-jays (*Aphelocoma californica*) do remember what types of food caches they hid, in which spatial locations, and how long ago [74]. Moreover, the birds form integrated memories about "what happened, where, and when" rather than encoding each of these three pieces of information separately [77].

Other researchers have argued about this definition, however. Eacott and colleagues, for example, have proposed that the "when" component simply serves as an occasion setter to identify episodic memories that occurred in different contexts, of which time is only one. Consequently they have argued that a better criterion for epsiodic-like memory is "what-where-which" rather than "what-where-when" because the "when" component is only one of a number of possible contexts or occasion setters [78]. Others, such as Zentall and colleagues [79], have argued that epsiodic recall happens automatically. In other words, at the time of encoding the information in an episodic memory, the subject does not normally know what information will need to be recalled at a later date. Zentall and colleagues give the example of what you ate for breakfast this morning. If you expect to be asked the question, you can encode an answer when you eat breakfast; and therefore when the expected question is asked, you only need to remember the prepared answer as opposed to having to recall the event itself, whereas if the question is unexpected you must cast your mind back to breakfast time in order to episodically recall the necessary information [79].

Similar to the case of episodic memory, it is possible to use behavioral criteria for the existence of forethought, but exactly what constitutes evidence for future planning is much debated. It is generally agreed that mental time travel into the future must be distinguished from other prospectively oriented but non-cognitive behaviors (such as those triggered by a seasonal cue). Three criteria are important: first, the behavior must be shown to be sensitive to consequences and the animals can, therefore, learn to adjust their responses appropriately, for example avoiding to cache in sites that are known to be subject to pilferage. Secondly, the behaviors must be oriented towards a future goal, independent of current goals. Finally, the behavior should involve true forethought, as opposed to instrumental conditioning in which the anticipatory act has previously been rewarded.

Although some primates [80,81] and corvids [82] take actions in the present based on their future consequences, these studies have not demonstrated reference to future motivational states independent of current ones [76], or without extensive reinforcement of the anticipatory act [83]. Here too studies of western scrub-jays have provided the key empirical work, capitalizing on the fact that food caching is prospective—the only benefit of caching now is in order to eat the food in the future. When given a novel opportunity to cache, the birds preferentially cached food in a room in which they were not given that food for breakfast relative to a food that they had received for breakfast in that room, when given these foods the evening before. It is important to note that the behavior is both a novel action (i.e. that no associative learning can have occurred) and is appropriate to a motivational state other than the one the animal is in at that moment. This then meets the requirements for future planning. One might argue that the jays simply cache according to a general heuristic to balance food sources, but this does not exclude the possibility that the cognitive processes that allow them to implement this heuristic involve some form of foresight [84].

Furthermore, studies have shown that when given two foods, A and B, the birds would cache more of food A relative to food B even if they are satiated on food A at the time of caching, once they have learned that when they get an opportunity to recover their caches

BOX 13.2

QUESTIONS FOR FUTURE RESEARCH

- Across vertebrate species, what specific aspects of knowledge of number, space and time are available at birth in the absence of specific experiences? What neural mechanisms are responsible for their operation?
- What are the evolutionary constraints on cognition from a biological point of view? To what extent do differences in neuroarchitecture impact upon the apparent functional similarities in behavior across distantly related species such as apes and crows?

- How can we use PCMs to identify sets of species to maximize the power of comparisons across small sets of species [99]?
- What experimental paradigms are appropriate for comparisons across a wider range of taxa?
- Do specific cognitive abilities arise in different ecological or social contexts and can PCMs be used for coevolutionary modeling?

they will be satiated on food B. This suggests that their caching decisions are motivated by what the birds want to eat at recovery rather than at caching [76]. These studies suggest that scrub-jays have the ability to take actions for the future, although it is far from clear whether they do so by mental time travel into the future.

Nonetheless, these studies suggest that some animals have the ability to take specific actions for the future. Recent work on nonhuman apes is substantiating this claim by showing that they can also take actions for future motivational needs [85,86]. At issue is whether these abilities are widely spread among the animal kingdom, or whether they are exclusive to corvids and apes, and thus a product of a rare convergent evolution and if so, what are the selective processes that were common to both corvids and apes and yet exclusive to them. Clearly more comparative studies across a greater range of species will be required to answer these types of questions (Box 13.2). Further work may also untangle the similarities and differences in the proximate mechanisms, given such intriguing similarities in cognition, yet divergence in the brain architecture. The bird brain has a very different structure to that of humans and all other mammals, bereft as it is of the six-layered structure of our neocortex, which has long been thought to provide the unique machinery for cognition [87].

CONCLUDING REMARKS

The careful selection of animal models provides exciting, novel perspectives on the development and evolution of human cognitive structure. We have reviewed evidence here from spatial, temporal and numerical cognition, all three of which are foundational cognitive domains ensuring basic vertebrate experience. In these domains, precocial animals can demonstrate how functional and complex cognition can be in place at birth without further specific experiential input. Taxonomically informed comparisons across related species allow us to identify the role of phylogeny in cognitive abilities and preferences. Finally, distantly related animal models often challenge what we might think are traits unique to our own species. Cases of convergent evolution invite us to identify equivalent evolutionary pressures, thus enabling the discovery of the proximate mechanisms that produce complex equifinal outcomes in two or more lineages. Cross-species comparative research, therefore, enables cognitive science go beyond the standard investigative toolbox and answer salient questions about the origins of the human mind and its capabilities.

GLOSSARY

Altricial

Species in which the young are relatively immobile after birth or hatching and must be cared for by adults.

Convergent Evolution

A process where similar characteristics evolve in unrelated groups of organisms, also called analogy.

Heritability (Narrow Sense)

Degree to which the individual phenotypes are determined by the additive effects of genes transmitted from the parents; mathematically it is expressed as the ratio of the additive genetic variance to the total phenotypic variance.

Homology/Homologous Evolution

Similar characteristics that are shared by groups of organisms due to descent from a common ancestor.

Model Organism

Species that are extensively studied with the expectation that conclusions drawn on the basis of the model species can be relevant to other organisms.

Phylogeny

The evolutionary history of a group of organisms or populations, usually described by a tree structure showing the hierarchy of relatedness between groups.

Phylogenetics

The modern field of evolutionary biology; uses a broad range of computational methods to construct trees and networks of how groups of organisms are related and how their characteristics evolve.

Precocial

Species in which the young are relatively mature and mobile soon after birth or hatching.

Taxa

A named population sharing similar characteristics, e.g., a species (singular: taxon).

References

[1] S.J. Shettleworth, Cognition, Evolution, and Behaviour, Oxford University Press (2010).

[2] L. Tommasi et al., Cognitive Biology, MIT Press, 2009.

[3] E.S. Spelke, K.D. Kinzler, Innateness, Learning, and Rationality, Child Dev. Perspect. 3 (2009) 96–98.

[4] E.J. Gibson, R.D. Walk, The "visual cliff", Sci. Am. 202 (1960) 64–71.

[5] E.S. Spelke, K.D. Kinzler, Core knowledge, Dev. Sci. 10 (2007) 89–96.

[6] G. Vallortigara et al., Visually inexperienced chicks exhibit spontaneous preference for biological motion patterns, PLoS Biol. 3 (2005) e208.

[7] E. Mascalzoni et al., Innate sensitivity for self-propelled causal agency in newly hatched chicks, Proc. Natl. Acad. Sci. U.S.A. 107 (2010) 4483–4485.

[8] G. Vallortigara, The Cognitive Chicken: Visual and Spatial Cognition in a Non-Mammalian Brain, in: E.A. Wasserman, T.R. Zentall, (Eds.), Comparative Cognition: Experimental Explorations of Animal Intelligence, Oxford University Press. (2006).

[9] G. Vallortigara, L. Regolin, Gravity bias in the interpretation of biological motion by inexperienced chicks, Curr. Biol. 16 (2006) R279–R280.

[10] A. Klin et al., Two-year-olds with autism orient to non-social contingencies rather than biological motion, Nature 459 (2009) 257–261.

[11] F. Simion et al., A predisposition for biological motion in the newborn baby, Proc. Natl. Acad. Sci. U.S.A. 105 (2008) 809–813.

[12] E.D. Jarvis et al., Avian brains and a new understanding of vertebrate brain evolution, Nat. Rev. Neurosci. 6 (2005) 151–159.

[13] K. Cheng, N.S. Newcombe, Is there a geometric module for spatial orientation? Squaring theory and evidence, Psychon. Bull. Rev. 12 (2005) 1–23.

[14] G. Vallortigara, Animals as natural geometers, in: L. Tommasi, et al. (Ed.), Cognitive Biology, MIT Press. (2009).

[15] S.A. Lee, E.S. Spelke, A modular geometric mechanism for reorientation in children, Cogn. Psychol. 61 (2010) 152–176.

[16] N.S. Newcombe, K.R. Ratliff, Explaining the development of spatial reorientation: Modularity-plus-language versus the emergence of adaptive combination, in: J. Plumert, J. Spencer, (Eds.), The Emerging Spatial Mind, Oxford University Press. (2007).

[17] K. Cheng, Whither geometry? Troubles of the geometric module, Trends Cogn. Sci. 12 (2008) 355–361.

[18] C. Chiandetti, G. Vallortigara, Experience and geometry: controlled-rearing studies with chicks, Anim. Cogn. 13 (2010) 463–470.

[19] M. Nardini et al., A viewpoint-independent process for spatial reorientation, Cognition 112 (2009) 241–248.

[20] T. Pecchia, G. Vallortigara, Reorienting strategies in a rectangular array of landmarks by domestic chicks (Gallus gallus), J. Comp. Psychol. 124 (2010) 147–158.

[21] A. Wystrach, G. Beugnon, Ants learn geometry and features, Curr. Biol. 19 (2009) 61–66.

[22] L. Lakusta et al., Impaired geometric reorientation caused by genetic defect, Proc. Natl. Acad. Sci. U.S.A. 107 (2010) 2813–2817.

[23] C.F. Doeller et al., Parallel striatal and hippocampal systems for landmarks and boundaries in spatial memory, Proc. Natl. Acad. Sci. U.S.A. 105 (2008) 5915–5920.

[24] T. Solstad et al., Representation of geometric borders in the entorhinal cortex, Science 322 (2008) 1865–1868.

[25] C. Chiandetti, G. Vallortigara, Is there an innate geometric module? Effects of experience with angular geometric cues on spatial re-orientation based on the shape of the environment, Anim. Cogn. 11 (2008) 139–146.

[26] R.F. Langston et al., Development of the spatial representation system in the rat, Science 328 (2010) 1576–1580.

[27] T.J. Wills et al., Development of the hippocampal cognitive map in preweanling rats, Science 328 (2010) 1573–1576.

[28] L. Regolin, G. Vallortigara, Perception of partly occluded objects by young chicks, Percept. Psychophys. 57 (1995) 971–976.

[29] P.J. Kellman, M.E. Arterberry, The Cradle of Knowledge, MIT Press, 1998.

[30] E. Valenza et al., Perceptual completion in newborn human infants, Child Dev. 77 (2006) 1810–1821.

[31] G. Vallortigara et al., Doing Socrates experiment right: controlled rearing studies of geometrical knowledge in animals, Curr. Opin. Neurobiol. 19 (2009) 20–26.

[32] J.E. Pyers, et al. Evidence from an emerging sign language reveals that language supports spatial cognition. Proc. Natl. Acad. Sci. U.S.A. 107, 12116–12120

[33] A.A. Brown et al., Growing in circles: rearing environment alters spatial navigation in fish, Psychol. Sci. 18 (2007) 569–573.

[34] L. Feigenson et al., Infants' discrimination of number vs. continuous extent, Cogn. Psychol. 44 (2002) 33–66.

[35] S. Cordes, E.M. Brannon, The relative salience of discrete and continuous quantity in young infants, Dev. Sci. 12 (2009) 453–463.

[36] L. Feigenson, A double-dissociation in infants' representations of object arrays, Cognition 95 (2005) B37–B48.

[37] R. Rugani et al., Is it only humans that count from left to right? Biol. Lett. 6 (2010) 290–292.

[38] R. Rugani et al., Discrimination of small numerosities in young chicks, J Exp. Psychol. Anim. Behav. Process 34 (2008) 388–399.

[39] R. Rugani et al., Arithmetic in newborn chicks, Proc. Biol. Sci. 276 (2009) 2451–2460.

[40] B. Diekamp et al., A left-sided visuospatial bias in birds, Curr. Biol. 15 (2005) R372–R373.

[41] A. Karmiloff-Smith, Beyond Modularity: A Developmental Perspective on Cognitive Science, The MIT Press, 1992.

[42] M. Mameli, P. Bateson, Innateness and the sciences, Biol. Philos. 21 (2006) 155–188.

[43] D. Gentner, Why We're So Smart, in: D. Gentner, S. Goldin-Meadow, (Eds.), Language in Mind: Advances in Study of Language and Thought, The MIT Press, pp. 195–235.

[44] H.M. Wellman et al., Meta-analysis of theory-of-mind development: The truth about false belief, Child Dev. 72 (2001) 655–684.

[45] E. Tulving, Episodic memory: from mind to brain, Annu. Rev. Psychol. 53 (2002) 1–25.

[46] R.W. Byrne, The Thinking Ape: Evolutionary Origins of Intelligence, Oxford University Press, 1995.

[47] W.T. Fitch et al., Social cognition and the evolution of language: constructing cognitive phylogenies, Neuron 65 (2010) 795–814.

[48] D.B.M. Haun, J. Call, Great apes' capacities to recognize relational similarity, Cognition 110 (2009) 147–159.

[49] D.B.M. Haun et al., Evolutionary psychology of spatial representations in the hominidae, Curr. Biol. 16 (2006) 1736–1740.

[50] D.B.M. Haun et al., Cognitive cladistics and cultural override in Hominid spatial cognition, Proc. Natl. Acad. Sci. U.S.A. 103 (2006) 17568–17573.

[51] C.P. Groves, Primate Taxonomy, Smithsonian Institution Press, 2001.

[52] E. Herrmann et al., Humans have evolved specialized skills of social cognition: The cultural intelligence hypothesis, Science 317 (2007) 1360–1366.

[53] A. Seed, M. Tomasello, Primate Cognition, Topics Cogn. Sci. 2 (2010) 407–419.

[54] J. Barth, J. Call, Tracking the displacement of objects: A series of tasks with great apes (*Pan troglodytes*, *Pan paniscus*, *Gorilla gorilla*, and *Pongo pygmaeus*) and young children (*Homo sapiens*), J. Exp. Psychol. Anim. B 32 (2006) 239–252.

[55] S. Okamoto-Barth, J. Call, Tracking and inferring spatial rotation by children and great apes, Dev. Psychol. 44 (2008) 1396–1408.

[56] D.C. Penn et al., Darwin's mistake: explaining the discontinuity between human and nonhuman minds, Behav. Brain Sci. 31 (2008) 109–130.

[57] M. Pagel, Inferring the historical patterns of biological evolution, Nature 401 (1999) 877–884.

[58] C. Boesch, What makes us human (*Homo sapiens*)? The challenge of cognitive cross-species comparison, J. Comp. Psychol. 121 (2007) 227–240.

[59] M. Tomasello, J. Call, Assessing the validity of ape–human comparisons: a reply to Boesch (2007), J. Comp. Psychol. 122 (2008) 449–452.

[60] P. Kanngiesser, J. Call, Bonobos, chimpanzees, gorillas, and orang utans use feature and spatial cues in two spatial memory tasks, Anim. Cogn. 13 (2010) 419–430.

[61] J.F. Cantlon et al., Beyond the number domain, Trends Cogn. Sci. 13 (2009) 83–91.

[62] D. Hanus, J. Call, Discrete Quantity Judgments in the Great Apes (*Pan paniscus*, *Pan troglodytes*, *Gorilla gorilla*, *Pongo pygmaeus*): The Effect of Presenting Whole Sets Versus Item-by-Item, J. Comp. Psychol. 123 (2007) 227–240.

[63] J. Halberda, L. Feigenson, Developmental change in the acuity of the "Number Sense": The approximate number System in 3-, 4-, 5-, and 6-year-olds and adults, Dev. Psychol. 44 (2008) 1457–1465.

[64] L. Feigenson et al., Core systems of number, Trends Cogn. Sci. 8 (2004) 307–314.

[65] E.M. Brannon, H.S. Terrace, Ordering of the numerosities 1 to 9 by monkeys, Science 282 (1998) 746–749.

[66] G. Martin-Ordas et al., Keeping track of time: evidence for episodic-like memory in great apes, Anim. Cogn. 13 (2010) 331–340.

[67] A. Seed et al., Intelligence in corvids and apes: a case of convergent evolution?, Ethology 115 (2009) 401–420.

[68] B. Hare, M. Tomasello, Human-like social skills in dogs? Trends Cogn. Sci. 9 (2005) 439–444.
[69] T. Suddendorf, M.C. Corballis, Mental time travel and the evolution of the human mind, Genet. Soc. Gen. Psychol. Monogr. 123 (1997) 133–167.
[70] W.A. Roberts, M.C. Feeney, The comparative study of mental time travel, Trends Cogn. Sci. 13 (2009) 271–277.
[71] Suddendorf, T., and Corballis, M.C. Behavioural evidence for mental time travel in nonhuman animals. Behav. Brain Res. 215 (2010) 292–298.
[72] D. Griffiths et al., Episodic memory: what can animals remember about their past? Trends Cogn. Sci. 3 (1999) 74–80.
[73] E. Tulving, Episodic and semantic memory, in: E. Tulving, W. Donaldson, (Eds.), Organisation of Memory, Academic Press, 1972, pp. 381–403.
[74] N.S. Clayton, A. Dickinson, Episodic-like memory during cache recovery by scrub jays, Nature 395 (1998) 272–274.
[75] R.R. Hampton et al., Rhesus monkeys (*Macaca mulatta*) demonstrate robust memory for what and where, but not for when, in an open-field test of memory, Learn Motiv. 36 (2005) 245–259.
[76] S.P. Correia et al., Western scrub-jays anticipate future needs independently of their current motivational state, Curr. Biol. 17 (2007) 856–861.
[77] N.S. Clayton et al., Can animals recall the past and plan for the future? Nat. Rev. Neurosci. 4 (2003) 685–691.
[78] M.J. Eacott, G. Norman, Integrated memory for object, place, and context in rats: a possible model of episodic-like memory? J. Neurosci. 24 (2004) 1948–1953.
[79] T.R. Zentall et al., Episodic-like memory: pigeons can report location pecked when unexpectedly asked, Behav. Processes 79 (2008) 93–98.
[80] N.J. Mulcahy, J. Call, Apes save tools for future use, Science 312 (2006) 1038–1040.
[81] M. Naqshbandi, W.A. Roberts, Anticipation of future events in squirrel monkeys (*Saimiri sciureus*) and rats (*Rattus norvegicus*): tests of the Bischof–Kohler hypothesis, J. Comp. Psychol. 120 (2006) 345–357.
[82] S.R. de Kort et al., The control of food-caching behavior by Western scrub-jays (*Aphelocoma californica*), J. Exp. Psychol. Anim. Behav. Process 33 (2007) 361–370.
[83] C.R. Raby et al., Planning for the future by western scrub-jays, Nature 445 (2007) 919–921.
[84] C.R. Raby, N.S. Clayton, Prospective cognition in animals, Behav. Processes 80 (2009) 314–324.
[85] M. Osvath, Spontaneous planning for future stone throwing by a male chimpanzee, Curr. Biol. 19 (2009) R190–R191.
[86] M. Osvath, H. Osvath, Chimpanzee (*Pan troglodytes*) and orangutan (*Pongo abelii*) forethought: self-control and pre-experience in the face of future tool use, Anim. Cogn. 11 (2008) 661–674.
[87] N.J. Emery, N.S. Clayton, The mentality of crows: convergent evolution of intelligence in corvids and apes, Science 306 (2004) 1903–1907.
[88] P.H. Harvey, M.D. Pagel, The Comparative Method in Evolutionary Biology, Oxford University Press, 1991.
[89] J. Felsenstein, Inferring Phylogenies, Sinauer Assoc, 2004.
[90] P. Lemey et al., (Ed.), The Phylogenetic Handbook: A Practical Approach to Phylogenetic Analysis and Hypothesis Testing, Cambridge University Press, 2004.
[91] J.J. Wiens, (Ed.), Phylogenetic Analysis of Morphological Data, Smithsonian Institution Press, 2000.
[92] M. Kennedy et al., Hop, step and gape: Do the social displays of the Pelecaniformes reflect phylogeny? Anim. Behav. 51 (1996) 273–291.
[93] Nunn, C.L. (in press) The Comparative Approach in Evolutionary Anthropology. University of Chicago Press.
[94] I. Capellini et al., Does sleep play a role in memory consolidation? A comparative test, PLoS One 4 (2009) e4609.
[95] S.M. Reader, K.N. Laland, Social intelligence, innovation, and enhanced brain size in primates, Proc. Natl. Acad. Sci. U.S.A. 99 (2002) 4436–4441.
[96] R. Mace, C.J. Holden, A phylogenetic approach to cultural evolution, Trends Ecol. Evol. 20 (2005) 116–121.
[97] M. Pagel, Human language as a culturally transmitted replicator, Nat. Rev. Genet. 10 (2009) 405–415.
[98] S.J. Lycett et al., Cladistic analyses of behavioural variation in wild *Pan troglodytes*: exploring the chimpanzee culture hypothesis, J. Hum. Evo. 57 (2009) 337–349.
[99] Arnold, C., and Nunn, C.L. Phylogenetic targeting of research effort in evolutionary biology. Am. Natural. 176 (2010) 601–12.
[100] Arnold, C., et al. (in press) The 10kTrees website: a new online resource for primate phylogeny. Evo. Anthrop.

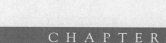

14

Evolutionary Foundations of the Approximate Number System

Elizabeth M. Brannon[*][†], *Dustin J. Merritt*[†]

[*]Department of Psychology and Neuroscience, Duke University, Durham,
USA; [†]Center for Cognitive Neuroscience, Duke University, Durham, USA

Summary

This chapter reviews the behavioral evidence for numerical capacities in animals. We show that animal number representations are ratio dependent, subject to the same numerical illusions as humans, illict semantic congruity effects, map across sensory modalities, enter into arithmetic computations, and support a precursor to the zero concept. The review illustrates that nonhuman animals share with humans a basic capacity to quantify the world around them that likely serves as a foundation for the rich and uniquely human mathematical mind.

Numbers and mathematics allow humans to build models that predict the timing and direction of the spread of oil from the 2010 BP oil disaster in the Gulf of Mexico, to calculate the cost of an international meeting in the south of France, and to build a sail boat and navigate around the world. No nonhuman animal is capable of any of these accomplishments. Where did these uniquely human cognitive capacities come from? Is the ability to store and manipulate numerical representations the exclusive domain of language-competent humans? Or, might we expect to see some of the building blocks and evolutionary antecedents of these abilities in animals?

In the last few decades, a wealth of data has emerged suggesting that dozens of animal species are capable of representing number and that they may even spontaneously attend to numerical cues in their natural environments (see Box 14.1). Although early research was fraught with issues of stimulus control and experimenter cueing, more recent work has made great efforts to eliminate these confounds.

© 2011 Elsevier Inc. All rights reserved.

BOX 14.1

UTILITY OF NUMBER

Why might a nonhuman animal need to represent number? Several studies examining animals in naturalistic settings suggest that representing number may enhance an animal's ability to survive and compete for resources. For example, mosquito fish join the numerically larger shoal to avoid predation and recent experimental studies show that mosquito fish can discriminate number independently of alternative cues, and may use number as a cognitive shortcut (Box 14.1 Fig. 1) [82,83]. Many different animal species may also use numerical representations when deciding how to solve territorial disputes. For example, several studies have shown that animals treat territorial incursions differently depending on the size of the invading group [84–86].

The above examples demonstrate that representing number may be useful. However, in many instances, number is confounded with other variables that may be more salient

or ecologically relevant to the animal. For example, a tree with 10 pieces of fruit will likely have a larger total amount of food than a tree with two pieces of fruit. In this case the amount of food is likely of greater import than the number of food morsels. In fact a prevalent view has been that animals may be capable of attending to number but only as a last resort when other more salient cues are not available [87].

Cantlon and Brannon [88] designed a laboratory task to experimentally ask whether rhesus monkeys use number only as a last-resort strategy. Monkeys were trained on a number match-to-sample task in which the sample and the correct choice could be matched by either number or by another non-numerical dimension such as shape, color, or surface area. For example, on training trials with the color *vs* shape condition, both the sample and correct choice might consist of four brown stars, whereas the incorrect answer might consist of

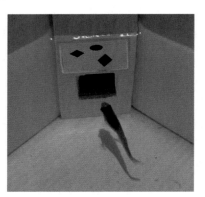

BOX 14.1 FIGURE 1 A mosquito fish was placed in a tank with two exits on opposite sides. Each exit was labeled with a numerical stimulus that contained either two or three items. Half of the fish were trained to choose the exit with 2 items, and the other half were trained to choose the exit with 3 items. Agrillo *et al.* [82] found that when non-numerical cues such as cumulative element surface area, total luminance, overall space occupied by the stimuli, and element size were controlled, the fish could still accurately choose the correct alternative. Photograph courtesy Christian Agrillo, University of Padova.

BOX 14.1 *(cont'd)*

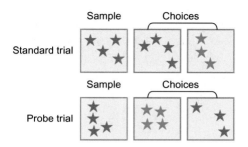

BOX 14.1 FIGURE 2 Example standard and probe trials during the color *vs* numerosity condition. During standard trials, the target matched the sample on both color and numerosity, whereas the distractor differed on both dimensions. Probe trials were non-differentially reinforced with one stimulus matching the sample's numerosity, and the other stimulus matching the sample's color [88].

three green stars (Box 14.1 Fig. 2). The correct answer could be matched either by number (four) or by color (brown). During probe trials, monkeys were given non-differentially reinforced trials where they could only match on one of the two dimensions. Thus, if the sample had four brown hearts, then the choices would contain four green stars and three brown stars. Results indicated that all monkeys were more likely to make a number match than a surface-area match. Monkeys did, however, prefer to match based on color or shape compared to number. Importantly, the monkeys' choices revealed that, in all conditions, they were tracking the numerosity of the sample even though this was not necessary during training. Specifically, the monkeys showed distance effects, whereby the probability that they would make a number match increased with the numerical disparity between the number match and the non-numerical match.

The above studies suggest that numerical representation may be useful to animals in many different ways; and, contrary to the last-resort hypothesis, the ability to represent numerical values may be a very natural component of most animal minds.

In this chapter, we focus on the behavioral evidence that animals represent number independently of other stimulus dimensions. We illustrate the psychophysical signatures of the approximate number system (ANS) shared by nonhuman animals and humans, and the arithmetic operations into which these representations enter. The review illustrates that nonhuman animals share with humans a basic capacity to quantify the world around them that likely serves as a foundation for the uniquely rich human mathematical mind.

SHARED SYSTEMS FOR NUMBER REPRESENTATION

Ratio Dependence

The hallmark of the ANS is that Weber's Law controls discrimination such that the ratio between numerosities determines how easily they are distinguished, e.g., [1–3]. Difficulty in discrimination increases as the ratio between numerosities approaches 1. Thus, the ANS does not support the same precision in discrimination made possible by symbolic number systems. With symbols for number, we can distinguish 342 from 343 as easily as we can distinguish 2 from 3. Without such a symbolic number system, animals are limited to the fuzzy representations supported by the ANS. Consequently, the ANS allows much more rapid and accurate discrimination of 2 from 4 than 32 from 34. Box 14.2 describes two alternative explanations for why discrimination in the ANS follows Weber's Law.

BOX 14.2

LINEAR VS LOGARITHMIC

The fact that animals, adults, and human infants all show evidence of ratio dependence in their number discriminations indicates that the internal representation of number is non-linearly related to objective number in some way. Two proposals have emerged to explain the relationship between objective and subjective number. According to the scalar variance proposal, numerosity is represented on a linear scale and ratio effects emerge because the noise that surrounds each mental magnitude increases in proportion to that magnitude (Box 14.2 Fig. 1, right) [29,89]. According to the logarithmic proposal, numerosity is represented on a logarithmic scale with a constant error variance surrounding each mental magnitude [90,91]. In this case, ratio effects

emerge because mental magnitudes become subjectively compressed as their objective magnitudes increase (Box 14.2 Fig. 1, left). These models differ in terms of how the underlying number scale is represented, but they predict the same behavioral signatures. Although the dominant view in the literature is that the internal number scale is logarithmically spaced Gibbon and Church [92] (see also [93]) argued that to adequately differentiate the logarithmic and linear with scalar variance hypotheses, it is necessary to use a task that required subjects to base their behavior on the difference between two points on a continuum rather than simply ordering or matching numerical values.

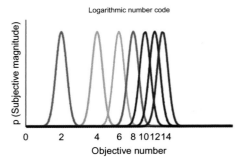 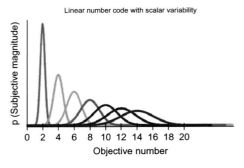

BOX 14.2 FIGURE 1   Two proposals used to explain numerical ratio effects. According to one proposal, subjective magnitudes maintain a constant error variance, and become logarithmically compressed as objective magnitude increases (e.g., [90], left). According to the scalar variance proposal, mental magnitudes are represented linearly with error variance increasing in proportion to the objective magnitude (e.g., [29], right). From [95].

When adult humans are tested in tasks that avoid verbal counting, they too show ratio-dependent number discrimination. In fact, animals and humans tested in parallel tasks often show remarkably similar patterns of performance. As shown in Fig. 14.1, when college students and monkeys were tested in a numerical ordering task, accuracy decreased and reaction time increased as the ratio between the two numerosities approached 1 [1,4]. Similarly, when humans and rats were required to produce a given number of lever or key presses, the number of presses was normally distributed around the target number, with the size of the distribution increasing linearly with the size of the target number [5–7].

Numerical Illusions

Non-verbal number judgments in adult humans are subject to a variety of different illusions such as the size–numerosity illusion [8], regular–random numerosity illusion, and the numerosity adaptation effect [9] (and see Chapter 12 in this volume). While most of these illusions have yet to be systematically explored in nonhuman animals, Beran [10] recently demonstrated that monkeys show the regular–random numerosity illusion (RRNI), and overestimate homogeneous numerical arrays that appear in regular arrangements (e.g., simple shapes) as opposed to random arrangements (Fig. 14.2) [11–13]. Beran trained monkeys

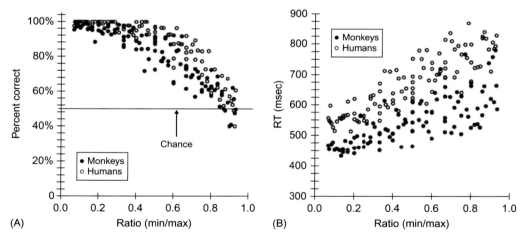

FIGURE 14.1 Monkeys and humans participated in a numerical ordering task. Accuracy (left) decreased and reaction time (right) increased as the ratio between the two numerical sets approached one. From [1,94].

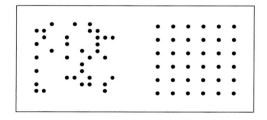

FIGURE 14.2 Stimuli used to test for the RRNI. Both humans and monkeys perceive randomly arranged dot patterns (left) as less numerous than regularly arranged dot patterns (right). From [10].

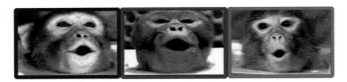

FIGURE 14.3   An example trial in which three animated monkey faces were presented with two or three simultaneous vocalizations. Monkeys looked longer when the number of faces matched the number of vocalizations. From [16].

to select the numerically larger of two numerically unequal arrays. He then presented probe trials where the two numerosities contained the same number of elements. The dots in one of the probe stimuli were arranged regularly in a matrix and the dots in the other stimulus were arranged randomly. Monkeys and humans reliably judged the regular patterns to be more numerous than the random patterns. The fact that number judgments are subject to some of the same visual illusions in rhesus monkeys and human adults supports the idea that the two species rely on a common representational system.

Cross-Modal Representations of Number

Number is abstract in that it is not bound to the physical or perceptual qualities of the stimulus. For example, three croissants and three iPhones differ in many important perceptual features, but they both share the common abstract feature of "threeness". Do animals appreciate the abstract numerical equivalence between sets perceived in different sensory modalities? Research addressing this topic has until recently been hard to interpret due to mixed results (e.g., [14] *vs* [15]). Jordan *et al.* [16] devised an ecologically relevant task to assess cross-modal mapping in rhesus monkeys. Monkeys heard choruses of two or three monkeys vocalizing while simultaneously viewing either two or three animated monkey faces on a computer screen (Fig. 14.3). The sound intensity of the choruses was equated and the videos were edited so that all mouth movements had a synchronous onset and offset. Monkeys looked longer at the screen that featured the number of faces that matched the number of vocalizing monkeys, suggesting that monkeys were able to match number across visual and auditory modalities. Human infants showed the same pattern of results when tested in parallel study with human faces and voices [17].

In a more direct test of monkeys' ability to cross-modally match based on number, Jordan, MacLean, and Brannon [18] trained three rhesus monkeys on a number match-to-sample task in which the monkeys were presented with a sample sequence of shapes or tones (Fig. 14.4). The monkeys were then required to choose the visual array that matched the number of sights or sounds in the sample. Monkeys performed above chance for both auditory and visual samples and their matching ability was dependent on the ratio between the numerosity of the correct match and the incorrect distractor. Furthermore, monkeys were just as accurate matching across sensory modalities (auditory–visual) as they were within a single modality (visual–visual), although there was a slight reaction-time cost. Similar studies by Barth and colleagues have shown that adults and preschool children can compare large arrays across sensory modalities and show little or no cost in accuracy [19,20].

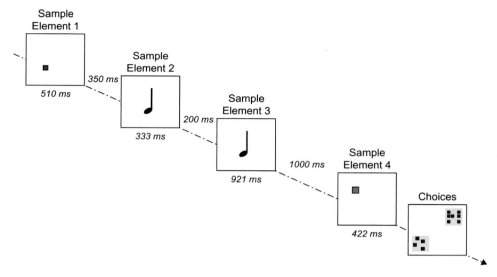

FIGURE 14.4 During cross-modal testing, rhesus monkeys were presented with a sequence of tones and shapes, followed by two sets of numerical arrays presented simultaneously on the screen. Cross-modal accuracy was equal to the accuracy obtained within modality. From [18].

The monkey face–voice matching study may or may not involve the ANS given that the experiment was limited to sets of two and three which could be handled by an alternative mechanism; however, the touch–screen version clearly showed ratio-dependence for a wide range of values and thus recruited the ANS. Thus, while auditory cortex and visual cortex are no doubt used to perceive the sound and sights presented to the monkeys, it seems likely that at subsequent processing stages the perceptual features of the arrays are either discarded or ignored.

Precursors to a Zero Concept

Zero is a special number in symbolic number systems for many reasons. First it serves as the additive identity for natural numbers such that when added to any element x in a set, the result remains x. Zero is a number that quantifies null sets and thus, unlike positive integers, it represents the absence rather than the presence of objects in the world. Does the ANS allow for the representation of empty sets as numerical values?

Research investigating the representation of zero in animals has met with mixed results. An African Grey Parrot, named Alex, was trained to verbally label empty sets, and a chimpanzee, named Ai, was trained to match empty sets to the Arabic numeral "0" [21–23]. However, in both cases the animals failed to show flexible use of the symbol and to transfer associations learned in one context to another.

Merritt, Rugani, and Brannon [24] suggest that rhesus monkeys represent empty sets as numerical values and that this ability may serve as a necessary prerequisite to a conceptual understanding of the symbol zero. They tested rhesus monkeys with empty sets that were inserted into two numerosity tasks with which the monkeys already had extensive experience. In the matching task, the monkeys were required to choose between two arrays based on the numerosity of a sample array. The sample arrays contained stimuli with 0, 1, 2, 3, 4, 6, 8, or 12 items and the two choice arrays contained the matching number of elements (target) and a different number of elements (distractor). The trials with empty sets (0 elements) were treated as probe trials and thus were non-differentially reinforced. Results indicated that monkeys were able to accurately match the empty sets, independently of background area and background color. Importantly, the monkeys showed numerical distance effects for empty sets and thus were more accurate at choosing the correct target array when the distractor array differed greatly from the target array in numerosity. The distance effect for empty sets suggests that monkeys were not treating the empty set as a qualitatively different picture-like stimulus, but rather, as a numerical value that could be compared with other numerical values (Fig. 14.5).

In a second experiment, monkeys were tested on a numerical ordering task. Monkeys were required to respond to pairs of numerical values in either ascending (red screen background) or descending (blue screen background) order. The monkeys were given non-differentially reinforced probe trials that contained an empty set paired with each of the other possible numerical values (1–9). For both ascending and descending trials, the monkeys were able to spontaneously place the empty set in the proper order with above chance accuracy. Further, as with the matching task, the monkeys showed distance effects that were comparable to those observed with the other numerical values (see also [25]). Collectively these data suggest that monkeys appreciate empty sets as values along the numerical continuum and suggest that a successful model of nonverbal numerical representation must be able to represent the absence of countable items [26,27].

Do humans show these same patterns? Although some data question whether zero is part of the approximate number system [28], very few studies have been conducted to test this question directly. Wellman and Miller [29] have shown that young children's understanding of zero lags behind that of the count-list integers, and that children do not fully grasp the cardinal and ordinal properties of zero until about age four. One reason may be that children have difficulty conceptualizing the symbol zero as a numerical value. But what

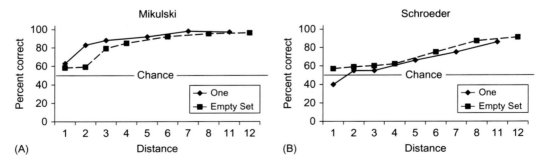

FIGURE 14.5 Accuracy as a function of the numerical distance between the target (i.e. correct match) and the distractor for two rhesus monkeys (A) Mikulski and (B) Schroeder. If empty sets were perceived as numerical values, then there should be a distance effect for the empty sets (dotted line) similar to that for the numerosity one (solid line). From [24].

if the symbolic component were removed? Would young children understand the cardinal and ordinal properties of empty sets prior to understanding these relationships with zero? In order to examine this, Merritt and Brannon (in preparation) tested four-year-old children using the same paradigm that was used to test rhesus monkeys [24]. Children responded to empty sets with above-chance performance and more importantly showed distance effects for empty sets in both tasks. This was true even among children who were unable to answer verbal questions about the ordinal relationships between zero and other numbers in the count-list. Overall, these findings demonstrate that the ANS can support representations of empty sets and these representations may serve as a precursor for the ability to represent symbolic zero.

THE RELATIONSHIP BETWEEN TIME, SPACE, AND NUMBER

It would be adaptive to represent time, spatial extent, and number in a single currency to allow arithmetic operations to combine variables across domains [30]. For example, many different animal species calculate the rate of return when making foraging decisions thus integrating over time and number [31].

Time and Number

A classic finding by Meck and Church [32] suggests that rats may automatically encode both time and number when trained to discriminate two stimuli for which the two dimensions provide redundant information (e.g., two events in 2s vs eight events in 8s). A stronger claim made by Meck and Church was that there was a quantitative equivalence between a unit of time and a single count. Rats were trained to classify stimuli as short or long (e.g., a constant tone that was 2 or 4s) and were then tested with sequences of 10–20 1-s-on/1-s-off white noise bursts. Despite the fact that the rats had been trained on a purely duration discrimination, they transferred to the number discrimination. Given that the duration of the test sequences was completely outside the range of the training durations the authors argued that successful transfer performance revealed that each countable event was psychologically equivalent to 200ms such that 10 events was equivalent to 2s and 20 events was equivalent to 4s.

More recent work, however, challenges these interpretations. Balci and Gallistel [33] showed that transfer performance may actually be mediated by cross-domain comparability of within domain proportions. They used the Meck and Church time–number bisection procedure and trained adult humans to classify two durations (2 or 4s) as short or long. The subjects were then tested with different numbers of light flashes (e.g., 5, 6, 7, 8, and 10 flashes) and required to classify the stimuli as short or long. Different groups of subjects were tested with different numerical ranges (i.e. 5–10 or 10–20). Transfer from duration to number was successful regardless of the absolute values with which subjects were tested. These results suggest that the subjects anchored their decisions to the range of values presented within each domain but did not actually make a direct comparison between magnitudes for duration and number. Thus, while it is possible that there is a single representational code for time and number at some point in the processing hierarchy, it is also possible that behavioral parallels and transfer across domains could instead reflect common comparison processes.

Space and Time

A related question is the degree to which variability in one dimension influences the judgments made about another dimension? In humans, there is an asymmetrical relationship between space and time, with spatial manipulations influencing judgments of time more than the reverse. Casasanto and Boroditsky [34] suggested that this asymmetry may be due to the fact that most languages have many more spatial metaphors for time than *vice versa*. But, what is the relationship between space and time in the mind of a nonverbal animal? Merritt, Casasanto, and Brannon [35] developed a new task that could be used with both monkeys and humans to assess whether temporal stimulus attributes influence judgments about spatial extent and *vice versa*. As expected, humans showed an asymmetrical pattern whereby space influenced time judgments more than the reverse. However, monkeys showed strong bidirectional and symmetrical influences of space and time on one another. The monkey findings are consistent with Walsh's [36] ATOM proposal (a theory of generalized magnitude) which suggests that time, space, and number are all represented by a common generalized magnitude system and also consistent with the possibility that language may be the driving force that creates an asymmetry between the perception of time and space.

Semantic Congruity

While ratio dependence is a behavioral signature of the ANS, the semantic congruity effect appears to be a universal hallmark of the wider class of all ordinal judgments. For example, when asked to compare the relative sizes of two small animals (e.g., termite *vs* roach), people respond more quickly when asked to choose the "smaller" item than when asked to choose the "larger" item. In contrast, when asked to compare two large animals (e.g., buffalo *vs* whale), people respond more quickly when asked to choose the "larger" compared to the "smaller" item. Thus, reaction time is faster when the question is congruent with the size of the comparators. This phenomenon, known as the semantic congruity effect, is robust and has been found in a variety of different prothetic dimensions including number [37,38], line length [39], brightness [40], distance between cities [41], animal intelligence [42], and animal size [43].

One explanation for the semantic congruity effect is that when two stimuli are compared on the basis of size or number, they are coded for magnitude (Small or Large) using symbolic or linguistic processes [44–46]. When the stimuli being compared differ greatly in magnitude, they are given different magnitude codes (e.g., small *vs* large). If asked "which is larger?" or "which is smaller?", these codes can then be quickly and easily matched to the form of the question. However, when the stimuli being compared are either both large or both small, then the magnitude codes for both stimuli will be similar to one another (e.g., Large and Large+ or Small and Small+, respectively). To answer an ordinal comparison question the codes must be translated from Small/Small+ to Small/Large (or Large/Large+ to Large/Small) so that one of the codes is consistent with the form of instruction. The reaction-time patterns that characterize the semantic congruity effect are the result of the added processing time necessary to translate these codes.

However, recent work with nonverbal animals casts doubt on this explanation, and suggests that semantic congruity is a more general feature of ordinal comparisons. Cantlon and Brannon [47] trained rhesus monkeys to make a conditional discrimination such that when

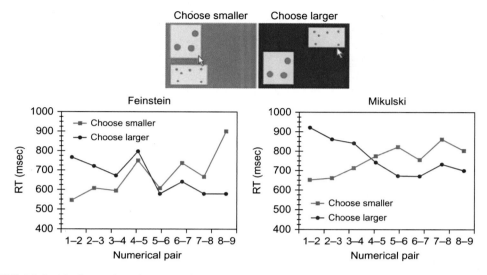

FIGURE 14.6 Monkeys selected numerical arrays in either ascending (red screen) or descending (blue screen) order. Both monkeys responded faster when the numerical value of the choices were congruent with the instructions (e.g., small values/choose smaller) than when they were incongruent (e.g., large values/choose smaller). From [47].

the screen background color was red, they were required to respond to pairs of numerical stimuli in ascending numerical order (e.g., two and then three) whereas when the background color was blue, they were required to select the stimuli in descending numerical order (e.g., three and then two). Figure 14.6 illustrates that both monkeys showed a semantic congruity effect. For relatively small pairs, the monkeys were faster when given the ascending cue compared to the descending cue (faster at responding 2 and then 3, compared to 3 and then 2). Likewise, when responding to relatively large pairs, the monkeys were faster when given the descending compared to the ascending cue (i.e. faster at responding 8 and then 7, compared to 7 and then 8).

The semantic congruity effect is subject to range effects in monkeys and adult humans alike, whereby a given set of values is treated as large or small depending on the context in which it is presented [43]. For example, 9 would be considered a "large" number within a range of 1–10, but a "small" number within a range of 1–10,000. Jones *et al.* [48] modified the paradigm used by Cantlon and Brannon [47], and manipulated the range of values. Like humans, the monkeys' performance was dependent on context. On average, when the pair 6:12 was presented within a range of 1–12, monkeys responded more quickly on descending trials (e.g., "choose larger") than on ascending trials (e.g., "choose smaller"). In contrast, when 6:12 was presented within a range of 6–72, monkeys responded more quickly on the ascending trials than on the descending trials.

ARITHMETIC REASONING

The ANS provides a simple avenue for performing arithmetic operations in a system analogous to histogram arithmetic [30]. In fact, studies with young children, adults, and nonhuman animals demonstrate that ANS representations enter into operations that are iso-morphic with ordering, addition, and subtraction [19,49–52].

Ordering

Numerical ordering is an operation that has been repeatedly demonstrated in nonhuman animals (e.g., Fig. 14.7). Many animal species, including chimpanzees [53–55], cebus monkeys [56,57], rhesus monkeys [58], horses [59], and elephants [60], can reliably pick a container with the greater number of food pieces. However, in these studies, it is often difficult to determine whether the animals are attending to the total amount of food, the duration of the baiting sequence, or the number of food items.

Other studies have used visual stimuli with elaborate controls to directly test whether animals are capable of ordering arrays on the basis of numerical attributes while ignoring the non-numerical continuous variables that often co-vary with number. These studies suggest that when non-numerical variables are dissociated from number, monkeys can easily attend to number. For example, a wide variety of primates (rhesus monkeys, baboons, cebus monkeys, squirrel monkeys, ringtail lemurs) are capable of extracting an abstract numerical ordinal rule such that when trained to order a subset of values (e.g., 1–4), can subsequently extend this rule to values outside the training range (e.g., 5–9) [61–64].

Addition and Subtraction

A few studies have shown that monkeys, lemurs, and even dogs track the number of objects behind a screen when they witness addition and subtraction events [25,65–70]. While these studies appear to reflect addition and subtraction operations analogous to that shown by human infants, it is unclear whether these studies tapped ANS representations or instead object-file representations given the exclusively small values tested (see Chapters 2, 15, and

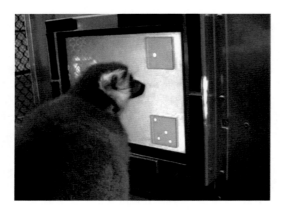

FIGURE 14.7 A ring-tailed lemur deciding which stimulus to choose in a numerical ordering task. In order to obtain reward, the lemur must select the stimulus containing the fewest number of elements first.

17 in this volume). However, Flombaum, Junge, and Hauser [71] found evidence of ratio-dependent number discrimination in free-ranging macaques on the island of Cayo Santiago. Monkeys that witnessed the operation 4 + 4 looked longer at outcomes of 4 compared to outcomes of 8 whereas monkeys that witness an 8 − 4 operation looked longer at outcome of 8 than an outcome of 4.

Other tasks that require more explicit choices also suggest that animals can track the total number of food items and compare these sums. In some of these studies the addends were all visible at the time of the choice whereas others required updating sets in memory [72–77]. For example, in one study chimpanzees watched as two different experimenters each dropped M&M candies into two opaque containers [74]. The chimpanzees reliably selected the container that contained the greater number of candies, suggesting that they could update their numerical representations in each cup as new items were added.

As mentioned earlier, food choice studies are subject to the criticism that animals may be attending to continuous variables and optimizing the amount of food they receive rather than the number of food morsels. To test for nonverbal addition while controlling for the myriad of possible non-numerical cues, Cantlon and Brannon [78] tested monkeys in a delayed-match-to-sample addition task (Fig. 14.8). Monkeys were shown two sample arrays separated in time by a brief delay and then presented with a choice between two arrays, one of which was the sum of the two sample arrays. Monkeys were trained with a few different problems and then tested with novel addends. Performance exceeded chance expectations on the novel problems and was dependent on the ratio between the correct sum and the incorrect distractor (Fig. 14.9A, B). In fact, monkeys and humans tested on the same task showed similar ratio-dependent performance, suggesting that both monkeys and humans can nonverbally add using the ANS (see also [19,49]).

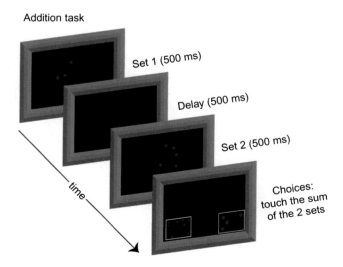

Addition task

Set 1 (500 ms)

Delay (500 ms)

Set 2 (500 ms)

Choices: touch the sum of the 2 sets

time

FIGURE 14.8 Monkeys and human participants added two sets of dots. The sets were presented sequentially, with each set separated by a brief delay. Next, two sets of dots were presented simultaneously, with one set equal to the sum of the two addends, and the other set serving as a distractor. From [78].

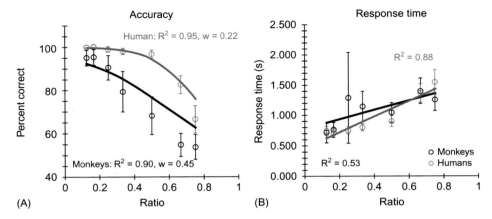

FIGURE 14.9 Accuracy (A) and reaction time (B) for humans (orange circles) and monkeys (black circles) as a function of ratio between the correct sum and the distractor choice. From [78].

BOX 14.3

QUESTIONS FOR FUTURE RESEARCH

Despite the recent advances in our understanding of the ANS in animals and its parallels in adult and developing humans, several important questions remain.

- Do animals possess separate systems for representing small and large sets as work with human infants elegantly demonstrates (e.g., Chapters 2 and 18 in this volume)? Why do some animals show set size limits in particular tasks [59,67,79,80], but not others [57,81,82]?
- What can animal models tell us about how symbols for number are learned? Are animals capable of using the same inductive processes used by humans to map magnitudes onto symbols? When animals are trained to map symbols to numerosities does this fundamentally change their underlying numerical representation? Or instead are precise numerical representations forever the beyond of nonhuman animals and only made possible by human language?
- How are number representations in animals related to representations of time or space? Are transfer studies simply showing abstract rule learning or do they in some cases reveal common representational codes for different quantitative domains?

CONCLUSIONS

The ability to understand and manipulate numbers is a hallmark of human cognition, but the data reviewed in this chapter show that such abilities are not unique to humans. Animals are capable of representing number independently of such non-numerical features as density, surface area, duration, and contour length. Moreover, these nonverbal representations of number enter into arithmetic computations such as ordering, addition, and subtraction. Many computations in the world require integrating information from multiple quantitative domains (e.g., number, time, and space). A challenge for further research is to determine at what level of the cognitive and neural processing stream these domains are distinct and when they are integrated (see Box 14.3). There is no doubt that animal models will be crucial for this enterprise (see Chapter 8 in this volume).

References

[1] J.F. Cantlon, E.M. Brannon, Shared system for ordering small and large numbers in monkeys and humans, Psychol. Sci. 17 (5) (2006) 402–407.

[2] L. Feigenson, S. Dehaene, E. Spelke, Core systems of number, Trends Cogn. Sci. 8 (7) (2004) 307–314.

[3] R. Gelman, C.R. Gallistel, Language and the origin of numerical concepts, Science 306 (5695) (2004) 441–443.

[4] M.J. Beran, Monkeys (*Macaca mulatta* and *Cebus apella*) track, enumerate, and compare multiple sets of moving items, J. Exp. Psychol. Anim. Behav. Process. 34 (1) (2008) 63–74.

[5] S. Cordes, R. Gelman, C. Gallistel, J. Whalen, Variability signatures distinguish verbal from nonverbal counting for both large and small numbers, Psychonomic Bull. Rev. 8 (4) (2001) 698–707.

[6] J.R. Platt, D.M. Johnson, Localization of position within a homogeneous behavior chain: Effects of error contingencies, Learn. Motiv. 2 (1971) 386–414.

[7] J. Whalen, C.R. Gallistel, R. Gelman, Nonverbal counting in humans: The psychophysics of number representation, Psychol. Sci. 10 (2) (1999) 130–137.

[8] M.H. Birnbaum, M. Kobernick, C.T. Veit, Subjective correlation and the size–numerosity illusion, J. Exp. Psychol. 102 (3) (1974) 537–539.

[9] D. Burr, J. Ross, A visual sense of number, Curr. Biol. 18 (6) (2008) 425–428.

[10] M.J. Beran, Quantity perception by adult humans (*Homo sapiens*), chimpanzees (*Pan troglodytes*), and rhesus macaques (*Macaca mulatta*) as a function of stimulus organization, Int. J. Comp. Psychol. 19 (4) (2006) 386–397.

[11] N. Ginsburg, Effect of item arrangement on perceived numerosity: Randomness vs. regularity, Percept. Mot. Skills 43 (1976) 663–668.

[12] N. Ginsburg, Perceived numerosity, item arrangement, and expectancy, Am. J. Psychol. 91 (1978) 267–273.

[13] N. Ginsburg, The regular–random numerosity illusion: rectangular patterns, J. Gen. Psychol. 103 (2d Half) (1980) 211–216.

[14] R.M. Church, W.H. Meck, The numerical attribute of stimuli, in: H.L. Roitblat, T.G. Bever, H.S. Terrace, (Eds.), Animal Cognition, Erlbaum, Hillsdale, NJ, 1984, pp. 445–464.

[15] H. Davis, M. Albert, Failure to transfer or train a numerical discrimination using sequential visual-stimuli in rats, Bull. Psychon. Soc. 25 (6) (1987) 472–474.

[16] K.E. Jordan, E.M. Brannon, N.K. Logothetis, A.A. Ghazanfar, Monkeys match the number of voices they hear to the number of faces they see, Curr. Biol. 15 (2005) 1–5.

[17] K. Jordan, E.M. Brannon, The multisensory representation of number in infancy. Pro. Natl. Acad. Sci. 103 (9) (2006) 3486–3489.

[18] K.E. Jordan, E.L. Maclean, E.M. Brannon, Monkeys match and tally quantities across senses, Cognition 108 (3) (2008) 617–625.

[19] H. Barth, N. Kanwisher, E. Spelke, The construction of large number representations in adults, Cognition 86 (3) (2003) 201–221.

[20] H. Barth, K. La Mont, J. Lipton, E.S. Spelke, Abstract number and arithmetic in preschool children, Proc. Natl. Acad. Sci. U.S.A. 102 (39) (2005) 14116–14121.

[21] I.M. Pepperberg, Grey Parrot (*Psittacus erithacus*) numerical abilities: addition and further experiments on a zero-like concept, J. Comp. Psychol. 120 (1) (2006) 1–11.

[22] I.M. Pepperberg, J.D. Gordon, Number comprehension by a grey parrot (*Psittacus erithacus*), including a zero-like concept, J. Comp. Psychol. 119 (2) (2005) 197–209.

[23] D. Biro, T. Matsuzawa, Use of numerical symbols by the chimpanzee (*Pan troglodytes*): Cardinals, ordinals, and the introduction of zero, Anim. Cogn. 4 (2001) 193–199.

[24] D.J. Merritt, R. Rugani, E.M. Brannon, Empty sets as part of the numerical continuum: conceptual precursors to the zero concept in rhesus monkeys, J. Exp. Psychol.: General 138 (2) (2009) 258–269.

[25] G.M. Sulkowski, M.D. Hauser, Can rhesus monkeys spontaneously subtract? Cognition 79 (3) (2001) 239–262.

[26] K. Wynn, Psychological foundations of number: numerical competence in human infants, Trends Cogn. Sci. 2 (8) (1998) 296–303.

[27] K. Wynn, W.C. Chiang, Limits to infants' knowledge of objects: The case of magical appearance, Psychol. Sci. 9 (6) (1998) 448–455.

[28] M. Brysbaert, Arabic Number Reading—on the Nature of the Numerical Scale and the Origin of Phonological Recoding, J. Exp. Psychol. Gen. 124 (4) (1995) 434–452.

[29] H.M. Wellman, K.F. Miller, Thinking about nothing: Developmental concepts of zero, Br. J. Dev. Psychol. 4 (1986) 31–42.

[30] C.R. Gallistel, R. Gelman, Preverbal and verbal counting and computation, Cognition 44 (1–2) (1992) 43–74.

[31] C.R. Gallistel, The Organization of Learning. Learning, Development, and Conceptual Change, MIT Press, Cambridge, Mass., 1990. viii, 648.

[32] W.H. Meck, R.M. Church, A mode control model of counting and timing processes, J. Exp. Psychol. Anim. Behav. Process. 9 (3) (1983) 320–334.

[33] F. Balci, C.R. Gallistel, Cross-domain transfer of quantitative discriminations: is it all a matter of proportion? Psychon. Bull. Rev. 13 (4) (2006) 636–642.

[34] D. Casasanto, L. Boroditsky, Time in the mind: using space to think about time, Cognition 106 (2) (2008) 579–593.

[35] D.J. Merritt, D. Casasanto, E.M. Brannon, Do monkeys think in metaphors? Representations of space and time in monkeys and humans, Cognition 117 (2010) 191–202.

[36] V. Walsh, A theory of magnitude: common cortical metrics of time, space and quantity, Trends Cogn. Sci. 7 (11) (2003) 483–488.

[37] W.P. Banks, M. Fujii, F. Kayra-Stuart, The locus of semantic congruity effects in comparative judgments, J. Exp. Psychol. Hum. Perception and Perform. 2 (1976) 435–447.

[38] R.S. Moyer, R.H. Bayer, Mental comparison and the symbolic distance effect, Cognit. Psychol. 8 (2) (1976) 228–246.

[39] W.M. Petrusic, J.V. Baranski, R. Kennedy, Similarity comparisons with remembered and perceived magnitudes: memory psychophysics and fundamental measurement, Mem. Cogn. 26 (5) (1998) 1041–1055.

[40] R.J. Audley, C.P. Wallis, Response instructions and the speed of relative judgments. I. Some experiments on brightness and discrimination, Br. J. Psychol. 55 (1964) 59–73.

[41] K.J. Holyoak, W.A. Mah, Cognitive reference points in judgments of symbolic magnitude, Cognit. Psychol. 14 (1982) 328–352.

[42] W.P. Banks, J. Flora, Semantic and perceptual processes in symbolic comparisons, J. Exp. Psychol. Human 3 (2) (1977) 278–290.

[43] C.G. Cech, E.J. Shoben, Context effects in symbolic magnitude comparisons, J. Exp. Psychol.. Learning, Memory, and Cognition 11 (2) (1985) 299–315.

[44] W.P. Banks, Encoding and processing of symbolic information in comparative judgments. The Psychology of Learn. Motiv., 11 (1977) 101–159.

[45] W.P. Banks, H.H. Clark, P. Lucy, The locus of the semantic congruity effect in comparative judgments, J. Exp. Psychol. Human 104 (1) (1975) 35–47.

[46] C.G. Cech, E.J. Shoben, M. Love, Multiple congruity effects in judgments of magnitude, J. Exp. Psychol. Learn. 21 (1990) 314–326.

[47] J. Cantlon, E.M. Brannon, Semantic congruity facilitates number judgments in monkeys, Proc. Natl. Acad. Sci. 102 (2005) 16507–16511.

[48] S.M. Jones, J.F. Cantlon, D.J. Merritt, E.M. Brannon, Context affects the numerical semantic congruity effect in rhesus monkeys (Macaca mulatta), Behav. Processes 82 (2) (2010) 191–196.

[49] H. Barth, K. La Mont, J. Lipton, S. Dehaene, N. Kanwisher, E. Spelke, Non-symbolic arithmetic in adults and young children, Cognition 98 (2006) 199–222.

[50] C.K. Gilmore, S.E. McCarthy, E.S. Spelke, Symbolic arithmetic knowledge without instruction, Nature 447 (7144) (2007) 589–591.

[51] C.K. Gilmore, S.E. McCarthy, E.S. Spelke, Non-symbolic arithmetic abilities and mathematics achievement in the first year of formal schooling, Cognition 115 (3) (2010) 394–406.

[52] P. Pica, C. Lemer, W. Izard, S. Dehaene, Exact and approximate arithmetic in an Amazonian indigene group, Science 306 (5695) (2004) 499–503.

[53] M.J. Beran, Chimpanzees (*Pan troglodytes*) respond to nonvisible sets after one-by-one addition and removal of items, J. Comp. Psychol. 118 (1) (2004) 25–36.

[54] M.J. Beran, M.M. Beran, Chimpanzees remember the results of one-by-one addition of food items to sets over extended time periods, Psychol. Sci. 15 (2) (2004) 94–99.

[55] M.J. Beran, T.A. Evans, E.H. Harris, Perception of food amount by chimpanzees based on the number, size, contour length, and visibility of items, Anim. Behav. 75 (2008) 1793–1802.

[56] T.A. Evans, M.J. Beran, E.H. Harris, D.F. Rice, Quantity judgments of sequentially presented food items by capuchin monkeys (*Cebus apella*), Anim. Cogn. 12 (1) (2009) 97–105.

[57] K. VanMarle, J. Aw, K. McCrink, L.R. Santos, How capuchin monkeys (*Cebus apella*) quantify objects and substances, J. Comp. Psychol. 120 (4) (2006) 416–426.

[58] M.D. Hauser, S. Carey, L.B. Hauser, Spontaneous number representation in semi-free-ranging rhesus monkeys, Proc. R. Soc., London 267 (2000) 829–833.

[59] C. Uller, J. Lewis, Horses (*Equus caballus*) select the greater of two quantities in small numerical contrasts, Anim. Cogn. 12 (5) (2009) 733–738.

[60] N. Irie-Sugimoto, T. Kobayashi, T. Sato, T. Hasegawa, Relative quantity judgment by Asian elephants (*Elephas maximus*), Anim. Cogn. 12 (1) (2009) 193–199.

[61] E.M. Brannon, H.S. Terrace, Ordering of the numerosities 1 to 9 by monkeys, Science 282 (5389) (1998) 746–749.

[62] E.M. Brannon, H.S. Terrace, Representation of the numerosities 1–9 by rhesus macaques (*Macaca mulatta*), J. Exp. Psychol. Anim. Behav. Process. 26 (1) (2000) 31–49.

[63] B.R. Smith, A.K. Piel, D.K. Candland, Numerity of a socially housed hamadryas baboon (*Papio hamadryas*) and a socially housed squirrel monkey (*Saimiri sciureus*), J. Comp. Psychol. 117 (2) (2003) 217–225.

[64] P.G. Judge, T.A. Evans, D.K. Vyas, Ordinal representation of numeric quantities by brown Capuchin monkeys (*Cebus apella*), J. Exp. Psychol. Anim. Behav. Process. 31 (1) (2005) 79–94.

[65] M.D. Hauser, P. MacNeilage, M. Ware, Numerical representations in primates, Proc. Natl. Acad. Sci. 93 (1996) 1514–1517.

[66] M. Hauser, S. Carey, Spontaneous representations of small numbers of objects by rhesus macaques: examinations of content and format, Cognit. Psychol. 47 (4) (2003) 367–401.

[67] M.D. Hauser, S. Carey, L.B. Hauser, Spontaneous number representation in wild rhesus monkeys, Proc. R. Acad. Sci. 93 (2000) 1514–1517.

[68] L.R. Santos, J.L. Barnes, N. Mahajan, Expectations about numerical events in four lemur species (*Eulemur fulvus, Eulemur mongoz, Lemur catta* and *Varecia rubra*), Anim. Cogn. 8 (4) (2005) 253–262.

[69] C. Uller, M. Hauser, S. Carey, Spontaneous representation of number in cotton-top tamarins (*Saguinus oedipus*), J. Comp. Psychol. 115 (3) (2001) 248–257.

[70] R.E. West, R.J. Young, Do domestic dogs show any evidence of being able to count? Anim. Cogn. 5 (3) (2002) 183–186.

[71] J.I. Flombaum, J.A. Junge, M.D. Hauser, Rhesus monkeys (*Macaca mulatta*) spontaneously compute addition operations over large numbers, Cognition 97 (3) (2005) 315–325.

[72] U.S. Anderson, T.S. Stoinski, M.A. Bloomsmith, M.J. Marr, A.D. Smith, T.L. Maple, Relative numerousness judgment and summation in young and old Western lowland gorillas, J. Comp. Psychol. 119 (3) (2005) 285–295.

[73] U.S. Anderson, T.S. Stoinski, M.A. Bloomsmith, T.L. Maple, Relative numerousness judgment and summation in young, middle-aged, and older adult orangutans (*Pongo pygmaeus abelii* and *Pongo pygmaeus pygmaeus*), J. Comp. Psychol. 121 (1) (2007) 1–11.

[74] M. Beran, Summation and numerousness judgements of sequentially presented sets of items by chimpanzees (*Pan troglodytes*), J. Comp. Psychol. 115 (2) (2001) 181–191.

[75] J. Call, Estimating and operating on discrete quantities in orangutans (*Pongo pygmaeus*), J. Comp. Psychol. 114 (2) (2000) 136–147.

[76] R. Pérusse, D.M. Rumbaugh, Summation in chimpanzees (*Pan troglodytes*): effects of amounts, number of wells, and finer ratios, Int. J. Primatol. 11 (5) (1990) 425–437.

[77] D.M. Rumbaugh, S. Savage-Rumbaugh, M.T. Hegel, Summation in the chimpanzee (*Pan troglodytes*), J. Exp. Psychol. Anim. Behav. Process. 13 (2) (1987) 107–115.

[78] J.F. Cantlon, E.M. Brannon, Basic math in monkeys and college students, PLoS Biol. 5 (12) (2007) e328.

[79] R. Rugani, L. Regolin, G. Vallortigara, Discrimination of small numerosities in young chicks, J. Exp. Psychol. Anim. Behav. Process. 34 (3) (2008) 388–399.

[80] C. Uller, R. Jaeger, G. Guidry, C. Martin, Salamanders (*Plethodon cinereus*) go for more: rudiments of number in an amphibian, Anim. Cogn. 6 (2) (2003) 105–112.

[81] K.P. Lewis, S. Jaffe, E.M. Brannon, Analog number representations in mongoose lemurs (*Eulemur mongoz*): evidence from a search task, Anim. Cogn. 8 (4) (2005) 247–252.

[82] R. Rugani, L. Fontanari, E. Simoni, L. Regolin, G. Vallortigara, Arithmetic in newborn chicks, Proc. Biol. Sci. 276 (1666) (2009) 2451–2460.

[83] C. Agrillo, M. Dadda, G. Serena, A. Bisazza, Use of number by fish, PLoS One 4 (3) (2009) e4786.

[84] M. Dadda, L. Piffer, C. Agrillo, A. Bisazza, Spontaneous number representation in mosquitofish, Cognition 112 (2) (2009) 343–348.

[85] K. McComb, C. Packer, A. Pusey, Roaring and numerical assessment in contests between groups of female lions, *Panthera leo*, Anim. Behav. 47 (1994) 379–387.

[86] M.L. Wilson, M.D. Hauser, R.W. Wrangham, Does participation in intergroup conflict depend on numerical assessment, range location, or rank for wild chimpanzees? Anim. Behav. 61 (2001) 1203–1216.

[87] D.M. Kitchen, Alpha male black howler monkey responses to loud calls: effect of numeric odds, male companion behaviour and reproductive investment, Anim. Behav. (2004) 125–139., 67 (2004) 125–139.

[88] H. Davis, J. Memmott, Autocontingencies: Rats count to three to predict safety from shock, Anim. Learn. Behav. 11 (1) (1983) 95–100.

[89] J.F. Cantlon, E.M. Brannon, How much does number matter to a monkey (*Macaca mulatta*)? J. Exp. Psychol. Anim. Behav. Process. 33 (1) (2007) 32–41.

[90] J. Gibbon, Scalar expectancy theory and Weber's Law in animal timing, Psychol. Rev. 84 (1977) 279–335.

[91] S. Dehaene, E. Dupoux, J. Mehler, Is numerical comparison digital—analogical and symbolic effects in 2-digit number comparison, J. Exp. Psychol. Human 16 (3) (1990) 626–641.

[92] S. Dehaene, The neural basis of the Weber–Fechner law: a logarithmic mental number line, Trends Cogn. Sci. 7 (4) (2003) 145–147.

[93] J. Gibbon, R.M. Church, Time Left—Linear versus logarithmic subjective time, J. Exp. Psychol. Anim. Behav. Process. 7 (2) (1981) 87–107.

[94] E.M. Brannon, C.J. Wusthoff, C.R. Gallistel, J. Gibbon, Numerical subtraction in the pigeon: Evidence for a linear subjective number scale, Psychol. Sci. 12 (3) (2001) 238–243.

[95] J.F. Cantlon, M.L. Platt, E.M. Brannon, Beyond the number domain, Trends Cogn. Sci. 13 (2) (2009) 83–91.

[96] J.F. Cantlon, S. Cordes, M.E. Libertus, E.M. Brannon, Comment on "Log or linear? Distinct intuitions of the number scale in Western and Amazonian indigene cultures", Science 323 (5910) (2009). p. 38.

Origins and Development of Generalized Magnitude Representation

Stella F. Lourenco*, Matthew R. Longo†

*Department of Psychology, Emory University, Atlanta, GA USA
†Department of Psychological Sciences, Birbeck, University of London, London, UK

Summary

Among the most fundamental of mental capacities is the ability to represent magnitude information such as physical size, numerosity, and duration. Accumulating evidence suggests that such cues are processed as part of a general magnitude system with shared *more vs less* representational structure. Here we review recent research with young children and preverbal infants suggesting that this system is operational from early in human life and may be far more general than currently believed. We present data suggesting that from early in development, the representation of magnitude extends across sensory modalities (e.g., vision and audition) and beyond the "big three" dimensions of spatial extent, number, and time. We also speculate about particular properties of the general magnitude system, including the potentially special role of space in grounding magnitude information.

Philosophers and scientists have long been interested in the human capacity to process magnitude. Questions such as "Which piece of pie is largest?" "How many guests are coming to the wedding?" and "Will my taxes take longer than two hours to finish?" illustrate the diversity of decisions that rest on the ability to represent magnitude in its many forms, among them being the dimensions of spatial extent, number, and time. Despite common empirical origins in psychophysical experiments [1–3], much research on the representation of magnitude exists in separate literatures, with claims of domain specificity prevalent in each (e.g., [4]). Debates on the nature and origins of quantitative reasoning reflect this approach. Some

© 2011 Elsevier Inc. All rights reserved.

investigators argue that infants discriminate sets of objects or sequences of events and perform simple arithmetic calculations such as addition and subtraction using number [5–9], whereas others suggest that these abilities are supported instead by spatial and/or temporal cues such as cumulative surface area (or contour length) and duration [10–14].

In other work, increasing attention has been paid to the psychological links among space, number, and time, and to the proposed existence of a *general magnitude system*, which processes magnitude information regardless of the specific dimension. This idea, as formalized by Walsh [15] and suggested previously by others [16,17], maintains that representations of different quantitative cues (e.g., physical size, numerosity, and duration) are, to some extent, undifferentiated and processed in a common code as generalized magnitude. The central characteristic of magnitude is the intrinsic "more than" *vs* "less than" structure of unequal stimulus values. Magnitude—whether it be the *size* of a piece of pie, the *number* of wedding attendees, or the *time* required to complete one's taxes—may be represented abstractly in terms of the more *vs* less relations or as some amount of "stuff." We would suggest that at the core of the general magnitude system is a (partly) shared currency of *more vs less stuff*. We use the notion of "stuff" to allow for inexactness in the representations, similar to that of the approximate number system [18] but applied more generally to both discrete and continuous quantities. While we do not distinguish in this review between discrete and continuous quantities, as both types involve magnitude, it is worth noting that there may be important differences between magnitude and other ordinal sequences. The more/less relations that characterize generalized magnitude information are inherently ordered. In contrast, ordinal sequences such as letters of the alphabet may exist without more/less relations, and, unless explicitly related to some dimension of magnitude (e.g., time), may not form part of this system (see below).

In the current review, we draw on recent behavioral research with children and infants to shed insight on the developmental origins of a general magnitude system. Much speculation has concerned these origins [15,19], but empirical data has only recently become available. We organize our review around three main issues, each treated in a separate section. In the first section, we focus on the associations among spatial extent, number, and time, as have been documented across early development. We refer to these dimensions as the "big three" because of their unambiguous more/less relations and their central importance in human cognition. In the second section, we turn to questions concerning the generality of a general magnitude system and its implications for development. Does this system extend to magnitudes beyond the big three, and across sensory modalities? In the third section, we turn to specific characteristics that may be fundamental to generalized magnitude representation, including the additional sense of space as location, as well as the development of its role in grounding and mentally organizing magnitude dimensions such as number and time.

THE BIG THREE: SPATIAL EXTENT, NUMBER, AND TIME

The notion of generalized magnitude representation has historical origins in philosophical writings [20–22]. Locke, for example, once argued for an intimate connection between space and time, suggesting that "expansion and duration do mutually embrace and comprehend each other… every part of space being in every part of duration, and every part of duration being in every part of expansion." Empirical support for such magnitude associations began emerging in the middle of the last century through the pioneering studies of Critchley [23] in neurology and

Piaget [24–26] in developmental psychology. Since then, accumulating evidence is suggestive of a shared representational code for at least the prototypical sources of magnitude information: spatial extent (e.g., physical size, length, height, and distance), number (whether symbolic or in non-symbolic form), and time (e.g., duration). In adult participants, cross-dimensional interactions between each pairing of space and number [27–29], space and time [30–32], and number and time [33,34] are now well documented (for reviews, see [15,35,36]).

As for so many cognitive domains, the developmental study of generalized magnitude representation begins with Piaget who observed that children often confused spatial extent with number [24] and time [25]. In the classic number conservation task, for example, Piaget asked children to judge the relative numerosity of two rows of objects that differed in length (see Fig. 15.1). Children between three and six years of age frequently judged longer rows as being greater in number, even when they actually had fewer (but, see [37]); they also claimed that the number of objects in a single row increased as the experimenter spread apart the objects. While such results have traditionally been taken as evidence for immature numerical

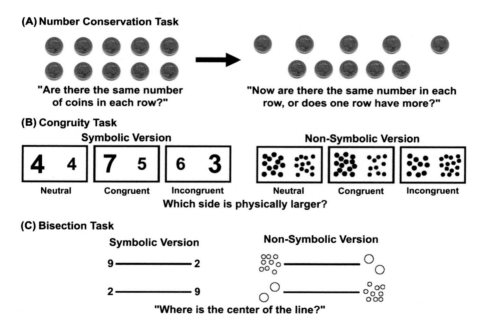

FIGURE 15.1 Three types of tasks (A: Number Conservation; B: Congruity; C: Bisection) used to show associations between space and number in children. (A) In the classic number conservation task, young children generally say that the longer row of coins is greater in numerical value (*right panel*), despite having previously answered that the two aligned rows contained an equal number of coins (*left panel*). (B) Symbolic (*left panel*) and non-symbolic (*right panel*) congruity tasks generally show interference and facilitation effects. When judging spatial extent, for example, numerical information both interferes with and facilitates spatial judgments. Relative to neutral conditions, participants (adults and children) are faster to respond in congruent conditions and slower in incongruent conditions. Reprinted with permission from [41]. (C) When asked to judge the perceived center of a physical line flanked by two numerical values, even children show systematic bias towards the larger value, whether numbers are presented symbolically (*left panel*) or in non-symbolic form (*right panel*), though effects are stronger for younger children in non-symbolic conditions. Such bisection tasks have been used to suggest that number affects the representation of length. Reprinted with permission from [43].

reasoning, several recent studies suggest instead that interference reflects a conceptual association between space and number, with bidirectional interactions. Indeed, both interference and facilitation effects have been reported in size congruity tasks with children as young as five to seven years, both with symbolic [38–40] and non-symbolic [41] stimuli (see Fig. 15.1). Other evidence for an association between space and number in childhood comes from bisection tasks. When flanked by numbers, adults' bisection judgments are systematically shifted towards the larger number [42]; five-year-olds, like older children and adults, judge the center of the line to be closer to the side of a larger numerical array [43] (see Fig. 15.1), suggesting that number affects the representation of length [44].

Since Piaget, others have focused on the association between space and time in school-aged children, with particular attention paid to the interactions between distance, duration, and speed [45–47]. The interactions with speed are particularly robust, perhaps not surprisingly given that calculations of speed, by definition, combine information about distance and duration. In a recent study, Casasanto and colleagues [48] examined distance and duration judgments by having children indicate which of two snails in a movie had traveled farther in space or longer in time. Clear cross-dimensional effects were observed, but they appeared to be stronger from space to time than *vice versa* (see below).

While less research has concerned the development of an association between number and time, evidence for such a connection has been reported in young children. In one study, numerical information interfered with five-year-olds' judgments of duration, even though they were explicitly told to ignore number [49]. Interestingly, despite more automatic access to number in both eight-year-olds and adults, numerical interference on temporal judgments decreased across development, suggesting that strategies such as explicit counting [49] may be effective in differentiating numerical and temporal magnitudes. There is also indirect evidence that temporal information may affect numerical reasoning. For example, preschoolers can detect numerical correspondence in audition and vision (e.g., three claps being equivalent to three objects), but only if rate and duration remain constant [50], suggesting that at least for young children, the processing of number is enhanced by temporal cues, as has been shown when spatial cues are congruent with numerical judgments (e.g., [12]).

Other research is consistent with a system of generalized magnitude representation that emerges as early as infancy. One line of evidence comes from comparisons of discrimination functions for spatial, numerical, and temporal stimuli. Discrimination sensitivity follows Weber's law, which holds that discriminability of unequal stimulus values varies as a function of the ratio difference. Using measures of reaction time and accuracy, discriminability of spatial extent (i.e. length and height), number, and duration [51–53] has been shown to increase in parallel from kindergarten into adulthood, even when accounting for developmental differences in processing speed [54]. Parallel discrimination functions have also been observed for these dimensions in the first year of life [7,55–58].

While parallel functions of discriminability are consistent with generalized magnitude representation, they can nevertheless be difficult to interpret. Greater discrimination sensitivity might be driven by developmental and experiential changes in, for example, perception, attention, and/or memory, none of which is specific to the general magnitude system. Consider changes in color discrimination and expertise effects on face processing. Over the first year of life, infants become sensitive to more colors because of maturation in the visual pathway [59], and with greater exposure to particular types of faces (e.g., gender and race), infants show increased sensitivity to faces with which they have greater expertise [60]. Increases in discriminablity for different stimuli can thus be driven by a variety of factors. In addition, discrimination functions for spatial extent, number, and time have only been observed for a restricted range of intensities, making it unclear whether parallel patterns of performance would generalize to non-tested intensities. Indeed, in the case of number, there are well-known range differences; infants, for example, have been shown to differentiate two *vs* three objects [61] but not eight *vs* twelve [7], despite identical ratios. In the case of temporal information, sub-second and supra-second ranges are even known to implicate distinct brain regions [62].

More direct evidence for the operation of a general magnitude system in infancy would involve showing *interactions* between different pairings of magnitude dimensions, as has been shown in adults (e.g., [27,30,33]) and older children (e.g., [24,26]). Recent studies have demonstrated such interactions, providing strong support for generalized magnitude representation by the end of the first year of life [63–65]. We conducted one of these studies [63], and our approach was modeled on the classic study of Meck and Church [17], in which rats were found to transfer associative learning from duration to number. We first taught nine-month-old infants that one magnitude (e.g., physical size) mapped systematically onto color/pattern cues; we then tested whether they generalized learning of these arbitrary mappings to other magnitudes (e.g., numerosity or duration). During habituation, infants might be shown, for example, that larger-sized rectangles were black with white stripes and that smaller rectangles were white with black dots (see Fig. 15.2). When subsequently tested with number, trials that maintained the mapping (i.e. congruent test trials) featured a larger numerical array with black/striped rectangles and a smaller numerical array with white/dotted rectangles; trials that violated the mapping (i.e. incongruent test trials) featured a larger numerical array with white/dotted rectangles and a smaller numerical array with black/striped rectangles (Fig. 15.2). The same logic was applied to duration (congruent test trials: longer-lasting objects as black/striped and shorter-lasting objects as white/dotted; incongruent test trials: longer-lasting objects as white/dotted and shorter-lasting objects as black/striped; Fig. 15.2). All combinations of size, numerosity, and duration were presented to infants, and for all, there was evidence of transfer across magnitude dimensions, as indicated by longer looking times to incongruent than congruent test trials (Fig. 15.2).

In another recent study, de Hevia and Spelke [65] tested the association between number and spatial extent in eight-month-old infants. Using a different procedure, they, too, showed transfer in infancy from one magnitude (i.e. numerosity) to another (i.e. length). Infants were visually habituated to continuous sequences of ascending or descending numerical values, and then during the test phase, presented with ascending and descending sequences of line lengths (see Fig. 15.2). Infants who habituated to ascending numbers, looked longer at descending lengths, and those who habituated to descending numbers, looked longer at ascending lengths (Fig. 15.2), suggesting that ordinal relations may have been coded with respect to more/less *generalized magnitude* (or *stuff*) rather than more/less *number*, which would allow for the observed generalization across visual stimuli. Srinivasan and Carey [64] have also provided converging evidence for an association between space and time in nine-month-olds, showing that congruent mappings between length and duration are easier to learn than incongruent ones.

Together, these findings suggest that generalized magnitude representation emerges by eight to nine months of age. In addition, they suggest that the associations among spatial extent, number, and time observed in the mature human organism are not mere

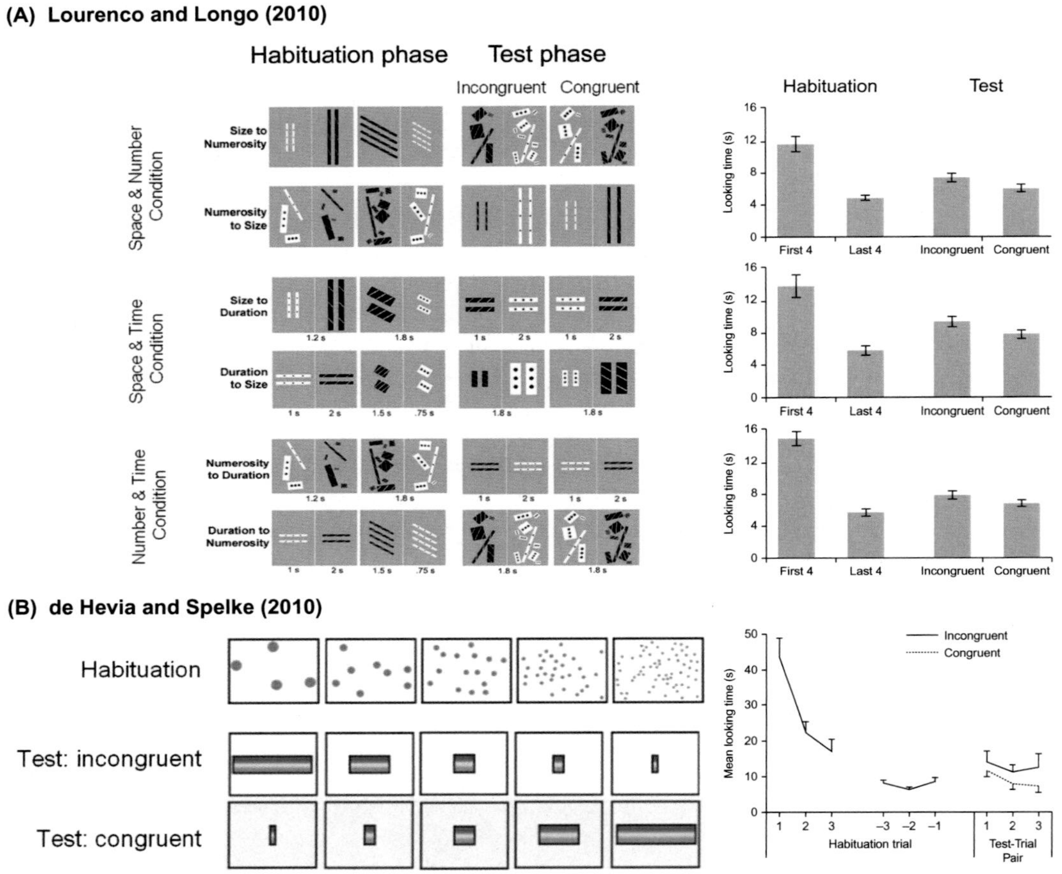

(A) Lourenco and Longo (2010)

(B) de Hevia and Spelke (2010)

FIGURE 15.2   Two recent studies (A: Lourenco & Longo, 2010; B: de Hevia & Spelke, 2010) showing magnitude-related associations in preverbal infants. (A) Stimuli and results for each of the conditions in Lourenco and Longo (2010). Each condition included two groups (Space & Number condition: size-to-numerosity and numerosity-to-size; Space & Time condition: size-to-duration and duration-to-size; Number & Time condition: numerosity-to-duration and duration-to-numerosity). Examples of stimuli used in habituation and test phases are shown (*left panel*). The test phase included incongruent and congruent trials. Results for each condition involve mean looking times (in seconds) for both phases, collapsed across group in each condition (*right panel*). In all conditions, looking times were significantly greater during incongruent than congruent test trials. Reprinted with permission from [63]. (B) Examples of stimuli (*left panel*) and results (*right panel*) in de Hevia and Spelke (2010). The habituation trial shown involves a sequence of ascending numerical values. Test trials involve sequences of decreasing line lengths (incongruent) and increasing line lengths (congruent). Results show that the mean looking times during incongruent test trials were significantly greater than during congruent test trials. Reprinted with permission from [65].

epiphenomenon of stimulus- or response-related conflation, but rather may reflect a fundamental underpinning of human cognition [64,65]. Much remains to be understood, however, about the development and nature of the general magnitude system. Do early associations reflect, for example, developmental differentiation or enrichment (see Box 15.1)? Is this

BOX 15.1

DEVELOPMENTAL TRAJECTORY OF THE GENERAL MAGNITUDE SYSTEM AS DIFFERENTIATION *VS* ENRICHMENT

While we acknowledge below that the task of characterizing development of the general magnitude system is complicated by various factors, here we suggest a distinction between increasing differentiation and increasing integration among magnitude dimensions. On one view, humans might begin life with a completely undifferentiated ("one-bit") representation of magnitude, which, with development, would become separated into more discrete dimensions [15]. On another view, generalized magnitude representation might arise over the course of development with exposure to correlational structure in the physical environment; and such associative learning may be further maintained by particular linguistic experiences such as exposure to metaphors, which highlight specific associations [64,108,115,139]. These views reflect two classic approaches to perceptual learning [140]: as proceeding via differentiation from an initially monolithic representation *vs* enrichment in which initially disparate dimensions become increasingly integrated. These views make opposite predictions about the expected developmental trajectory of generalized magnitude representation, suggesting an important area for future research. On the differentiation view, conceptual associations as observed via, for example, cross-dimensional

transfer should be strongest earlier in life, whereas on the enrichment view, these effects would increase in strength over development. Others have recently made similar distinctions concerning neural development. Cohen Kadosh and colleagues [35], for example, differentiate two types of neural change (see also [141]); one involves an increase in neural specialization with greater selectivity of activation and the other involves an increase in shared neural areas for highly similar dimensions, a type of neural economy.

Development is of course a highly complex process, and developmental accounts that emphasize either only increasing (conceptual or neural) differentiation or only increasing (conceptual or neural) integration are likely to be incomplete. Characterizing development of the general magnitude system is also likely to be complicated by the fact that the representation of *more vs less stuff* may constitute a distributed system with different classes of magnitude (stuff) which interact in complex ways (see [64] for a distinction between dimensions involving structural similarity *vs* functional overlap). Other complexities may emerge for associations and dissociations among magnitudes that occur at different stages of processing (see [36] for a distinction between input and comparison stages) and for different mental operations [35].

system limited to the big three magnitudes, or does it incorporate other dimensions such as pitch and luminance? Does cross-dimensional transfer operate primarily across visual stimuli, as used in recent studies, or does it extend across sensory modalities, as has been shown for number where infants match numerical value across vision and audition [66–68]? We turn to questions of generality in the next section.

BEYOND THE BIG THREE MAGNITUDES AND CROSS-MODAL TRANSFER

The defining feature of generalized magnitude representation is the more *vs* less ordering of unequal stimulus values. That is, for any pair of unequal values, one member of the pair always has more "stuff" and the other has less. It is this shared ordinal structure that serves as the mechanism by which magnitudes such as the big three are united and that may serve to support cross-dimensional comparisons from early in human life. Before considering how dimensions of magnitude beyond the big three might be represented by the general magnitude system, it is worth reiterating the distinction made above between magnitude and other ordinal sequences. While the more/less relations that characterize generalized magnitude representation are inherently ordered, ordinal structure can exist in the absence of magnitude. Indeed, magnitude and order are not synonymous and their relation is asymmetric, with magnitude implying order but order not implying magnitude, though this distinction can be complicated by contextual factors. Consider, for example, letters of the alphabet, for which there is a clear ordering from A to Z. Technically speaking, letters such as C and T are not characterized in terms of their more/less relations; that is, C is no more or less than T. And, yet, if considered in terms of their distances relative to some other letter (e.g., the distance between C and A is less than that between T and A) or in terms of temporal information (e.g., C comes earlier than T in the alphabet sequence), magnitude is clearly present. Existing evidence on the relation between magnitudes such as number and ordinal sequences such as letters are mixed [69–72], perhaps in part because it may be difficult to find ordinal sequences that are truly magnitude free (see Box 15.2). We thus discuss in this section only cases for which magnitude is more clearly delineated, even if the more and less ends of a continuum are not (see below).

Much of the recent research on magnitude representation has concentrated on *prothetic* dimensions [73]—those for which the polarity of more *vs* less is intrinsically determined. The big three magnitudes represent prothetic cues with a clear zero point, which marks where no magnitude exists and which may serve to unambiguously specify direction, namely, the more/less ends of a continuum. While there are countless other experiences that can be organized according to their magnitude (more/less) relations, many of these lack intrinsic polarity and have been referred to as *metathetic* dimensions [73,74]. Consider luminance—does darker or lighter gray represent the "more" end on the continuum? If luminance is defined with respect to black, the more end should be darker; if defined with respect to white, more is lighter (or "brighter"). Are such metathetic dimensions also represented by the general magnitude system? In a truly general system of magnitude representation, the lack of intrinsic polarity may have little functional impact, so long as one direction is operationally specified. Metathetic dimensions with arbitrarily imposed polarity may operate much like prothetic ones. But what about more complex stimuli for which magnitude is only one of many available cues? In this section, we distinguish between several classes of magnitude dimensions, and review recent research with adults, children, and infants demonstrating striking parallels in discriminability and cross-dimensional transfer regardless of class (see also [35,36,75]).

School-aged children (six to nine years of age) show distance effects when making judgments of relative luminosity [54], paralleling those observed in adulthood [76,77]. As with discrimination judgments of physical size, number, and duration (see above), reaction times

BOX 15.2

QUESTIONS FOR FUTURE RESEARCH

- Does language play a role in shaping the general magnitude system? There are at least two ways in which linguistic experience might affect generalized magnitude representation. One is that linguistic metaphors, which highlight directional associations (e.g., from space to time but not *vice versa*), may change initially symmetrical connections into asymmetrical ones [48]. Another possibility is that language may serve to delineate polarity for metathetic dimensions where more/less direction is not intrinsic [74,90].

- The more and less ends of the luminance continuum have been shown to vary across development; young children appear to represent darker as "more" and a significant proportion of adults represent lighter (or brighter) as "more" [74,78]. What might account for these developmental and individual differences? Does such variability extend to other metathetic dimensions?

- The dissociation between near and far space is well known [142–144], and recent research suggests that in adult humans, representations of number [145] and time [146] vary as a function of these relations. What are the developmental origins of the near/far space dissociation, and to what extent does it apply to other magnitude dimensions?

- In Western culture, the mental number line is oriented from left to right [110,111,147]. In speakers of Semitic languages such as Arabic and Hebrew, however, increasing numerical value is represented in the opposite direction,

from right to left [130,148]. This variation has been tied to reading/writing direction as well as counting practices [110,130]. Does the spatial orientation of other magnitudes (e.g., duration and emotional expression) show similar cultural variation, and does the spatial grounding of magnitude dimensions depend on culture-specific experiences?

- Siegler and colleagues suggest that whereas young children appear to represent number along a compressive scale, older children and adults rely on a linear scale [149,150]. More recent evidence, however, suggests that adults in Western culture have access to both compressive and linear scales of number, switching flexibly between the two depending on task demands [151,152]. Do other dimensions of magnitude follow similar developmental, cultural, and task-related coordination of linear and compressive scales?

- Dyscalculia (known as a mathematical learning disability) is generally regarded as a developmental deficit of numerical processing [4,153,154]. To what extent are other magnitudes processed deficiently? Is the general magnitude system sufficiently malleable to withstand and compensate for deficits in one or more dimension?

- What is the relation between generalized magnitude representation and other, non-magnitude related, ordinal sequences? Existing evidence is mixed; for example, some studies show spatial organization and neural activation of letters similar to that for number [69,70], whereas others show differentiation [71,72]. What might

---

BOX 15.2   *(cont'd)*

account for the inconsistencies? Do similarities between letters and numbers, when they exist, reflect generalized magnitude representation? Do differences reflect unique characteristics for each stimulus type?

- How does generalized magnitude representation relate to other phenomena such as synesthesia [79,155] and sound symbolism [156–159]? Do synesthetic and sound-symbolic experiences involving magnitude dimensions implicate the general magnitude system, or do they reflect unique phenomena supported by distinct conceptual and neural mechanisms (cf. [90])?

- Walsh and colleagues [15,75] suggest that associations among spatial extent, number, and time are grounded in shared relevance for action, with convergence among these dimensions having evolved for the purpose of supporting sensory-motor transformations. In contrast, Cantlon and colleagues [36] have suggested that, rather than action, these dimensions share an evolutionarily "primitive" mechanism. These different, though not necessarily incompatible, views indicate the need for future research to investigate the developmental and evolutionary origins of generalized magnitude representation.

---

are shorter, and error rates lower, as luminosity differences between stimuli increase. In addition, direct interactions between luminance and size have been reported in younger children, with both preschoolers [78] and toddlers [74] associating larger objects with darker stimuli and smaller objects with lighter ones. Interestingly, whereas adults with synesthesia employ the same mapping as that of typically-developing children [79], the pattern for typical adults is less consistent, with a significant proportion mapping "lighter" or "brighter" onto larger size [74,80], greater number [81], and longer duration [82]. Importantly, however, there appears to be within-subject stability for these mappings [74,83], suggesting that while the processing of luminance may involve the general magnitude system, the exact manner in which it is incorporated may differ across individuals.

Pitch is another dimension lacking intrinsic polarity [84]. Yet, as with luminance, existing data suggest that pitch too may be treated as generalized magnitude information. In adults, clear distance effects are found for pitch discrimination [76,85], although nonlinear patterns of discrimination have been reported for complex (musical) tones [85]. Using measures such as heart rate, sucking, and head-turning, several older studies [86–88] reported distance effects for pitch in infants; and a recent experiment confirms sensitivity to ordinal relations of pitch by showing that at six months of age, infants treat relative pitch as more salient than absolute pitch in melodies [89].

Cross-dimensional interactions between pitch and other magnitude dimensions provide more direct evidence for generalization beyond the big three. Classic work by Marks and colleagues [77,90,91] demonstrated that adults associate higher pitch with brightness, light colors, and even sharp edges; sharpness, as discussed below, can be conceptualized with respect to more/less relations. More recent research also reveals a link between pitch and vertical height in space, with adults mapping higher pitch onto "up" spatial positions (i.e.

greater height) and lower pitch onto less vertical height [92]. Evidence of early developmental origins for these mappings comes from studies with young preschoolers; two-and-a-half-year-olds, for example, expect lighter and smaller objects to produce higher pitched sounds, although the association between pitch and size appears to be less robust than that between pitch and luminance [78].

A recent study [94] revealed that by three to four months of age, infants make associations between pitch and visuospatial height as well as between pitch and pointedness (see also [93]), with congruity effects that parallel those observed in adults. Preverbal infants preferred to look at mappings between higher frequency and greater height than between higher frequency and less height; they also spent more time looking at a mapping between higher frequency and greater pointedness than between higher frequency and less pointedness (i.e. smoother object). We suggest that these mappings may reflect generalized magnitude representation. With respect to pointedness, *pointed vs smooth* represent a natural polarity imposed by constraints in the physical world. For example, if object A is less pointy than object B, then A will also be smoother than B. This implication, however, is not symmetric; if A is less smooth than B, it is not necessarily pointier; it might be, for example, full of holes. Thus, on a continuum of pointedness, pointed reflects the *more* end and smooth the *less* end, with a perfectly smooth object perhaps even considered the zero point (between concave objects on the one hand and convex ones on the other).

That higher pitch is mapped onto greater visuospatial height and greater pointedness in both infants and adults suggests that higher pitch represents the *more* end of the pitch continuum and lower pitch the *less* end. However, higher pitch has also been shown to map onto smaller size [78], suggesting that there may be combinations in which lower pitch represents the *more* end and higher pitch the *less* end. Recent research with adults confirms that whereas higher pitch maps systematically onto "more" for both height and luminance, it maps systematically onto "less" for both physical size and number [95]. Yet, so long as polarity is somehow specified and there is internal consistency, more/less relations may align across dimensions (see also [36] who propose a distinction based on the stage of processing), allowing generalized magnitude representation to accommodate flexibly to developmental changes (as with luminance) and to variation depending on the combination of dimensions (as with pitch).

Other research suggests that more complex social stimuli may also involve some processing by the general magnitude system. In adults, comparisons of relative social status are accompanied by activation in posterior parietal cortex, particularly the intraparietal sulcus (IPS) [96]—a putative neural locus of the general magnitude system [15]—similar to that reported for prothetic dimensions [80,97–100], as well as for metathetic magnitudes such as luminance [80] and pitch [101]. In children (three, five, and eight years old), recent research points to associations between facial expression and temporal processing [102], with angry faces judged as lasting longer than neutral faces, as has also been observed in adulthood [103] and having been interpreted as reflecting acceleration of an internal clock in response to heightened arousal of negatively valenced stimuli. The temporal over-estimation of angry faces is reminiscent of recent data showing that larger numbers are judged as lasting longer than smaller numbers [33,82], and we would suggest that in addition to the difference in valence, angry faces involve more emotional expression than neutral faces [104]. The effect of emotion on duration judgments may thus reflect generalized magnitude representation, with more emotional expression associated with longer duration.

Much research has concentrated on the specific pairings of spatial extent, numerical value, and temporal information, with some investigators even arguing for privileged associations, such as between space and number [65,80], space and time [64], or number and time [17,58]. Given the multitude of associations, which include metathetic dimensions and social stimuli, we suggest that generalized magnitude representation may arise from a basic organizational structure of *more vs less*, widely applicable across a variety of magnitude dimensions and modalities (and perhaps relying on shared neural resources). Even when there is an arbitrary imposition of polarity and when magnitude exists alongside other cues, cross-dimensional transfer has been observed for different classes of dimensions and at different developmental time points, suggesting a general magnitude system that extends beyond the big three and across at least visual and auditory modalities from early in human life.

While various dimensions beyond the big three may form part of the general magnitude system, it is critical to note that not all more *vs* less relations are necessarily created equal or that there is a single code for representing amount of "stuff." While conceptual and behavioral implications of more/less ordering may be functionally similar for different classes of magnitude, there will likely be unique experiential and neural processes supporting distinctions among them. Indeed, development changes for pitch and luminance (described above) are suggestive of some fundamental distinctions. One important difference is that for dimensions such as pitch there may be a translation to *more vs less stuff* that occurs with reference, or in comparison, to some other dimension (e.g., one of the big three), rather than from the perception of the specific dimension itself (cf. [105,106]). In a recent review, Bueti and Walsh [75] suggested that generalized magnitude representation likely exists as a distributed system and not a single area in, for example, the IPS. Consistent with this possibility is neural evidence showing involvement of similar parietal and frontal regions for prothetic [80,97–100], metathetic [80,101], and more complex social dimensions [96]. Cohen Kadosh and colleagues [35] recently suggested a system of overlapping and distinct populations of neurons (see also [80]). Even within the big three, it is clear that whereas some neurons code for multiple magnitude dimensions (e.g., number and length), others do not [107].

PARTICULARS OF THE GENERAL MAGNITUDE SYSTEM

In this section, we address two questions that relate to specific properties characterizing generalized magnitude representation. The first concerns the extent to which magnitude associations are symmetric so as to produce bidirectional transfer. Recent research suggests that pairings between, for example, spatial extent and time, may be asymmetric, with cross-dimensional transfer applying more strongly from space to time than *vice versa* [48,108]. The second issue concerns whether the space dimension may have a special (foundational) role as the primary grounding of the general magnitude system (see [109] for a discussion of how space may structure numerical representations). In one sense, space exists as magnitude, and spatial extent has been shown to interact from early in life with other magnitude dimensions, including number [38–41,63], duration [25,48,63], luminance [78], and pitch [94]. In another sense, however, space provides location information and may serve to mentally organize magnitude cues such as numerical value in a reliable direction [109–111].

That spatial variables such as length and distance influence duration judgments more than the reverse has been reported across development, both in adults [108] and school-aged children [48]. Asymmetrical transfer has also been documented for spatial extent and number, with physical size and cumulative surface area having a greater influence on numerical judgments than *vice versa* [29,112]. Asymmetries are consistent with theories of conceptual metaphor [113,114], which argue that abstract concepts such as number and time are structured in terms of more concrete concepts such as space. People are consequently more likely to talk (and think) about number and time using spatial terms than the reverse [108,115].

Recent findings in preverbal infants reveal bidirectional associations among spatial, numerical, and temporal cues [63]. That these associations include transfer from more "abstract" (number and duration) to more "concrete" (spatial extent) information (e.g., [65]) argues against the exclusive role of conceptual metaphor (or linguistic conflation) in creating associations, asymmetric or otherwise. Of course, another possibility is that experience with metaphor shapes initially symmetrical associations to reflect directional relations highlighted in language or experience in the physical world. This possibility, however, is at odds with accumulating evidence of bidirectional interactions over development. For space and time, greater distances are associated with longer durations, with basically symmetrical transfer; perceived distance increases as a function of temporal separation for sequentially presented stimuli (known as the *Tau effect*) and perceived duration increases as function of spatial separation (known as the *Kappa effect*) [30–32]. Furthermore, the finding that number is more likely to influence duration judgments than *vice versa* in both adults [34] and children [49] is not predicted by theories based on metaphor, since number, like temporal information, is considered an abstract experience.

Asymmetrical effects could certainly be taken as evidence against generalized magnitude representation, since one might argue that shared representations of *more vs less stuff* should not differentially affect the specific dimensions involved. This type of logic, however, can be problematic, and we would urge that investigators use other approaches to address this issue (see [35] for one possibility concerning dissociations at the level of mental operations such as arithmetic). Asymmetries within the general magnitude system could easily arise from stimulus- or task-related factors, or differences in discriminability either within or across magnitude dimensions. In the case of spatial extent, for example, there is within dimension variability, with infants appearing more sensitive to individual element size [116] than to cumulative surface area [5,9] (but see [10,11]). There are also well known "size effects," which show that discrimination sensitivity depends on the magnitude of stimulus values; holding distance across stimulus values constant, discriminability decreases with increasing magnitude. At least some variation in discriminability may also reflect earlier developmental differences and differential experience with particular stimuli. In young children, acuity for duration is worse than that for spatial extent [40,51] and number [51]. And asymmetries between space and number in preschoolers may be largely due to inexperience with symbolic notation; when non-symbolic dot arrays (instead of Arabic numerals) are used, there are clear effects of numerical information on judgments of cumulative surface area [41]. These examples illustrate that asymmetrical transfer does not itself provide evidence against generalized magnitude representation, but, rather, may reflect dimensional properties and/or developmental differences in acuity.

Accumulating evidence suggests that space may be represented in two distinct ways in the general magnitude system, as information about *where* something is and as information about *how much* there is. The focus of the discussion above was on space as magnitude, with spatial extent cues such as physical size, height, length, and distance all referring to some amount of (i.e. how much) stuff. Here we discuss space as location, with spatial information serving to organize magnitude in a consistent manner. For number, it is well documented that Western adults mentally represent increasing numerical value from left to right, the so-called "mental number line." When making parity (odd/even) judgments, adults respond faster to smaller numbers (e.g., 1 and 2) on the left side of space and to larger numbers (e.g., 8 and 9) on the right, known as the SNARC (Spatial–Numerical Association of Response Codes) effect (e.g., [110,117,118]). Other evidence for the spatial organization of number comes from research showing that numerical value biases spatial attention, with adults detecting left- and right-side targets faster following small and large number primes, respectively [111,120–122].

Recent research on the representation of duration and emotional expression suggests that space may serve a fundamental organizational role, extending beyond number to magnitude information more generally. Western adults underestimate the amount of time that stimuli remain on screen when presented on the left side of space and overestimate when on the right [123]. They are also faster (and more accurate) when responding to shorter (or earlier) durations with their left hand and to longer (or later) durations with their right [124,125]. Similar left-to-right mental organization was recently shown for emotional expression, with Western adults responding faster to faces depicting greater emotion (whether happy or angry in expression) on the right side of space and to faces depicting less emotion on the left [104,126]. The magnitude of emotional expression was even found to bias spatial attention in leftward and rightward directions on a target detection task [127], as has been shown for number (e.g., [111]). Together, these data suggest that, like number, other magnitudes may be mentally organized in a consistent spatial direction, with increasing stimulus values oriented from left to right.

Studies with children suggest that the spatial organization of number and other magnitudes emerges over development with exposure to cultural conventions such as reading/writing direction [128–130] and counting practices [131,132]. Evidence for innate spatial organization of magnitude, as perhaps predicted by hemispheric-specific lateral biases [133,134], is lacking. Initial research designed to examine the development of the mental number line used parity judgments of Arabic numerals (as has been done with adults [110]) and found that children did not appear to represent number spatially until approximately nine years of age [135]. More recent studies confirm that younger children may not access numerical value in left-to-right orientation unless more/less relations are explicitly processed [136]. With explicit magnitude judgments (e.g., "Is the target number larger than 5?"), seven-year-olds show evidence of spatially oriented numerical representations, suggesting that spatial organization supports the instantiation of magnitude and may depend on direct access to the general magnitude system.

Other recent research provides evidence that the spatial orientation of number may emerge even earlier, following experience with the counting routine. By four to five years of age, American children reliably count arrays of objects from left to right and this strategy increases reliably over the school years [131,132]. Using a location task, Opfer and colleagues [131] found that preliterate preschoolers were more accurate at finding hidden objects when the locations were labeled using number words in a left-to-right *vs* right-to-left order, suggesting that the spatial organization of number may emerge, at least in part, from experience with counting in which common practice highlights a specific orientation. Other research has revealed that this orientation may be culture specific (e.g., left-to-right for English speakers and right-to-left for Arabic speakers) and may emerge in the school years for temporal information [128].

Taken together, these findings suggest that numerical magnitude is characterized by spatial organization, and at least in Western culture, involves left-to-right orientation. The specific orientation appears to emerge in the early preschool years with exposure to counting practices, and perhaps strengthened and extending to other magnitudes (e.g., time) with increasing exposure to more general spatial-attentional experiences such as reading/writing direction [110,128,129,135,136]. In this section, we distinguished between two senses of space—space as magnitude and space as location information. The latter sense should not be confused with the former, in which more/less structure is shared with other magnitudes such as number and time. As location, space may serve to organize various types of magnitude (e.g., number, time, and emotional expression), but is not itself magnitude per se. While direct evidence on the function of spatial organization is lacking, grounding magnitude dimensions in a common mental orientation may serve to further unite the dimensions, perhaps facilitating transfer across distinct forms of perceptual inputs.

CONCLUSIONS

Why might we represent magnitude in generalized form? And why might such a system emerge so early in development? One answer is that it makes adaptive sense. Many dimensions of magnitude, especially the big three, are highly correlated in the physical world. Bigger spaces tend to hold more objects than smaller spaces, and more objects usually take more time to put away. Representing different dimensions of magnitude with a partly shared vocabulary—more *vs* less stuff—might constitute a powerful learning mechanism, allowing information from one dimension to be used in making predictions about others. It is also the case that a system of generalized magnitude representation may be highly economical both with respect to conceptual and neural resources [137,138]. In this review, we presented evidence for early-developing associations among spatial extent, number, and time, as well as for generalized magnitude representation that extends beyond the big three. Such evidence provides reason to doubt strong claims of domain-specificity for dimensions such as number and has important implications for the debate on the origins of quantitative reasoning, which presupposes that at least the big three are conceptually dissociable. While the distinctions among magnitude dimensions may be salient to researchers, they may be less so in the mind of the young child. It is possible that any continuously varying stimulus dimension will naturally be conceptualized in terms of *more vs less stuff*, even if this involves a metaphorical leap or the arbitrary and idiosyncratic delineation of polarity. Given the myriad of magnitude dimensions, however, such a system would undoubtedly need limits and it will be up to future research to uncover whether these are imposed by developmental experiences or by various conceptual and neural constraints.

Acknowledgments

This work was supported by a grant from the Eunice Kennedy Shriver National Institute of Child Health and Human Development (NICHD, HD059993) and a Scholar award from the John Merck Fund to Stella F. Lourenco.

References

[1] F. Attneave, Dimensions of similarity, Am. J. Psychol. 63 (1950) 516–556.

[2] E.Z. Rothkopf, A measure of stimulus similarity and errors in some paired-associate learning tasks, J. Exp. Psychol. 53 (1957) 94–101.

[3] R.N. Shepard, Stimulus and response generalization: tests of a model relating generalization to distance in psychological space, J. Exp. Psychol. 55 (1958) 509–523.

[4] B. Butterworth, Developmental dyscalculia, in: J.I.D. Campbell (Ed.), Handbook of Mathematical Cognition, Psychology Press, pp. 455–467.

[5] E.M. Brannon et al., Number bias for the discrimination of large visual sets in infancy, Cognition 93 (2004) B59–B68.

[6] K. Wynn, Addition and subtraction by human infants, Nature 358 (1992) 749–750.

[7] F. Xu, E.S. Spelke, Large number discrimination in 6-month-old infants, Cognition 74 (2000) B1–B11.

[8] K. McCrink, K. Wynn, Large-number addition and subtraction by 9-month-old infants, Psychol. Sci. 15 (2004) 776–781.

[9] S. Cordes, E.M. Brannon, Discrimination of continuous quantities in 6-month-old infants: using number is just easier, Child Dev. 79 (2008) 476–489.

[10] M.W. Clearfield, K.S. Mix, Number versus contour length in infants' discrimination of small visual sets, Psychol. Sci. 10 (1999) 408–411.

[11] K.S. Mix et al., Multiple cues for quantification in infancy: is number one of them? Psychol. Bull. 128 (2002) 278–294.

[12] L. Rousselle et al., Magnitude comparison in preschoolers: what counts? Influence of perceptual variables, J. Exp. Child Psychol. 87 (2004) 57–84.

[13] M.W. Clearfield, K.S. Mix, Infant use continuous quantity — not number — to discriminate small visual sets, J. Cogn. Dev. 2 (2001) 243–260.

[14] L. Feigenson et al., Infants' discrimination of number vs. continuous extent, Cogn. Psychol. 44 (2002) 33–66.

[15] V. Walsh, A theory of magnitude: common cortical metrics of time, space and quantity, Trends Cogn. Sci. 7 (2003) 483–488.

[16] C.R. Gallistel, R. Gelman, Preverbal and verbal counting and computation, Cognition 44 (1992) 43–74.

[17] W.H. Meck, R.M. Church, A mode control model of counting and timing processes, J. Exp. Psychol. Anim. Behav. Proc. 9 (1983) 320–334.

[18] S. Dehaene et al., Sources of mathematical thinking: behavioral and brain-imaging evidence, Science 284 (1999) 970–974.

[19] L. Feigenson, The equality of quantity, Trends Cogn. Sci. 11 (2007) 185–187.

[20] I. Kant, Critique of Pure Reason, Macmillan, 1787/1929.

[21] J. Locke, An Essay Concerning Human Understanding, Clarendon Press, 1690/1975.

[22] E. Mach, The Analysis of Sensations, 1886/1956.

[23] M. Critchley, The Parietal Lobes, Edward Arnold & Co., 1953.

[24] J. Piaget, The Child's Conception of Number, Routledge & Kegan Paul, 1941/1952.

[25] J. Piaget, The Child's Conception of Time, Routledge & Kegan Paul, 1946/1969.

[26] J. Piaget, B. Inhelder, The Child's Conception of Space, Routledge & Kegan Paul, 1948/1956.

[27] A. Henik, J. Tzelgov, Is three greater than five: the relation between physical and semantic size in comparison tasks, Mem. Cogn. 10 (1982) 389–395.

[28] J. Tzelgov et al., Automatic and intentional processing of numerical information, J. Exp. Psychol. Learn., Mem. Cogn. 18 (1992) 166–179.

[29] F. Hurewitz et al., Sometimes area counts more than number, Proc. Natl. Acad. Sci. USA 103 (2006) 19599–19604.

[30] J. Cohen et al., Interdependence of temporal and auditory judgments, Nature 174 (1954) 642–644.

[31] Y.L. Huang, B. Jones, On the interdependence of temporal and spatial judgments, Percept. Psychophys. 32 (1982) 7–14.

[32] J.C. Sarrazin et al., Dynamics of balancing space and time in memory: tau and kappa effects revisited, J. Exp. Psychol. Hum. Percept. Perform. 30 (2004) 411–430.

[33] M. Oliveri et al., Perceiving numbers alters time perception, Neurosci. Lett. 438 (2008) 308–311.

[34] V. Dormal et al., Numerosity-duration interference: a Stroop experiment, Acta Psychol. 121 (2006) 109–124.

[35] R. Cohen Kadosh et al., Are numbers special? An overview of chronometric, neuroimaging, developmental and comparative studies of magnitude representation, Prog. Neurobio. 84 (2008) 132–147.

[36] J.F. Cantlon et al., Beyond the number domain, Trends Cogn. Sci. 13 (2009) 83–91.

[37] R. Gelman, M.F. Tucker, Further investigations of the young child's conception of number, Child Dev. 46 (1975) 167–175.

[38] O. Rubinsten et al., The development of internal representations of magnitude and their association with Arabic numerals, J. Exp. Child Psychol. 81 (2002) 74–92.

[39] L. Girelli et al., The development of automaticity in accessing number magnitude, J. Exp. Child Psychol. 76 (2000) 104–122.

[40] X. Zhou et al., Chinese kindergartners' automatic processing of numerical magnitude in stroop-like tasks, Mem. Cogn. 35 (2007) 464–470.

[41] T. Gebuis et al., Automatic quantity processing in 5-year olds and adults, Cogn. Proc. 10 (2009) 133–142.

[42] M. Calabria, Y. Rossetti, Interference between number processing and line bisection: a methodology, Neuropsychologia 43 (2005) 779–783.

[43] M.D. de Hevia, E.S. Spelke, Spontaneous mapping of number and space in adults and young children, Cognition 110 (2009) 198–207.

[44] M.D. de Hevia et al., Numbers and space: a cognitive illusion? Exp. Brain Res. 168 (2006) 254–264.

[45] I. Levin, Interference of time-related and unrelated cues with duration comparisons of young children: analysis of Piaget's formulation of the relation of time and speed, Child Dev. 50 (1979) 469–477.

[46] R.S. Siegler, D.D. Richards, The development of speed, time, and distance concepts, Dev. Psychol. 15 (1979) 288–298.

[47] R. Stavy, D. Tirosh, How Students (Mis)-Understand Science and Mathematics, Teachers College Press, 2000.

[48] D. Casasanto et al., Space and time in the child's mind: evidence for a cross-dimensional asymmetry, Cogn. Sci. 34 (2010) 387–405.

[49] S. Droit-Volet et al., Time and number discrimination in a bisection task with a sequence of stimuli: a developmental approach, J. Exp. Child Psychol. 84 (2003) 63–76.

[50] K.S. Mix et al., Do preschool children recognize auditory–visual numerical correspondences? Child Dev. 67 (1996) 1592–1608.

[51] S. Droit-Volet et al., Time, number and length: similarities and differences in discrimination in adults and children, Quart. J. Exp. Psychol. 61 (2008) 1827–1846.

[52] J. Halberda, L. Feigenson, Developmental change in the acuity of the "number sense": the approximate number system in 3-, 4-, 5-, and 6-year-olds and adults, Dev. Psychol. 44 (2008) 1457–1465.

[53] E.M. Duncan, C.E. McFarland, Isolating the effects of symbolic distance and semantic congruity in comparative judgments: an additive-factors analysis, Mem. Cogn. 8 (1980) 612–622.

[54] I.D. Holloway, D. Ansari, Domain-specific and domain-general changes in children's development of number comparison, Dev. Sci. 11 (2008) 644–649.

[55] E.M. Brannon et al., Temporal discrimination increases in precision over development and parallels the development of numerosity discrimination, Dev. Sci. 10 (2007) 770–777.

[56] M.E. Libertus, E.M. Brannon, Stable individual differences in number discrimination in infancy, Dev. Sci. (in press).

[57] J.S. Lipton, E.S. Spelke, Origins of number sense. Large-number discrimination in human infants, Psychol. Sci. 14 (2003) 396–401.

[58] K. vanMarle, K. Wynn, Six-month-old infants use analog magnitudes to represent duration, Dev. Sci. 9 (2006) F41–F49.

[59] A.M. Brown, Development of visual sensitivity to light and color vision in human infants: a critical review, Vis. Res. 30 (1990) 1159–1188.

[60] D.J. Kelly et al., The other-race effect develops during infancy: evidence of perceptual narrowing, Psychol. Sci. 18 (2007) 1084–1089.

[61] S. Cordes, E.M. Brannon, The relative salience of discrete and continuous quantity in young infants, Dev. Sci. 12 (2009) 453–463.

[62] C.V. Buhusi, W.H. Meck, What makes us tick? Functional and neural mechanisms of interval timing, Nat. Rev. Neurosci. 6 (2005) 755–765.

[63] S.F. Lourenco, M.R. Longo, General magnitude representation in human infants, Psychol. Sci. 21 (2010) 873–881.

[64] M. Srinivasan, S. Carey, The long and the short of it: on the nature and origin of functional overlap between representations of space and time, Cognition 116 (2010) 217–241.

[65] M.D. deHevia, E.S. Spelke, Number–space mapping in human infants, Psychol. Sci. 21 (2010) 653–660.

[66] P. Starkey et al., Detection of intermodal numerical correspondences by human infants, Science 222 (1983) 179–181.

[67] K.E. Jordan, E.M. Brannon, The multisensory representation of number in infancy, Proc. Natl. Acad. Sci. USA. 103 (2006) 3486–3489.

[68] V. Izard et al., Newborn infants perceive abstract numbers, Proc. Natl. Acad. Sci. USA. 106 (2009) 10382–10385.

[69] W. Fias et al., Processing of abstract ordinal knowledge in the horizontal segment of the intraparietal sulcus, J. Neurosci. 27 (2007) 8952–8956.

[70] W. Gevers et al., The mental representation of ordinal sequences is spatially organized, Cognition 87 (2003) B87–B95.

[71] E. Turconi et al., Electrophysiological evidence for differential processing of numerical quantity and order in humans, Cogn. Brain Res. 21 (2004) 22–38.

[72] M. Zorzi et al., The spatial representation of numerical and non-numerical sequences: evidence from neglect, Neuropsychologia 44 (2006) 1061–1067.

[73] S.S. Stevens, On the psychophysical law, Psychol. Rev. 64 (1957) 153–181.

[74] L.B. Smith, M.D. Sera, A developmental analysis of the polar structure of dimensions, Cogn. Psychol. 24 (1992) 99–142.

[75] D. Bueti, V. Walsh, The parietal cortex and the representation of time, space, number and other magnitudes., Philos. Trans. R. Soc. Lond., B 364 (2009) 1831–1840.

[76] R.N. Shepard, Toward a universal law of generalization for psychological science, Science 237 (1987) 1317–1323.

[77] J.C. Stevens, L.E. Marks, Cross-modality matching of brightness and loudness, Proc. Natl. Acad. Sci. USA. 54 (1965) 407–411.

[78] C. Mondloch, D. Maurer, Do small white balls squeak? Pitch-object correspondences in young children, Cogn. Affect. Behav. Neurosci. 4 (2004) 133–136.

[79] R. Cohen Kadosh et al., Small is bright and big is dark in synaesthesia, Curr. Biol. 17 (2007) R834–R835.

[80] P. Pinel et al., Distributed and overlapping cerebral representations of number, size, and luminance during comparative judgments, Neuron 41 (2004) 983–993.

[81] R. Cohen Kadosh et al., When brightness counts: the neuronal correlate of numerical–luminance interference, Cereb. Cortex 18 (2008) 337–343.

[82] B. Xuan et al., Larger stimuli are judged to last longer, J. Vis. 7 (10) (2007) 2.

[83] R. Cohen Kadosh, A. Henik, A common representation for semantic and physical properties: a cognitive–anatomical approach, Exp. Psychol. 53 (2006) 87–94.

[84] S.S. Stevens et al., A scale for the measurement of the psychological magnitude of pitch, J. Acoust. Soc. Am. 8 (1937) 185–190.

[85] R. Cohen Kadosh et al., Mental representation: what can pitch tell us about the distance effect? Cortex 44 (2008) 470–477.

[86] W.K. Berg, Habituation and dishabituation of cardiac responses in 4-month-old, alert infants, J. Exp. Child Psychol. 14 (1972) 92–107.

[87] L.W. Olsho et al., Preliminary data on frequency discrimination in infancy, J. Acoust. Soc. Am. 71 (1982) 509–511.

[88] S.J. Wormith et al., Frequency discrimination by young infants, Child Dev. 46 (1975) 272–275.

[89] J. Plantinga, L.J. Trainor, Memory for melody: infants use a relative pitch code, Cognition 98 (2005) 1–11.

[90] L.E. Marks, Bright sneezes and dark coughs, loud sunlight and soft moonlight, J. Exp. Psychol. Hum. Percept. Perform. 8 (1982) 177–193.

[91] L.E. Marks, On cross-modal similarity: the perceptual structure of pitch, loudness, and brightness, J. Exp. Psychol. Hum. Percept. Perform. 15 (1989) 586–602.

[92] E. Rusconi et al., Spatial representation of pitch height: the SMARC effect, Cognition 99 (2006) 113–129.

[93] D.J. Lewkowicz, G. Turkewitz, Intersensory interaction in newborns: modification of visual preferences following exposure to sound, Child Dev. 52 (1981) 827–832.

[94] P. Walker et al., Preverbal infants' sensitivity to synaesthetic cross-modality correspondences, Psychol. Sci. 21 (2010) 21–25.

[95] Z. Eitan, R. Timmers, Beethoven's last piano sonata and those who follow crocodiles: cross-domain mappings of auditory pitch in a musical context, Cognition 114 (2010) 405–422.

[96] J.Y. Chiao et al., Neural representations of social status hierarchy in human inferior parietal cortex, Neuropsychologia 47 (2009) 354–363.

[97] E. Eger et al., A supramodal number representation in human intraparietal cortex, Neuron 37 (2003) 719–725.

[98] P. Maquet et al., Brain activation induced by estimation of duration: a PET study, NeuroImage 3 (1996) 119–126.

[99] M. Piazza et al., Tuning curves for approximate numerosity in the human intraparietal sulcus, Neuron 44 (2004) 547–555.

[100] M. Piazza et al., A magnitude code common to numerosities and number symbols in human intraparietal cortex, Neuron 53 (2007) 293–305.

[101] N.E. Foster, R.J. Zatorre, A role for the intraparietal sulcus in transforming musical pitch information, Cereb. Cortex 20 (2010) 1350–1359.

[102] S. Gil et al., Anger and time perception in children, Emotion 7 (2007) 219–225.

[103] S. Droit-Volet et al., Perception of the duration of emotional events, Cogn. Emot. 18 (2004) 849–858.

[104] K.J. Holmes, S.F. Lourenco, Spatial organization of magnitude in the representation of number and emotion, in: N.A. Taatgen, H. van Rijn (Eds.), Proceedings of the 31st Annual Conference of the Cognitive Science Society, Cognitive Science Society, pp. 2402–2407.

[105] K.J. Holyoak, W.A. Mah, Semantic congruity in symbolic comparisons: evidence against an expectancy hypothesis, Mem. Cogn. 9 (1981) 197–204.

[106] W.P. Banks et al., Semantic congruity and expectancy in symbolic judgments, J. Exp. Psychol. Hum. Percept. Perform. 9 (1983) 560–582.

[107] O. Tudusciuc, A. Nieder, Neuronal population coding of continuous and discrete quantity in the primate posterior parietal cortex, Proc. Natl. Acad. Sci. USA 104 (2007) 14513–14518.

[108] D. Casasanto, L. Boroditsky, Time in the mind: using space to think about time, Cognition 106 (2008) 579–593.

[109] E.M. Hubbard et al., Interactions between number and space in parietal cortex, Nat. Rev. Neurosci. 6 (2005) 435–448.

[110] S. Dehaene et al., The mental representation of parity and number magnitude, J. Exp. Psychol. Gen. 122 (1993) 371–396.

[111] M.H. Fischer et al., Perceiving numbers causes spatial shifts of attention, Nat. Neurosci. 6 (2003) 555–556.

[112] V. Dormal, M. Pesenti, Numerosity–length interference: a Stroop experiment, Exp. Psychol. 54 (2007) 289–297.

[113] G. Lakoff, M. Johnson, Metaphors We Live By, University of Chicago Press, 1980.

[114] G. Lakoff, R. Núñez, Where Mathematics Comes from: How the Embodied Mind Brings Mathematics into Being, Basic Books, 2000.

[115] L. Boroditsky, Metaphoric structuring: understanding time through spatial metaphors, Cognition 75 (2000) 1–28.

[116] E.M. Brannon et al., The development of area discrimination and its implications for number representation in infancy, Dev. Sci. 9 (2006) F59–F64.

[117] J. Castronovo, X. Seron, Semantic numerical representation in blind subjects: the role of vision in the spatial format of the mental number line, Quart. J. Exp. Psychol. 60 (2007) 101–119.

[118] H.C. Nuerk et al., The universal SNARC effect: the association between number magnitude and space is amodal, Exp. Psychol. 52 (2005) 187–194.

[119] W. Fias et al., Parietal representation of symbolic and nonsymbolic magnitude, J. Cogn. Neurosci. 15 (2003) 47–56.

[120] M. Ranzini et al., Neural mechanisms of attentional shifts due to irrelevant spatial and numerical cues, Neuropsychologia 47 (2009) 2615–2624.

[121] G. Galfano et al., Number magnitude orients attention, but not against one's will, Psych. Bull. Rev. 13 (2006) 869–874.

[122] J. Ristic et al., The number line effect reflects top-down control, Psych. Bull. Rev. 13 (2006) 862–868.

[123] C.M. Vicario et al., Relativistic compression and expansion of experiential time in the left and right space, PLoS One 3 (2008) e1716.

[124] M. Ishihara et al., Horizontal spatial representations of time: evidence for the STEARC effect, Cortex 44 (2008) 454–461.

[125] A. Vallesi et al., An effect of spatial–temporal association of response codes: understanding the cognitive representations of time, Cognition 107 (2008) 501–527.

[126] K.J. Holmes, S.F. Lourenco, Emotional expression, like number, is mentally organized in left-to-right orientation, (under review).

[127] S.F. Lourenco, K.J. Holmes, The magnitude of emotional expression biases spatial attention, (under review).

[128] B. Tversky et al., Cross-cultural and developmental trends in graphic productions, Cogn. Psychol. 23 (1991) 515–557.

[129] S. Zebian, Linkages between number concepts, spatial thinking, and directionality of writing: the SNARC effect and the reverse SNARC effect in English and Arabic monoliterates, biliterates, and illiterate Arabic speakers, J. Cogn. Cult. 5 (2005) 165–190.

[130] S. Shaki, M.H. Fischer, Reading space into numbers: a cross-linguistic comparison of the SNARC effect, Cognition 108 (2008) 590–599.

[131] J.E. Opfer et al., Early development of spatial–numeric associations: evidence from spatial and quantitative performance of preschoolers, Dev. Sci. 13 (2010) 761–771.

[132] D. Briars, R.S. Siegler, A featural analysis of preschoolers' counting knowledge, Dev. Psychol. 20 (1984) 607–618.

[133] G. Geminiani et al., Analogical representation and language structure, Neuropsychologia 33 (1995) 1565–1574.

[134] B. Landau, Multiple geometric representations of objects in languages and language learners, in: P. Bloom, et al. (Ed.), Language and Space, MIT Press, pp. 317–363.

[135] D.B. Berch et al., Extracting parity and magnitude from Arabic numerals: developmental changes in number processing and mental representation, J. Exp. Child Psychol. 74 (1999) 286–308.

[136] M.S. Van Galen, P. Reitsma, Developing access to number magnitude: a study of the SNARC effect in 7- to 9-year-olds, J. Exp. Child Psychol. 101 (2008) 99–113.

[137] S. Dehaene, Evolution of human cortical circuits for reading and arithmetic: the neuronal recycling hypothesis, in: S. Dehaene, et al., (Ed.), From Monkey Brain to Human Brain, MIT Press, pp. 133–157.

[138] S. Dehaene, L. Cohen, Cultural recycling of cortical maps, Neuron 56 (2007) 384–398.

[139] D. Gentner, Metaphor as structure mapping: the relational shift, Child Dev. 59 (1988) 47–59.

[140] J.J. Gibson, E.J. Gibson, Perceptual learning; differentiation or enrichment? Psychol. Rev. 62 (1955) 32–41.

[141] M.H. Johnson, Functional brain development in humans, Nat. Rev. Neurosci. 2 (2001) 475–483.

[142] W.R. Brain, Visual disorientation with special reference to lesions of the right cerebral hemisphere, Brain 64 (1941) 244–272.

[143] P.W. Halligan, J.C. Marshall, Left neglect for near but not far space in man, Nature 350 (1991) 498–500.

[144] M.R. Longo, S.F. Lourenco, On the nature of near space: effects of tool use and the transition to far space, Neuropsychologia 44 (2006) 977–981.

[145] M.R. Longo, S.F. Lourenco, Bisecting the mental number line in near and far space, Brain Cogn. 72 (2010) 362–367.

[146] P. Zäch, P. Brugger, Subjective time in near and far representational space, Cogn. Behav. Neurol. 21 (2008) 8–13.

[147] M.R. Longo, S.F. Lourenco, Spatial attention and the mental number line: evidence for characteristic biases and compression, Neuropsychologia 45 (2007) 1400–1407.

[148] S. Shaki et al., Reading habits for both words and numbers contribute to the SNARC effect, Psych. Bull. Rev. 16 (2009) 328–331.

[149] R.S. Siegler, J.E. Opfer, The development of numerical estimation: evidence for multiple representations of numerical quantity, Psychol. Sci. 14 (2003) 237–243.

[150] R.S. Siegler, J.L. Booth, Development of numerical estimation in young children, Child Dev. 75 (2004) 428–444.

[151] S.F. Lourenco, M.R. Longo, Multiple spatial representations of number: evidence for co-existing compressive and linear scales, Exp. Brain Res. 193 (2009) 151–156.

[152] A. Viarouge, et al., Number line compression and the illusory perception of random numbers, Exp. Psychol. (in press).

[153] T. Iuculano et al., Core information processing deficits in developmental dyscalculia and low numeracy, Dev. Sci. 11 (2008) 669–680.

[154] M. Piazza et al., Developmental trajectory of number acuity reveals a severe impairment in developmental dyscalculia, Cognition 116 (2010) 33–41.

[155] E.M. Hubbard et al., What information is critical to elicit interference in number–form synaesthesia? Cortex 45 (2009) 1200–1216.

[156] E. Sapir, A study in phonetic symbolism, J. Exp. Psychol. 12 (1929) 225–239.

[157] W. Köhler, Gestalt Psychology, second ed., Liveright, 1929/1949.

[158] L.C. Nygaard et al., Sound to meaning correspondences facilitate word learning, Cognition 112 (2009) 181–186.

[159] V. Kovic et al., The shape of words in the brain, Cognition 114 (2010) 19–28.

REPRESENTATIONAL CHANGE AND EDUCATION

Introduction, by Elizabeth M. Brannon

The quantification of space, time, and number allows human civilizations to build airplanes, construct atlases of the world, create economies, and model the future. Since Socrates and Plato, philosophers have pondered where such abstract and intangible concepts come from, and whether nature or nurture is more dominant in their emergence. To fully understand the human mind it is necessary to explore the developmental building blocks of human cognition and how thought changes over development. Only with a developmental perspective can we come to understand which aspects of cognition are universal and which are products of education and culture. The last section of this book explores the development of concepts of space, time and number and how education and language transform these foundational intuitions. Some of the authors focus on specifying the preverbal building blocks of adult cognition by asking how the infant mind is predisposed to view the spatial, temporal and numerical aspects of the world and others ask how these initial intuitions are transformed over development into adult conceptions.

Manuella Piazza, **Elizabeth Spelke**, and **Brian Butterworth** each flesh out a unique position on how preverbal numerical concepts give rise to symbolic mathematical abilities. **Piazza** offers us an account by which the approximate number system (ANS) serves as the foundation for constructing symbolic numerical thinking. She argues against Susan Carey's influential proposal that object file representations function as the critical substrate for children to begin to make meaning of the integer list. A central argument, for Piazza, is that vestiges of the ANS can be seen in symbolic number judgments in children and adults, long after children learn the meaning of number words. She argues that, in contrast, there are no traces

245

of the limitations of the object file system in numerical judgments beyond infancy.

Butterworth approaches the question of the foundations of symbolic number from the lens of clinical disorder. He asks whether dyscalculia, a specific learning disability in math, reflects a deficiency in a core system for representing number. Butterworth argues that the foundational system for arithmetic that is damaged in dyscalculics consists of a numerosity coding scheme whereby each value is represented as a set of discrete individuals. This system allows precision akin to the object-file system but it is not limited in its capacity. Butterworth contends that the ANS is inadequate as a foundational capacity for arithmetic learning because it cannot support precise arithmetic and that object-files are inadequate because they are by definition unordered and limited in capacity. He argues that dyscalculic data are largely consistent with an impairment in numerosity coding in that dyscalculics have difficulty with enumeration, addition, and finger arithmetic.

Finally, **Spelke** proposes that the critical ingredient for children's conceptual change in the domains of space and number is the integration of two core systems within each domain. In the case of number, Spelke turns to Karen Wynn's classic finding that children slowly learn the first few number words and their mapping to numerosities, but that somewhere around age 3.5 or 4 years the child makes an induction and comes to comprehend the meaning of all the numbers in their count list. For Spelke, it is language that allows children to integrate their two core number systems. As the child comes to understand that object-file representations $(1 + 1 + 1)$ and approximate number representations (~3) map onto the same words this allows them to grasp the successor principle and complete the mapping of ANS representations onto all the words within their number list.

In the case of natural geometry Spelke similarly argues that there are two core systems. One allows us to navigate and use the geometry of the world to reorient in space. The second system represents the shapes of 2D visual forms and moveable objects and captures the relations between length and angle that are invariant over changes in size. The important thesis offered by Spelke is that language is the catalyst that integrates the core systems within each domain and allows conceptual change and the emergence of human-specific culturally dependent systems of knowledge.

Veronique Izard, Pierre Pica, Stanislas Dehaene, Danielle Hinchey and **Elizabeth Spelke** expand upon one of the two core systems of geometry, that which is dedicated to representing small manipulable objects and 2D displays. The paper describes experiments with the Munduruku of Amazonian Brazil, and illustrates how relative length and angle, in contrast to sense, seem to have a privileged status in form perception. The paper also explores how more abstract geometrical concepts such as infinite lines or parallelism seem to be universal cross-culturally but nevertheless likely to be dependent on education.

While language is Spelke's catalyst for representational change, it shapes cognition in a more direct sense for **Lera Boroditsky**. Boroditsky argues that we construct representations of abstract domains like time by using concrete dimensions such as space. She shows us how the language we speak and the metaphors we use influence both our verbal and nonverbal perceptions of time. In one dramatic example, the Pormpuraaw languages of aboriginal Australia appear to be void of relational spatial terms such as left and right and instead rely on absolute directional terms such as "the boy is a little west of the fire." Her work illustrates how even fundamental abstractions such as time and space can be dramatically shaped by culture and language.

Finally, **Robert Siegler**'s paper is representative of a field of research that asks whether early educational interventions can have lasting influences on children's mathematical abilities. His work suggests that an intervention that helps construct linear representations of number can boost early numerical knowledge and help close the achievement gap between low and high-income children. He provides dramatic evidence that playing board games with linear number lines has positive and lasting consequences for young children's number concepts.

Of necessity we limited the scope of our conference and book and thus were unable to cover the myriad of other interactions between culture, education and the representations of space, time and number that are exemplified by the work of scholars such as Rochel Gelman, John Anderson, and Martha Alibali. Work by these researchers and many others demonstrates the tremendous representational challenges children face in learning to represent rational numbers as fractions, learning to solve algebraic equations and the variety of strategies that children attempt as they move through the educational system. Although work presented in and outside this book shows how culture and education can transform representations of space, time and number it also shows how the fundamental magnitude representations described by Charles R. Gallistel in the very first chapter of this book, continue to support our quantitative mind throughout the lifespan.

Foundational Numerical Capacities and the Origins of Dyscalculia*

Brian Butterworth

Institute of Cognitive Neuroscience, University College London, London, UK

Summary

One important cause of very low attainment in arithmetic (dyscalculia) appears to be a core deficit in an inherited foundational capacity for numbers. According to one set of hypotheses, arithmetic is built on an inherited system responsible for representing approximate numerosities (ANS). On one account, this is supported by a system for representing exactly a small number (≤ 4) of individual objects. For these approaches, the core deficit in dyscalculia lies in either of these systems. An alternative proposal holds that the deficit lies in an inherited system for sets of objects and operations on them (Numerosity Coding), on which arithmetic is built. I argue that a deficit in Numerosity Coding, not in the ANS or the small number system, is responsible for dyscalculia. Nevertheless, the critical tests will involve both longitudinal studies and intervention, and these have yet to be carried out.

WHY ARE PEOPLE BAD AT LEARNING ARITHMETIC?

Low numeracy is a serious handicap for individuals and a major cost for nations (see [1] for relevant data in the United Kingdom). It makes individuals less employable, is a risk of depression in adulthood, and lowers lifetime earnings significantly. In the United Kingdom about 25% of adults have poor functional numeracy [2]. Low arithmetical attainment has

*Reprinted from Trends in Cognitive Sciences, Vol 14, Brian Butterworth, Foundational numerical capacities and the origins of dyscalculia, pg 534–541, 2010, with permission from Elsevier.

BOX 16.1

FACTORS ASSOCIATED WITH POOR ARITHMETICAL LEARNING

The available evidence suggests that there are several factors underlying low numeracy. For example, low socio-economic status, minority ethnic status, and gender can all be associated with lower mathematics attainment (see [87] for a review). Although it is difficult to assess the role of poor or inappropriate teaching, the fact that the introduction of detailed new national primary school strategy for numeracy in the UK has had only a minor and possibly non-significant effect on numeracy for the studied group is indicative [1]. Even relatively simple tasks, that depend relatively little on the quality of educational experience, such as comparing the magnitudes of two single-digit numbers, or enumerating a small array of objects, show wide variation (see [13,14] for reviews).

This evidence suggests that individual cognitive characteristics play a major role in variation in individual attainment. For example, there is evidence to suggest that IQ and working memory contribute to arithmetical attainment [10]. In fact, the usual definitions of dyscalculia (or equivalent constructs) use a discrepancy between arithmetical attainment and IQ as a criterion (see Table 16.2 and [7]).

Many authors, but most influentially Piaget, have argued that understanding concepts of number and arithmetic are premised on general cognitive abilities, especially reasoning with class inclusion, transitive inference and quantitative seriation, and the way the child applies reasoning to interactions with the environment [31]. More recently, Gardner coupled arithmetic with logic into one out of seven types of intelligence (termed "Logical–mathematical") [88]. On this approach, difficulties or disabilities in learning arithmetic would necessarily be associated with difficulties or disabilities in reasoning and cognitive domains that support it, including, presumably, working memory. More strongly, if these domain-general capacities are sufficient to learn arithmetic, then the prediction would be that dyscalculics will all have a deficit in a domain-general ability. However, the data presented in the main text argue strongly against this conclusion.

been attributed in the past to a deficit in general cognitive abilities such as working memory [3] and executive function [4], and there is evidence that these factors do affect arithmetical learning as well as scholastic attainment more generally [3]. Many social and cognitive factors are known to affect arithmetic learning (see Box 16.1). This means that the presenting symptoms can be very varied, and the underlying causes difficult to identify.

Arithmetical difficulties and disabilities frequently co-occur with other developmental disorders, especially reading and digit span deficits and Attention Deficit Hyperactivity Disorder (for a recent review, see [5]). Individuals seriously affected, those classified with "developmental dyscalculia" [6] or "mathematics learning disability" [7] (see Table 16.1), which both identify the same construct, have a modal prevalence of about 6.5% [8].

Several strands of recent evidence argue that very low arithmetical attainment can be an isolated deficit. For instance, several studies have found it in learners matched for IQ

TABLE 16.1 Definitions of Dyscalculia and Equivalent Constructs

DSM-IV [84]	**Mathematics disability**. The child must substantially underachieve on a standardized test relative to the level expected given age, education, and intelligence and must experience disruption to academic achievement or daily living
International Classification of Diseases—10 [85]	**Specific disorder of arithmetical skills**. A specific impairment in arithmetical skills that is not solely explicable on the basis of general mental retardation or of inadequate schooling.
Department for Education and Skills UK [86]	**Dyscalculia**. A condition that affects the ability to acquire arithmetical skills. Dyscalculic learners may have difficulty understanding simple number concepts, lack an intuitive grasp of numbers, and have problems learning number facts and procedures. Even if they produce a correct answer or use a correct method, they may do so mechanically and without confidence

and working memory [9]. Recent evidence suggests that factors specific to the domain of numbers and arithmetic make a major independent contribution to low arithmetical attainment. In a longitudinal study by Geary and colleagues, tests of understanding the numerosity of sets and of estimating the position of a number on a number line, are two important predictors of "Low Achieving" in mathematics, affecting some 50% of the sample, and "Mathematics Learning Disability", affecting about 7% of the sample [10]. Kovas and colleagues, in a sample of 1500 pairs of monozygotic and 1375 pairs of dizygotic seven-year-old twins, found in multivariate genetic analysis that about 30% of the genetic variance was specific to mathematics [11]. In a study of the first degree relatives of dyslexic probands, a principal component analysis revealed that numerical abilities constituted a separate factor, with reading-related and naming-related being the two other principal components [12].

Taken together, these studies raise the possibility that difficulties and disabilities in learning arithmetic could arise from a selective impairment in a domain-specific capacity. Indeed, recent reviews have proposed that developmental dyscalculia follows from a "core deficit" in this domain-specific capacity [5,6,9,13,14].

DOMAIN-SPECIFIC FOUNDATIONAL CAPACITIES FOR ARITHMETIC

Here I briefly outline proposals for a domain-specific capacity for numbers, before discussing whether this capacity is foundational for acquiring arithmetic.

A foundational capacity for numbers is revealed in human infants' ability to discriminate on the basis of the numerosity of a display (e.g., [15]) and to match numerosities across modalities (e.g., [16]), which suggests that the capacity is not tied to one modality and implies a relatively abstract understanding of numerosity.

There is also extensive evidence from converging sources of specialized neural networks for numerical processing and calculation. Neurological damage has identified the left parietal lobe as a critical area in calculation, in particular, the left angular gyrus [17]. There is also evidence from case studies that the right parietal lobe is specifically involved in rapid enumeration [18]. Novel arithmetical problems, word problems, and reasoning about arithmetic involve the prefrontal cortex [19]. Functional neuroimaging confirms a role for the left

TABLE 16.2   Typical Development of Whole Number Competencies in Arithmetic

Age	Typical study
0;0	Can discriminate on the basis of small numerosities
0;4	Can add and subtract one
0;11	Discriminates increasing from decreasing sequences of numerosities
2;0	Begins to learn sequence of counting words
	Can do one-to-one correspondence in a sharing task
2;6	Recognizes that number words mean more than one ("grabber")
3;0	Counts out small numbers of objects
	Can recognize transformations that affect number
3;6	Can use the cardinality principle to establish numerosity of set
4;0	Can use fingers to aid adding
5;0	Can add small numbers without being able to count out sum
5;6	Understands commutativity of addition
6;0	Piagetian "Conservation of number"
6;6	Understands complementarity of addition and subtraction
7;0	Retrieves some arithmetical facts from memory

(After [29].)

angular gyrus in calculation (see [20] for a review), especially for the retrieval of arithmetical facts [21], while simple number tasks, such as magnitude comparison, typically show a bilateral intraparietal sulcus (IPS) implementation (e.g., [20,22–24]). Simple enumeration is frequently found most prominently in the right IPS (rIPS) [25].

The existence of specialized neural networks for numerical processing is perhaps most clearly revealed in primate studies showing that number-related neural activity in monkeys carrying out numerical tasks occurs in brain networks homologous to those activated in humans carrying out similar tasks (see [26] for a review).

To be foundational, representations of numbers must be able to enter into arithmetical operations. Formally, arithmetic is interpretable in terms of manipulations on sets [27,28], and much of early learning is based on physically manipulating sets of objects (see [29] for a review). Therefore, representations have to be able to enter into set-based operation. This will involve both number-abstraction (that is, the capacity to represent the numerosity of a set) from number-reasoning (that is, the capacity to deploy number representations in arithmetical operations) [30]. The typical development of arithmetical competencies for whole numbers is given in Table 16.2. Therefore, the relevant foundational capacities must be able to represent numerosities of sets abstractly (independently of the properties of the objects in the set) and must be able to carry out arithmetical operations upon them—specifically, the standard school operations of adding, subtracting, multiplying and dividing. Of course, arithmetic, even in primary school (K-6) involves fractions and decimals as well as whole number.

As preconditions, foundational capacities for number reasoning must be able to establish the numerical equivalence or non-equivalence of two sets through one-to-one correspondence, and to distinguish transformations that do and do not affect numerosity. These requirements, already prefigured by Piaget [31], constitute benchmarks against which to evaluate theoretical accounts of the foundational capacities supporting the development of arithmetic.

THE APPROXIMATE NUMBER SYSTEM

While there is little doubt that we share with many nonhuman species a system for estimating and comparing approximate numerosities [26,32], it remains to be clarified what role this system plays in the development of arithmetic. The Approximate Number System (ANS) is one system of "core knowledge" of numbers [32]. According to this approach, number-abstraction processes extract some kind of "summary statistics" from a scene (which, in principle, could be in a modality other than visual) that is separate from the processes implicated in analog quantity estimation (how many objects *vs* how much stuff), but is nevertheless mapped onto analog magnitude representations.

The strongest claim is that "this nonverbal quantification system seems to constitute the phylogenetic and ontogenetic foundation of all further, more elaborate numerical skills" ([26], p.186), which presumably includes arithmetic. In a number of studies, Spelke and colleagues have correlated children's performances on tasks involving approximate arithmetic with tasks involving symbolic arithmetic. The method used to assess the functioning of the ANS is typically non-symbolic number comparison, where the larger of two random arrays of objects, dots or squares systematically varied for area, is selected. Either the accuracy of the response, or its speed, is used to determine individual "numerical acuity". These scores are then correlated with performance on symbolic tasks [33]. Recent studies report a correlation between numerical acuity and mathematics attainment [34,35] (see also Chapter 17 in this volume).

However, there are problems with ANS as a foundational capacity for arithmetic learning. First, the ANS system is primarily concerned with number-abstraction, and not at all with number reasoning. It is unclear how approximate numerosities, or their analog representations, satisfy the two basic preconditions of arithmetical reasoning (see above). First, one-to-one correspondence cannot be carried out with approximate sets to establish their equality or inequality. Second, the effects of different types of transformations cannot be determined on approximate sets. Therefore, adding one or subtracting one may not be detectable. In any event, the idea that these transformations should affect numerosity cannot be captured by this kind of representation. On the other hand, transformations that do not affect numerosity may well affect estimations or judgments made by the ANS. It is known, for example, that the nature of the objects to be enumerated [36] and their visual crowding reduces accuracy of numerical estimation [37]. A third problem is that approximate numerosities are held to be represented logarithmically [38], hence making the use of this representation in addition and subtraction problematic.

A main prediction from the ANS hypothesis is that dyscalculics will have a deficit in approximate number tasks. ANS theory implies that approximate numerosities and symbolic numbers (e.g., 8 and eight) are mapped onto an analog magnitude system that supports number comparison tasks. Thus, symbolic number comparison performance should index underlying numerical representations, and hence a foundational capacity relevant to arithmetical capability.

Recent studies have correlated ability to discriminate approximate numerosities with low arithmetical attainment (e.g., [33–35]). On the other hand, some research has failed to find this association. For example, approximate numerosity comparison did not discriminate typical from low-numeracy seven-year-olds [39], six- to eight-year-olds [40], or nine-year-olds [41]. However, it is worth noting that symbolic number comparison using digits rather than arrays of objects *is* associated with arithmetical performance in children of six to eight years [40].

In any event, correlations, as we know, are not the cause, and it is unclear whether poor performance on ANS tasks is the cause or the consequence of poor arithmetical abilities. It is at least plausible that more work with numbers will lead to both a better performance on number comparison tasks and a better performance on arithmetic. It is worth noting that better counting skills are correlated with better *approximate* estimation [42]: again more number work may lead to improvements in many areas of number skills.

THE SMALL NUMEROSITY SYSTEM

Arithmetic is about exact numbers, and to be foundational, representations of exact numbers need to be developed. How do approximate representations (of the type the ANS hypothesis proposes) develop into the sequence of numerosities, each with a unique successor?

One possibility is to exploit our ability to represent small numerosities without serial enumeration and with a high degree of precision; this is called "subitizing" (for a review, see [43]; but see [44]). It has therefore been proposed that the perceptual system underlying subitizing that keeps track of a small number (≤ 4) of individual objects [45] can have "numerical content" [46]. The argument is that there are distinct states of this system for individuating 1, 2, 3, or 4 objects [46]. This enables inference about adding or subtracting 1, 2, or 3 objects. Given that each state is distinct, the child will learn that distinct states of the system are associated with distinct number words: "one" with one object, "two" with two objects, "three" with three objects [46].

Carey uses the concept of "bootstrapping" (a form of induction), so that a child infers from what she knows about the small numbers to large numbers [46]. Thus when she hears "five" in a numerical context, and the approximate numerosity of *about fiveness* is active, she will figure out that the word must refer to an exact numerosity—like one, two, three, and four—and therefore conclude that the word "five" refers not to approximately five but to exactly five (see [47,48] for assessments of this argument).

Recently Carey and colleagues have introduced a new notion called "Enhanced parallel individuation", where the contents of the small number system are treated as a set [49]. This process is called "set based quantification", and is charged with enabling the set-based properties of arithmetic to be carried out. This appears to go beyond the two core systems of ANS plus the small number system by introducing a third core system for both number abstraction and number reasoning that are not available in the former.

A main prediction arising from bootstrapping is that dyscalculics will suffer from a deficit in the subitizing range. Although there is some evidence that the small number system is impaired in dyscalculic learners, typically, enumerating the entire range from 1 to 9 is also impaired [9]. Even if a selective deficit in small numerosities is observed in dyscalculics and others with delayed counting and arithmetic, this may be because subitizing enables early counters to check the result of their counting [50,51].

A second prediction from the small number hypothesis is that language impairments will affect number vocabulary which, in turn, should affect the development of exact number concepts. However, studies of children with Specific Language Impairment (SLI) suggest that they are unimpaired on number comparison and tasks of numerical estimation [52]. Even more strikingly, they outperform learners matched for language-matched controls on nonverbal number tasks [53], suggesting that the grasp of the counting word sequence, on which they are generally poorer, is not the main driver of magnitude representation. However, they perform more poorly on many arithmetical tasks that depend on fact retrieval and more complex arithmetical procedures (see [54] for a review).

NUMEROSITY CODING

Piaget, maintained that "the concept of number" by which he meant cardinal number, is based on sets [31]. However, he thought that conservation of number under numerosity-irrelevant transformations, was only possible at about the age of four years when a particular stage in logical reasoning had been reached [31].

Since then, many studies have indicated that human infants can use the numerosity of visual arrays as a discriminative stimulus (e.g., [15]). Moreover, infants can select collections of objects and treat them as a single unit [55,56]. These findings suggest that the idea of treating a collection of objects as a set may be present early in ontogeny. What this would mean is that a set can be the kind of object that can itself take a property. This property need not be something common to the objects in the set, but could be a property of the set itself. One such property is its numerosity (a psychological way of talking about the logical concept of cardinality). Studies of infant behavior suggest that these properties can be intermodal and therefore relatively abstract in the sense that the property of a set (e.g., *eightness*) is not the property of any member of the set [16,57].

The hypothesis that humans inherit a capacity to quantify over sets is not new. This was essentially the proposal of Gelman and Gallistel in 1978 [30], who hypothesized that precounting children, like many other species, possess "numerons", an ordered sequence of numerosity concepts—e.g., the numeron for *one*, the numeron for *two* and so on. Learning to count is essentially a developmental process of learning to associate an ordered sequence of counting words with an ordered sequence of numerons. The concept of *fiveness* pre-exists acquiring the knowledge that the word "five" refers to the numerosity *fiveness*.

More recently, Halberda and Feigenson have suggested that the "concept set is required and that this notion cannot come from object tracking, the approximate number system, or language ... Conceiving of a set requires representing the hierarchical relationship between individual items and the larger structure into which they are bound" ([58], p. 655). There is also evidence showing that numerosity processing in the brain is distinct from the processing of continuous quantity, and that the numerosity of sets of objects distributed in time are processed by the same mechanisms as sets distributed in space [59].

This conceptualization has been captured in a neural network model called the "numerosity code" [60,61]. The idea here is that mental representation of numerosities is a discrete set of neuron-like elements. Metaphorically, *oneness* is represented by one element, *twoness* by two elements, and so on (see Fig. 16.1). There is thus a step change from

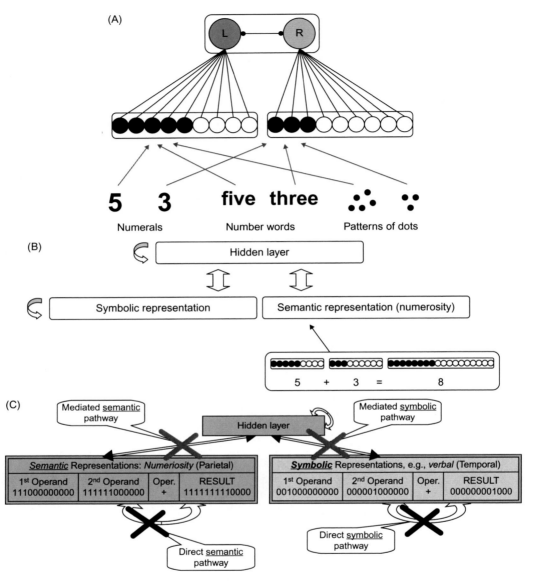

FIGURE 16.1 **Numerosity coding.** (A) This panel shows the structure of numerosity coding in a neural network model [60,61]. Numeral, verbal and non-symbolic numbers are mapped onto an internal code that represents each numerosity as a set of discrete "neurons". For number comparison, each set contributes activation proportional to the number of neurons activated to a binary (in this example) decision procedure with reciprocal inhibition between nodes. Reaction times are modeled as the number of cycles for the decision process to settle into one state. This provides a good fit to human reaction time data [60]. Reproduced, with permission, from [68]. (B) The same internal coding can be used as part of a system for addition. Reproduced, with permission, from [68]. (C) To model verbal coding of addition facts, a symbolic route consists of arbitrary codes for the operands so that contribution of this coding can be evaluated. Reproduced with permission from [61]. The distinction between semantic and symbolic coding enables modeling of the effects of neural damage by reducing the connections between addends and sums. Network performance is worse the greater the damage, but the effect is greater when the connections within the semantic network are damaged. This reflects the findings with acquired dyscalculic patients, where parietal lobe lesions affecting numerosity representation, impairs addition and subtraction, while damage to temporal lobe language areas affect mappings from symbolic input to output but not knowledge of arithmetic facts and procedures [62].

one numerosity to the next, unlike in the ANS. Although discrete, this kind of representation can capture parametrically number comparison accuracy and reaction time data, and also arithmetical accuracy and reaction time data including the well-known "problem size effect" in which reaction times increase with size of the sum [60,61] (see Glossary). Notice that the model includes a standard decision procedure used widely in neural network modeling.

A main prediction arising from the numerosity coding hypothesis is that dyscalculics will suffer from a deficit in enumerating sets. Although this may sound like a simple extension of small number coding, no upper limit or a role for attention is assumed. In fact, several studies of dyscalculia have shown this in group studies (e.g., [9]) and in individual cases (e.g., [41]).

The numerosity coding hypothesis further predicts that impaired numerosity representations will affect addition. The effects of impaired representations of numerosity on addition within the neural network model have been simulated [62]. Both semantic representations (numerosities) and symbolic representations are included in the model, since it has been claimed that addition facts are represented as non-semantic verbal formulae [63]. In verbal representations, the form of the representation is arbitrary with respect to the magnitude of the addends or the results. The main result was that damaging even a relatively small proportion of the connections between the numerosity representations of addends and result affected accuracy, while damaging the symbolic connections had a much smaller effect, whether the answer was symbolic or semantic.

Numerosity coding also enables, though it does not entail, the ability to use fingers in arithmetic since it provides a set of elements that can be put in one-to-one correspondence with a set of fingers. The link between fingers and arithmetic is close in both development and the brain. Damage to the left angular gyrus has long been known to affect both in Gerstmann's Syndrome [64], and recent research has shown that using transcranial magnetic stimulation over the angular gyrus will interfere with both [65]. It is not clear how either the ANS or the small number system could support the one-to-one relationship between the set of fingers (or other body-parts) and the set involved in arithmetic.

A final prediction arising from the numerosity coding hypothesis is that poor finger representations in the brain (finger agnosia) will be associated with poor arithmetical skills. The link between fingers and numbers was described 90 years ago by Gerstmann, who observed the frequent co-occurrence of finger agnosia, dyscalculia, left–right disorientation and apraxia, following damage to the angular gyrus, A developmental form of this syndrome has been documented and poor finger gnosis in young learners is known to predict poor arithmetic [66]. Moreover, poor representations of numerosity may also hinder the development of finger use in early arithmetic, even where the learner has good finger representations, since the mapping between fingers and numerosities will be obscure. This hypothesis has still to be tested.

THE ROLE OF LANGUAGE

The counting words, or what Carey calls "the integer list", are held to play "a special role" in the emergence of exact arithmetic during child development [46]. Thus, a critical test of the role of language in arithmetical development is whether language impairments cause arithmetical disabilities. It is claimed that the role of language is to refine approximate representations through bootstrapping and the regular association of the counting word with a particular approximate numerosity. If that is the case, then language impairments should affect very simple numerical tasks, such as comparing numerosities or enumerating sets. Children with SLI invariably show slower and less accurate verbal counting, held to be the key element in the transition from approximate to exact representations of number. However, these learners are as good as age-matched controls on number comparison, and indeed on number reasoning, and superior to younger language-matched controls [67].

Nevertheless, symbolization of numerosities is undoubtedly important in both individual arithmetical skills and those of humans collectively since it can be used to think about numbers and to communicate facts about them [47]. Moreover symbolization supports syntax, which in turn supports reasoning about large and small numbers that one has never before experienced, and perhaps cannot know by direct experience. This may be particularly important in understanding fractions, decimals and division more generally. On this account, the development of arithmetical skills and knowledge could be affected by low language competence even when mental representation of numbers is intact. This does seem to be the case [67,68].

As noted above, children can attain normal levels on non-symbolic comparison tasks, yet be impaired on symbolic digit comparison. Noël and colleagues have proposed that this may reflect a failure to link intact number concepts with their symbolic representations, which they suggest is at the root of dyscalculia [39]. However, as noted above, basic number concepts as measured by non-symbolic comparison tasks can also be defective, so linkage failure cannot be the whole story.

THE NEURAL BASIS OF DYSCALCULIA

Can studies of neural differences in structure or activation in dyscalculics decide among the foundational hypotheses? Structurally, reduced gray matter in dyscalculics has been observed in areas known to be involved in basic numerical processing, in the left IPS [69],

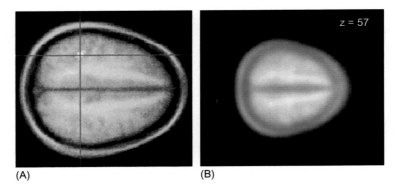

(A)   (B)

FIGURE 16.2 **Structural abnormalities in dyscalculic brains.** Structural abnormalities in young dyscalculic brains suggesting a critical role for the IPS. As noted in the text, both left and right IPS are implicated, possibly with a greater role for left IPS in older learners. (A) This panel shows a small region of reduced gray matter density in left IPS in adolescent dyscalculics. Reproduced with permission from [69]. (B) This panel shows right IPS reduced grey matter density in nine-year-olds. Reproduced with permission from [70].

BOX 16.2

METHODOLOGICAL PROBLEMS

- Developmental hypotheses need longitudinal studies to determine whether the measures employed are stable over time. That is, if a learner is in a slow group at age five years, will he or she still be in the slow group at 11 years or older? If they are not, that will be unhelpful for predicting outcomes in the long-term.
- Stability of measures need to be contrasted with their changes over time. Learners get faster and better as they get older. What are the typical and atypical trajectories of these changes?
- Are the slowest or lowest group at age five years simply delayed or are they qualitatively different on the basic measures? For example, will the parameters of their enumeration or number comparison performance always differ from their peers?

- Most studies use a single measure of underlying capacity, which might lead to artifacts. It is critical to deploy convergent measures, determined by theory.
- Studies assume that graded differences in underlying capacity will lead to graded differences in arithmetical attainment. However, it may be that the underlying capacity only needs to be "good enough". (The Matisse effect: having color blindness will prevent you being the next Matisse, but normal color vision will not ensure that you are.)
- Studies of number-reasoning are needed to complement studies of number-abstraction.
- Prevalence studies should use a "gold standard" criterion based on stable predictive measures.

in the right IPS [70], and in the IPS bilaterally [71] (see Fig. 16.2). Moreover, there seem to be differences in the connectivity between relevant regions as revealed by diffusion tensor imaging tractography [71].

Activation differences in non-symbolic number comparison in young learners have also been observed in the right IPS [72] and symbolic abnormalities in the left IPS [73]. The reason for these apparently conflicting findings is not yet clear. Two considerations may in time clarify the picture. First, the organization of numerical activity may change with age [74], shifting from right dominance to left dominance [75] as representations of numerosity link up with language [25]. Second, there may turn out to be residual specializations in the two parietal lobes, with the right specializing in subitizing and estimation [76,77], and the left in symbolic processing and calculation. If this is correct, longitudinal studies that combine neuroimaging with careful tests of basic numerical capacities may reveal different developmental trajectories depending on the locus of the neural abnormality. However, since the representations of approximate numerosities, exact numerosities and their symbols occupy overlapping neural systems [23,78], these cannot yet decide among hypotheses.

INTERVENTION

The efficacy of interventions designed to strengthen purported foundational capacities would constitute a critical test of the hypotheses discussed in preceding sections. For the ANS, as Piazza and colleagues note, their "findings lend support to remediation programs for developmental dyscalculia that include exercises aimed at retraining the core non-symbolic sense of number and to cement its links to the symbols used to denote it" ([79], p.39). The intervention they cite as appropriate is the *Number Race* game [80], a digital environment found to be effective in promoting basic number skills [81]. However, this game uses relatively small exact numerosities rather than approximate numerosities. It would be interesting to see if training to improve the Weber fraction in approximate comparison improves arithmetic, as the ANS account would predict.

Other attempts to use digital media have also focused on exact rather than approximate numerosities in numerical tasks involving some very simple arithmetic [82]. Similarly, the use of board games to promote numerical understanding have used small exact numerosities based on dice and counting, with the aim of moving children away from approximate numerosities represented logarithmically to a linear representation [83]. This preliminary evidence supports the idea that numerosity coding is foundational; however, systematic tests using approximate numerosities have yet to be attempted.

CONCLUDING REMARKS

In summary, although the evidence is not yet conclusive, it appears that the ANS and small number systems are not sufficient to support the typical development of arithmetical skills. A system that represents sets, their numerosities, and the effects of transformations on

---

BOX 16.3

PRIORITIES FOR FUTURE RESEARCH

- Establish developmental trajectories of key measures.
- Determine whether different aspects of number-abstraction processes are critical at different stages in the development of arithmetic.
- Implement tests of number-reasoning appropriate for different ages or stages.

- Use targeted interventions to help those with low arithmetical attainment and to test hypotheses about the domain-specific precursors to arithmetic.
- Establish the heritability of basic capacities using twin studies.

these sets appears to be required. Numerosity coding is such a system and there is extensive evidence that young humans possess it. However, we have only just begun to collect the critical evidence from longitudinal and intervention studies of the developmental trajectory of typical and atypical learners. Definitive answers are therefore not yet available (see also Box 16.3).

GLOSSARY

Approximate Numerosity Tasks

Tasks involving "clouds" of dots (or other objects) typically too numerous to enumerate exactly in the time available. One common task is comparing two clouds of dots. Also used are addition and subtraction tasks where the solution is compared with a third cloud of dots. (The term Approximate Arithmetic is sometimes used when an exact answer is not available or not needed: e.g., is 73 + 98 closer to 180 or to 130?)

Cardinality Principle

In the development of counting, understanding that the last word in the count represents the number of objects in the set counted.

Distance Effect

Number comparison, symbolic or non-symbolic, is slower and more error-prone, as number magnitudes are more similar. See Fig. 16.1.

IPS

Intra-parietal sulcus. This is the brain area for core number processing: simple enumeration, estimation, subitizing, and comparison. Functional specialization of the left and right IPS develops with time and experience.

Numerosity

The number of objects in a set.

Problem Size Effect

Arithmetical problems involving larger numbers are harder than those involving smaller numbers, even for highly practiced sums and multiplications. Explanations of the effect vary.

Weber's Law, Weber Fraction, and Numerical Acuity

The psychologist, Ernst Weber, stated "equal relative increments of stimuli are proportional to equal increments of sensation." That is, the difference threshold depends on the proportional not the absolute difference between two quantities. The Weber *fraction* means the proportional difference that is reliably detected. So the smaller the Weber fraction, the better the discrimination between two quantities. "Numerical acuity" refers to the Weber fraction of two approximate numerosities.

Acknowledgments

I am grateful for helpful comments and discussions with Randy Gallistel, Justin Halberda, and Sashank Varma, and comments on the manuscript from three anonymous referees.

References

[1] J. Gross, The Long Term Costs of Numeracy Difficulties, Every Child Chance Trust, KPMG, London, 2009.

[2] J. Bynner, S. Parsons, Does Numeracy Matter More? National Research and Development Centre for Adult Literacy and Numeracy, Institute of Education, London, 2005.

[3] S.E. Gathercole, S.J. Pickering, C. Knight, Z. Stegmann, Working memory skills and educational attainment: evidence from national curriculum assessments at 7 and 14 years of age, Appl. Cogn. Psychol. 18 (2004) 1–16.

[4] R. Bull, K.A. Espy, S. Wiebe, Short-term memory, working memory and executive functioning in preschoolers: longitudinal predictors of mathematical achievement at age 7, Dev. Neuropsychol. 33 (2008) 205–228.

[5] O. Rubinsten, A. Henik, Developmental Dyscalculia: heterogeneity might not mean different mechanisms, Trends Cogn. Sci. 13 (2009) 92–99.

[6] B. Butterworth, Developmental dyscalculia, in: J.I.D. Campbell (Ed.), Handbook of Mathematical Cognition, Psychology Press, Hove, 2005, pp. 455–467.

[7] M.M.M. Mazzocco, Defining and differentiating mathematical learning disabilities and difficulties, in: D.B. Berch, M.M.M. Mazzocco (Eds.), Why is Math so Hard for Some Children? The Nature and Origins of Mathematical Learning Difficulties and Disabilities, Paul H Brookes Publishing Co., Baltimore, MD, 2007, pp. 29–47.

[8] R.S. Shalev, Prevalence of developmental dyscalculia, in: D.B. Berch, M.M.M. Mazzocco (Eds.), Why is Math so Hard for Some Children? The Nature and Origins of Mathematical Learning Difficulties and Disabilities, Paul H Brookes Publishing Co., Baltimore, MD, 2007, pp. 49–60.

[9] K. Landerl, A. Bevan, B. Butterworth, Developmental dyscalculia and basic numerical capacities: a study of 8–9 year old students, Cognition 93 (2004) 99–125.

[10] D.C. Geary, D.H. Bailey, A. Littlefield, P. Wood, M.K. Hoard, L. Nugent, First-grade predictors of mathematical learning disability: a latent class trajectory analysis, Cogn. Dev. 24 (2009) 411–429.

[11] Y. Kovas, C. Haworth, P. Dale, R. Plomin, The genetic and environmental origins of learning abilities and disabilities in the early school years, Monogr. Soc. Res. Child Dev. 72 (2007) 1–144.

[12] G. Schulte-Körne, A. Ziegler, W. Deimel, J. Schumacher, E. Plume, C. Bachmann, et al., Interrelationship and familiality of dyslexia related quantitative measures, Ann. Hum. Genet. 71 (2007) 160–175.

[13] B. Butterworth, V. Reigosa Crespo, Information processing deficits in dyscalculia, in: D.B. Berch, M.M.M. Mazzocco (Eds.), Why is Math so Hard for Some Children? The Nature and Origins of Mathematical Learning Difficulties and Disabilities, Paul H Brookes Publishing Co., Baltimore, MD, 2007, pp. 65–81.

[14] A.J. Wilson, S. Dehaene, Number sense and developmental dyscalculia, in: D. Coch, K.W. Fischer, G. Dawson, (Eds.), Human Behavior, Learning and the Developing Brain, The Guilford Press, New York City NY, 2007

[15] P. Starkey, R.G. Cooper, Jr, Perception of numbers by human infants, Science 210 (1980) 1033–1035.

[16] K.E. Jordan, E.M. Brannon, The multisensory representation of number in infancy, Proc. Nat. Acad. Sci. U.S.A. 103 (2006) 3486–3489.

[17] L. Cipolotti, N. van Harskamp, Disturbances of number processing and calculation, second ed., in: R.S. Berndt (Ed.), Handbook of Neuropsychology, vol. 3, Elsevier Science, Amsterdam, 2001, pp. 305–334.

[18] E.K. Warrington, M. James, Tachistoscopic number estimation in patients with unilateral lesions, J. Neurol. Neurosur. Psychiat. 30 (1967) 468–474.

[19] A.R. Luria, The Higher Cortical Functions in Man, Basic Books, New York, 1966.

[20] S. Dehaene, M. Piazza, P. Pinel, L. Cohen, Three parietal circuits for number processing, Cogn. Neuropsychol. 20 (2003) 487–506.

[21] R.H. Grabner, D. Ansari, K. Koschutnig, G. Reishofer, F. Ebner, C. Neuper, To retrieve or to calculate? Left angular gyrus mediates the retrieval of arithmetic facts during problem solving, Neuropsychologia 47 (2009) 604–608.

[22] M. Piazza, V. Izard, P. Pinel, D. Le Bihan, S. Dehaene, Tuning curves for approximate numerosity in the human intraparietal sulcus, Neuron 44 (2004) 547–555.

[23] M. Piazza, P. Pinel, D. Le Bihan, S. Dehaene, A magnitude code common to numerosities and number symbols in human intraparietal cortex, Neuron 53 (2007) 293–305.

[24] P. Pinel, S. Dehaene, D. Rivièinel, D. Le Bihan, Modulation of parietal activation by semantic distance in a number comparison task, NeuroImage 14 (2001) 1013–1026.

[25] M. Piazza, A. Mechelli, C.J. Price, B. Butterworth, Exact and approximate judgements of visual and auditory numerosity: an fMRI study, Brain Res. 1106 (2006) 177–188.

[26] A. Nieder, S. Dehaene, Representation of number in the brain, Ann. Rev. Neurosci. 32 (2009) 185–208.

[27] M. Giaquinto, Concepts and calculation, Math. Cogn. 1 (1995) 61–81.

[28] M. Giaquinto, Knowing numbers, J. Philoso. XCVIII (2001) 5–18.

[29] B. Butterworth, The development of arithmetical abilities, J. Child Psychol. Psychiat. 46 (2005) 3–18.

[30] R. Gelman, C.R. Gallistel, The Child's Understanding of Number, 1986 Edition, Harvard University Press, Cambridge, MA, 1978.

[31] J. Piaget, The Child's Conception of Number, Routledge & Kegan Paul, London, 1952.

[32] L. Feigenson, S. Dehaene, E. Spelke, Core systems of number, Trends Cogn. Sci. 8 (2004) 307–314.

[33] C.K. Gilmore, S.E. McCarthy, E.S. Spelke, Non-symbolic arithmetic abilities and mathematics achievement in the first year of formal schooling, Cognition 115 (2010) 394–406.

[34] J. Halberda, M.M.M. Mazzocco, L. Feigenson, Individual differences in non-verbal number acuity correlate with maths achievement, Nature 455 (2008) 665–668.

[35] M. Piazza, A. Facoetti, A.N. Trussardi, I. Berteletti, S. Conte, D. Lucangeli, et al., Developmental trajectory of number acuity reveals a severe impairment in developmental dyscalculia, Cognition 116 (2010) 33–41.

[36] G.A. Alvarez, P. Cavanagh, The capacity of visual short-term memory is set both by visual information load and by number of objects, Psychol. Sci. 15 (2004) 106–111.

[37] D.G. Pelli, K.A. Tillman, The uncrowded window of object recognition, Nat. Neurosci. 11 (2008) 1129–1135.

[38] S. Dehaene, The neural basis of the Weber–Fechner law: a logarithmic mental number, Trends Cogn. Sci. 7 (2004) 145–147.

[39] L. Rousselle, M.-P. Noël, Basic numerical skills in children with mathematics learning disabilities: a comparison of symbolic vs non-symbolic number magnitude processing, Cognition 102 (2007) 361–395.

[40] I.D. Holloway, D. Ansari, Mapping numerical magnitudes onto symbols: the numerical distance effect and individual differences in children's mathematics achievement, J. Exp. Child Psychol. 103 (2009) 17–29.

[41] T. Iuculano, J. Tang, C. Hall, B. Butterworth, Core information processing deficits in developmental dyscalculia and low numeracy, Dev. Sci. 11 (2008) 669–680.

[42] H. Barth, A. Starr, J. Sullivan, Children's mappings of large number words to numerosities, Cogn. Dev. 24 248–264.

[43] M. Piazza, V. Izard, How humans count: numerosity and the parietal cortex, Neuroscientist 15 (2009) 261–273.

[44] J. Ross, Visual discrimination of number without counting, Perception 32 (2003) 867–870.

[45] M. Piazza, Neurocognitive start-up tools for symbolic number representations, Trends Cogn. Sci. (in press).

[46] S. Carey, On the origin of concepts, Daedalus (2004) 59–68.

[47] R. Gelman, B. Butterworth, Number and language: how are they related? Trends Cogn. Sci. 9 (2005) 6–10.

[48] L.J. Rips, A. Bloomfield, J. Asmuth, From numerical concepts to concepts of number, Behav. Brain Sci. 31 (2008) 623–642.

[49] M. Le Corre, S. Carey, One, two, three, four, nothing more: an investigation of the conceptual sources of the verbal counting principles, Cognition (2007), doi:10.1016/j.cognition.2006.10.005.

[50] K.L. Koontz, D.B. Berch, Identifying simple numerical stimuli: processing inefficiencies exhibited by arithmetic learning disabled children, Math. Cogn. 2 (1996) 1–23.

[51] K.C. Fuson, Children's Counting and Concepts of Number, Springer Verlag, New York, 1988.

[52] C. Donlan, The early numeracy of children with specific language impairments, in: A.J. Baroody, A.D. Dowker (Eds.), The Development of Arithmetic Concepts and Skills: Constructing Adaptive Expertise, Lawrence Erlbaum Associates, Mahwah, NJ, 2003, pp. 337–358.

[53] T. Koponen, R. Mononen, P. Rasanen, T. Ahonen, Basic numeracy in children with specific language impairment: heterogeneity and connections to language, J. Speech Lang. Hear. Res. 49 (2006) 58–73.

[54] C. Donlan, Mathematical development in children with specific language impairments, in: D.B. Berch, M.M.M. Mazzocco (Eds.), Why is Math so Hard for Some Children? The Nature and Origins of Mathematical Learning Difficulties and Disabilities, Paul H Brookes Publishing Co., Baltimore, MD, 2007, pp. 151–172.

[55] L. Feigenson, J. Halberda, Infants chunk object arrays into sets of individuals, Cognition 91 (2004) 173–190.

[56] K. Wynn, P. Bloom, W.C. Chiang, Enumeration of collective entities by 5-month-old infants, Cognition 83 (2002) B55–B62.

[57] J.F. Cantlon, M.E. Libertus, P. Pinel, S. Dehaene, E.M. Brannon, K.A. Pelphrey, The neural development of an abstract concept of number, J. Cogn. Neurosci. 21 (2009) 2217–2229.

[58] J. Halberda, L. Feigenson, Set representations required for the acquisition of the "natural number" concept, Behav. Brain Sci. 31 (2008) 655–656.

[59] F. Castelli, D.E. Glaser, B. Butterworth, Discrete and analogue quantity processing in the parietal lobe: a functional MRI study, Proc. Nat. Acad. Sci. 103 (2006) 4693–4698.

[60] M. Zorzi, B. Butterworth, A computational model of number comparison, in: M. Hahn, S.C. Stoness (Eds.), Proceedings of the Twenty First Annual Meeting of the Cognitive Science Society, LEA, Mahwah, NJ, 1999.

[61] M. Zorzi, I. Stoianov, C. Umilta, Computational modelling of numerical cognition, in: J.I.D. Campbell (Ed.), Handbook of Mathematical Cognition, Psychology Press, Hove, 2005, pp. 67–84.

[62] I. Stoianov, M. Zorzi, C. Umiltà, The role of semantic and symbolic representations in arithmetic processing: insights from simulated dyscalculia in a connectionist model, Cortex 40 (2004) 194–196.

[63] S. Dehaene, N. Molko, L. Cohen, Arithmetic and the brain, Curr. Opin. Neurobiol. 14 (2004) 218–224.

[64] J. Gerstmann, Syndrome of Finger Agnosia: disorientation for right and left, agraphia and acalculia, Arch. Neurol. Psychiat. 44 (1940) 398–408.

[65] E. Rusconi, V. Walsh, B. Butterworth, Dexterity with Numbers: rTMS over left angular gyrus disrupts finger gnosis and number processing, Neuropsychologia 43 (2005) 1609–1624.

[66] M.-P. Noel, Finger gnosia: a predictor of numerical abilities in children? Child Neuropsychol. 11 (2005) 413–430.

[67] C. Donlan, R. Cowan, E.J. Newton, D. Lloyd, The role of language in mathematical development: Evidence from children with specific language impairments, Cognition 103 (2007) 23–33.

[68] R. Cowan, C. Donlan, E. Newton, D. Lloyd, Number skills and knowledge in children with specific language impairment, J. Educ. Psychol. 97 (2005) 732–744.

[69] E.B. Isaacs, C.J. Edmonds, A. Lucas, D.G. Gadian, Calculation difficulties in children of very low birthweight: a neural correlate, Brain 124 (2001) 1701–1707.

[70] S. Rotzer, K. Kucian, E. Martin, M.v. Aster, P. Klaver, T. Loenneker, Optimized voxel-based morphometry in children with developmental dyscalculia, NeuroImage 39 (2008) 417–422.

[71] E. Rykhlevskaia, L.Q. Uddin, L. Kondos, V. Menon, Neuroanatomical correlates of developmental dyscalculia: combined evidence from morphometry and tractography, Front. Hum. Neurosci. 3 (2009) 1–13.

[72] G.R. Price, I. Holloway, P. Räsänen, M. Vesterinen, D. Ansari, Impaired parietal magnitude processing in developmental dyscalculia, Curr. Biol. 17 (2007) R1042–R1043.

[73] C. Mussolin, A. De Volder, C. Grandin, X. Schlögel, M.-C. Nassogne, M.-P. Noël, Neural correlates of symbolic number comparison in developmental dyscalculia, J. Cogn. Neurosci. 22 (2009) 860–874.

[74] D. Ansari, Effects of development and enculturation on number representation in the brain, Nat. Rev. Neurosci. 9 (2008) 278–291.

[75] S.M. Rivera, S.M. Reiss, M.A. Eckert, V. Menon, Developmental changes in mental arithmetic: evidence for increased functional specialization in the left inferior parietal cortex, Cereb. Cortex 15 (2005) 1779–1790.

[76] D. Ansari, I.M. Lyons, L. van Eimeren, F. Xu, Linking visual attention and number processing in the brain: the role of the temporo-parietal junction in small and large symbolic and nonsymbolic number comparison, J. Cogn. Neurosci. 19 (2007) 1845–1853.

[77] P. Vetter, B. Butterworth, B. Bahrami, A candidate for the attentional bottleneck: set-size specific modulation of the right TPJ during attentive enumeration, J. Cogn. Neurosci. 23 (2010) 728–736.

[78] R. Cohen Kadosh, V. Walsh, Numerical representation in the parietal lobes: abstract or not abstract? Behav. Brain Sci. 32 (2009) 313–328.

[79] M. Piazza, A. Facoetti, A.N. Trussardi, I. Berteletti, S. Conte, D. Lucangeli, et al., Developmental trajectory of number acuity reveals a severe impairment in developmental dyscalculia, Cognition 116 33–41.

[80] A. Wilson, S. Dehaene, P. Pinel, S. Revkin, L. Cohen, D. Cohen, Principles underlying the design of "The Number Race", an adaptive computer game for remediation of dyscalculia, Behav. Brain Funct. 2 (2006).

[81] P. Räsänen, J. Salminen, A.J. Wilson, P. Aunioa, S. Dehaene, Computer-assisted intervention for children with low numeracy skills, Cogn. Dev. 24 (2009) 450–472.

[82] B. Butterworth, D. Laurillard, Low numeracy and dyscalculia: identification and intervention, ZDM Math. Educ. (2010).

[83] G.B. Ramani, R.S. Siegler, Promoting broad and stable improvements in low-income children's numerical knowledge through playing number board games, Child Dev. 79 (2008) 375–394.

[84] American Psychiatric Association, Diagnostic and Statistical Manual of Mental Disorders, fourth ed., American Psychiatric Association, Washington, DC, 1994.

[85] World Health Organization, International Classification of Diseases—10, tenth ed., World Health Organization, Geneva, Switzerland, 1994.

[86] Guidance to Support Pupils with Dyslexia and Dyscalculia, Department of Education and Skills, London, 2001.

[87] J.M. Royer, R. Walles, Influences of gender, ethnicity, and motivation on mathematical performance, in: D.B. Berch, M.M.M. Mazzocco (Eds.), Why is Math so Hard for Some Children? The Nature and Origins of Mathematical Learning Difficulties and Disabilities, Paul H Brookes Publishing Co., Baltimore, MD, 2007.

[88] H. Gardner, Frames of Mind: The Theory of Multiple Intelligences, Basic Books, New York, 1983.

Neurocognitive Start-Up Tools for Symbolic Number Representations*

Manuela Piazza

INSERM, U562, Cognitive Neuroimaging Unit, CEA/SAC/DSV/DRM/Neurospin
Center, Gif-sur-Yvette, France, Center for Mind/Brain Sciences and Dipartimento di
Scienze della Cognizione e della Formazione University of Trento, Rovereto, Italy

Summary

Attaching meaning to arbitrary symbols (i.e. words) is a highly complex and lengthy process. In the case of numbers, it was previously suggested that this process is grounded on two early preverbal systems for numerical quantification, the approximate number system (ANS or "analogue magnitude"), and the object tracking system (OTS or "parallel individuation"), which children are equipped with prior to symbolic learning. Each of these systems is based on dedicated neural circuits, characterized by specific computational limits, and undergoes a separate developmental trajectory. Reviewing the available cognitive and neuroscientific data, I argue that the evidence is more consistent with a crucial role for the ANS, rather than the OTS, in the acquisition of abstract numerical concepts that are uniquely human.

Current theories of cognitive development posit that knowledge acquisition is based on a limited set of "core knowledge" systems, defined as domain-specific representational priors which guide and constrain the cultural acquisition of novel representations [1,2]. This notion fits well with a recent proposal that cultural learning takes place by a partial reconversion ("cortical recycling") of a limited number of cerebral circuits initially selected

*Reprinted from Trends in Cognitive Sciences, Vol 14, Manuela Piazza, Neurocognitive start-up tools for symbolic number representations, pg 542–551, 2010, with permission from Elsevier.

to support evolutionary relevant functions, but sufficiently plastic for changing their coding scheme and acquiring new functions [3]. The combination of these two ideas defines the notion of a "neurocognitive start-up tool". In the specific case of number, I review the features of two preverbal systems for numerical quantification, the approximate number system (ANS) and the object tracking system (OTS), and critically assess their role in cultural learning of symbolic numbers. Although the evidence is as yet inconclusive, I will argue that the currently available cognitive and neural data are more consistent with a foundational role of the ANS, but not the OTS, in the acquisition of more elaborate numerical concepts.

THE APPROXIMATE NUMBER SYSTEM

Approximate number, much like color or shape, is a basic feature of the environment to which animals appear wired to attend to: spontaneous extraction of the approximate number of objects in sets is reported in several species, both in the wild and in more controlled laboratory settings (see [4] for a review). For example, macaque monkeys spontaneously match the approximate number of individuals they see to the number of individuals' voices they hear [5], and also sum up visual and auditory stimuli to estimate their total number, without previous training [6]. The evolutionary relevance of such ability is clear: appreciation of number (e.g., of in-group *vs* out-group members) can be crucial for social behavior [7,8], foraging [9], and reproductive strategies [10]. Although not precise, number representations in nonhuman animals can be mentally combined to perform complex operations such as comparison, addition, and subtraction across sets [11,12]. In humans, a similar spontaneous detection of the approximate number of objects in sets, even across different sensory modalities, is reported surprisingly early, since the very first hours of life [13]: newborn babies habituated for some minutes to auditory sequences of a given number (e.g., six syllables), look longer to subsequently presented numerically matching visual sets (e.g., six dots) than to non-numerically matching sets (e.g., 18 dots). However, they fail with sets numerically differing by smaller ratios, for example, six *vs* 12 elements. This suggests a shared evolutionarily ancient innate system for approximate number: the ANS.

The most important defining feature of the ANS is that it represents number in an approximate and compressed fashion, in such a way that two sets can be discriminated only if they differ by a given numerical ratio, according to Weber's law (see Glossary). Weber's law (as first demonstrated by Fechner [14]) can be accounted for by postulating a logarithmic relation between the physical stimulus and its internal representation. Most current models of the internal representation of number assume that such logarithmic relation comes from the compressed nature of the internal representation of numerosity itself, which for some takes the form of equally spaced mental magnitudes with increasing noise [15], and for others of logarithmically spaced mental magnitudes with fixed noise [16,17]. Taking a rather different perspective, still others have suggested that the origin of the weberian nature of numerosity compression is to be found in the computational processes engaged during the judgment of relative numerical magnitude [18]. Although theoretically possible, this hypothesis is not supported by neuroimaging data which show a weberian neural response to number even in conditions in which subjects do not perform any explicit computations on the stimuli but simply observe sets of different number [19].

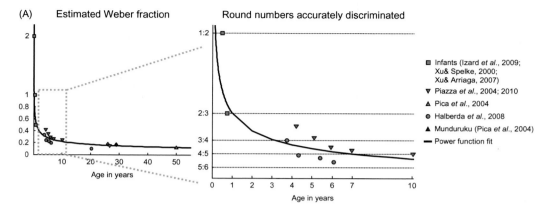

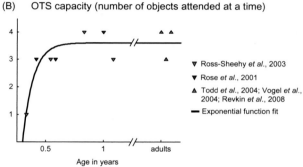

FIGURE 17.1 **ANS and OTS development**. (A) Estimated Weber fractions (measuring ANS acuity) are reported from different studies as a function of subjects' age. In the inset (right) Weber fractions are expressed as the two closest round numbers accurately discriminated in the age range between 0 and 10. (B) Estimated OTS capacities are reported from different studies as a function of subjects' age.

Irrespective of the specific model of the internal representation of number assumed, the Weber fraction, indicating the smallest variation to a number that can be readily perceived (see Glossary), can be safely taken as an index of ANS acuity. Interestingly, ANS acuity is variable across individuals, and this variability is present from very early in life [20–22]. Moreover, it is not stable across the life span but increases consistently during development [22,23], and most dramatically during the first years of life: while newborns can discriminate sets differing by a minimal numerical ratio of 1:3 at birth, at six months their acuity increases to 1:2, and to 2:3 around nine to 12 months of age [20,24,25]. Between the third and the fourth year, children can reliably discriminate between sets with a 3:4 ratio, and may become sensitive to an adult-like 7:8 ratio around 20 years of age [22,23] (see Fig. 17.1).

Neuroimaging techniques have extensively investigated the neuronal underpinnings of the ANS in humans. Converging results using passive fixation [19], as well as tasks like numerosity comparison [26], or approximate calculation [27] using dot patterns or sequentially presented stimuli [28] consistently point to regions in the mid-intraparietal sulcus as the source of approximate number representations in both adults and infants (Fig. 17.2; for recent reviews, see [29,30]).

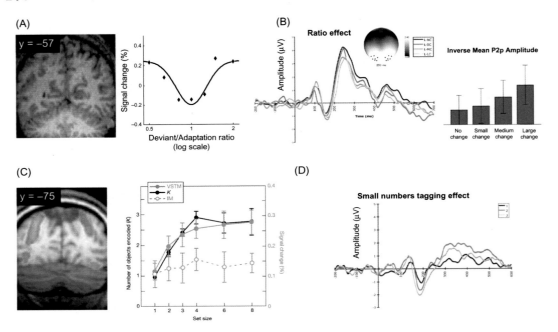

FIGURE 17.2 **The neural basis of the ANS and the OTS.** (A) Mid-Parietal regions showing weberian responses to non-symbolic numerical quantity in an fMRI number adaptation experiment investigating the neural underpinning of the ANS in human adults. Adaptation stimuli were sets with a fixed number of dots, while deviant stimuli, presented rarely, were sets of variable number along a continuum spanning from half to double the adaptation values. Parietal activation for deviant numerical stimuli was a direct function of the ratio between the deviant and the adaptation number, according to Weber's law [19]. (B) ERP recordings of activity evoked by numerically deviant stimuli embedded in sequences of repeated numerically fixed stimuli (EEG adaptation) characterize the time-course of brain activation associated with the ANS, showing that parietal electrodes are modulated by the ratio between the deviant and the adaptation number at about 250 ms after stimulus onset (at the level of the N1 to P2p transition zone) [48]. (C) Posterior parietal regions whose activity shows OTS signature (linearly increasing response for sets with 1 to 3–4 items and leveling off thereafter) in an fMRI visual short-term memory (VSTM) experiment [39] . Subjects were shown sets of one to eight colored dots and, after a short retention period were subsequently asked to detect a change in color of one of the items. Paralleling behavioral responses, measured as the estimated number (K) of encoded colored discs at each set size, posterior parietal activation shows a set-size limit at about three to four items. The same regions did not show the same response when subjects were performing an iconic memory (IM) task consisting of detecting the presence of a given color in the same displays used for the VSTM. (D) Electrophysiological signatures of the OTS. ERP recordings of activity evoked by numerically deviant stimuli embedded in sequences of repeated numerically fixed stimuli (EEG adaptation) show that the amplitude of an early (150 ms post-stimulus) negative peak (N1), over parietal electrodes is modulated by the number of items for sets of one to four items only [48].

THE OBJECT TRACKING SYSTEM

The OTS is a mechanism by which objects are represented as distinct individuals that can be tracked through time and space. This core system for representing objects centers on the spatio-temporal principles of cohesion (objects move as bounded wholes), continuity (objects move on connected, unobstructed paths), and contact (objects do not interact at a distance). These principles allow human infants as well as other animals to perceive object boundaries, and to predict when objects will move and where they will come to rest (see [1]).

BOX 17.1

THE APPROXIMATE NUMBER SYSTEM AND THE OBJECT TRACKING SYSTEM: TWO DIFFERENT SYSTEMS?

For quite some time there has been a debate on whether subitizing and the OTS truly reflect a mechanism dedicated to small sets, or whether they rather reflect the ANS, which, due to its weberian nature, codes for small numbers with a higher precision than for larger numbers [49,94]. More recently, however, behavioral evidence for a non-estimation-like process responsible for subitizing has been reported: first, in dual task conditions, attentional manipulations affect subitizing but not estimation [91]; second, in the small 1–4 subitizing range, the variability of the estimates (or coefficient of variation, see glossary, under "scalar variability") is substantially lower than the one in the large 10–40 range, even when the ratios between numbers is identical across ranges; finally, the inter-individual variability in subitizing span and in large numerosity estimation precision does not correlate across subjects [34]. Interestingly, the absence of correlation between the ANS and the OTS has been recently replicated in infants as young as nine months [20]. Further behavioral support for the distinction between the ANS and the OTS comes from studies on young infants mainly conducted by Feigenson and colleagues (see [51] for a review). First, for small sets falling within the limits of the OTS (<4), but not for large sets, when certain such features (such as surface area or contour length) are pitted against number, infants sometimes more automatically attend to those and thus fail to respond to number. Second, if, of two sets to be compared or matched, one falls within the OTS capacity (e.g., <4 objects) and the other one beyond (>4 objects), they also fail to attend to number, or need extremely large numerical ratios to succeed [95]. This suggests that the OTS may be automatically recruited whenever the number of items falls within its limits, and on some occasions may even mask the ANS, thus interfering with otherwise perfectly feasible numerical operations.

One of the defining properties of this system is that it is limited in capacity to three to four individuals at a time. This property has been confirmed using several different tasks, such as visual short-term memory tasks, whereby simple features (such as color or orientation) of a small, limited number of objects can be accurately retained in memory ("visuo-spatial short-term memory SPAN") [31], or multiple-object tracking tasks, whereby a small number of moving items can be tracked in parallel throughout the display ("multiple objects tracking capacity") [32]. The existence of the OTS is also evident in enumeration tasks: subjects can determine the number of objects in small collections of three or four items with very high accuracy and high speed, even in conditions of very briefly presented or masked stimuli (a phenomenon called "subitizing"; see Glossary) [33,34]. For sets with more than three or four items, enumeration is only possible either via exact counting, which implies a serial scanning of the display, or via approximate estimation, which falls under the computational constraints of the ANS, thus reflecting Weber law's through scalar variability (see Glossary and Box 17.1).

Similar to the ANS, the OTS is also variable across individuals [21,34,35], and is also subject to maturation: using preferential looking paradigms researchers have shown that the capacity limit of the OTS develops quickly over the first year of life, such that, while at six months the OTS capacity is limited to a single object, its capacity reaches an adult-like limit of three to four items at about 12 months [36–38] (see Fig. 17.1). The neural underpinnings of the OTS are much less clearly defined, but seem to be distinct from the neural substrates of the ANS. Several neuroimaging studies using object tracking tasks report capacity-limited neural activation, paralleling behavioral measures, in the posterior parietal and occipital regions bilaterally [35,39–42], while others associate subitizing to regions of the right temporo-parietal junction [43,44]. Neuropsychological studies indicate a critical role of posterior parietal cortex in the OTS, as the inability to track multiple items in parallel (a disorder called simultanagnosia [45]) typically emerges following lesions to the bilateral posterior parietal cortex [46]. Interestingly, simultanagnosic patients also seem to have a restricted subitizing range (at approximately two items) [47]. EEG recordings also support a separation between the neural signatures of the ANS and OTS. For example, using an adaptation paradigm, Hyde and colleagues showed that the amplitude of an early (150ms post-stimulus) negative peak (N1), centered over the parietal cortex, was modulated by the absolute number of elements in the display for small numbers, while the amplitude of a later (250ms post-stimulus) positive peak (P2p), also centered over the parietal cortex, showed an ANS signature in that it was modulated by the ratio of change in the large number range, regardless of the absolute number of objects presented [48]. Event-related potential (ERP) source reconstruction was not performed in this study, and this does not allow any conclusions on anatomical dissociation between the ANS and the OTS. In sum, although somewhat inconsistently across studies, the OTS seems to be associated with regions of the posterior parietal and occipital cortices that do not seem to overlap with regions involved in the ANS. The electrophysiological signatures of the two systems also appear to be distinct.

THE ROLE OF THE ANS AND THE OTS IN THE ACQUISITION OF SYMBOLIC NUMBER REPRESENTATIONS

Most existing proposals of the acquisition of symbolic number (here the term "symbolic numbers" stands for positive integers) claim that the symbols for numbers acquire meaning by being mapped onto the pre-existing core quantity representations: some proposals highlight the role of the ANS [15,17,49], others the role of the OTS [2,50], while others consider the combination of the two systems as crucial [1,51] (see [52] for a concise review of the different positions, [53] for a stand-alone provocative proposal that neither the ANS nor the OTS play any role in learning symbolic numbers, and Chapter 16 in this volume for the proposal of an innate representation of large exact number).

In this paper, I focus on the question of whether the ANS and OTS are foundational (i.e. act as start-up tools) in symbolic number acquisition. In critically reviewing the existing cognitive and neuroscientific literature, I will assess two criteria which are definitional for a neurocognitive start-up system [3]:

1. Their integrity should be a necessary (albeit not sufficient) condition for efficient learning. Thus, early impairments in a foundational system should systematically lead to specific learning difficulties (in this case, dyscalculia).

2. Their computational constraints should predict speed and ease of cultural knowledge acquisition in children, and they may be observed even in adults after successful learning.

EVIDENCE FOR A FOUNDATIONAL ROLE OF THE ANS IN SYMBOLIC NUMBER PROCESSING

Traces of the ANS Signature in Symbolic Number Processing

Behavioral Evidence

Traces of the ANS signature in symbolic number processing appear to arise almost as soon as children acquire symbolic numbers: in an elegant series of studies Gilmore and colleagues showed that four- to five-year-old kindergarteners, although they had not yet been taught the principles of exact calculation, solve simple arithmetical operations on large symbolic two-digit numbers relying on an approximate, ratio-dependent representation of quantity, and they do so spontaneously [54]. Moreover, and crucially, performance on non-symbolic numerical tasks (measuring ANS acuity) predicts children's mastery of number words and symbols as well as performance in school-level mathematics tasks some months later, and is independent of achievement in reading or general intelligence ([55], but see [56] for failure to observe such correlation in six- to eight-year-old children). As children undergo formal mathematical training, they solve symbolic numerical tasks with high precision. However, traces of the ANS remain discernible even in adulthood. For example, Moyer and Landauer [57] established early on that when adults are asked to determine which of two symbolic numbers (Arabic digits or number words) is larger, they are faster and make fewer errors when their ratio is high. Symbolic ratio effects also emerge in priming contexts, in that the speed of processing of a target number (digit or number word) is directly influenced by the numerical distance to a prime number [58,59]. Such symbolic priming effects are already present in first graders, and their size remains stable across development [60]. This suggests a rapid crystallization of the internal representation of symbolic numbers according to an internal scale which inherits some of the key properties of the scale governing the pre-existing representation of approximate quantity (i.e. that of being approximate and compressed).

Neuroimaging Evidence

Complementary evidence that symbolic numbers map onto a core quantity code comes from neuroimaging studies showing a format invariant parietal response to numerical quantity. First, the same parietal brain regions and similar ERP responses are modulated by the distance and magnitude effects for both Arabic digits and non-symbolic numerical quantities [61–63]. Second, and more importantly, quantity-related responses of the mid-intraparietal cortex *transfer* across symbolic and non-symbolic formats. Thus, in an adaptation paradigm, the parietal response to quantity is proportional to numerical ratio between novel and repeated quantities even when they are represented in different formats [64]. Interestingly, this effect is not fully bidirectional (especially in the left hemisphere): while adaptation to dots extends to Arabic digits, the opposite does not occur. A similar asymmetric effect is reported by an fMRI "decoding" study by which a multi-voxel pattern classifier

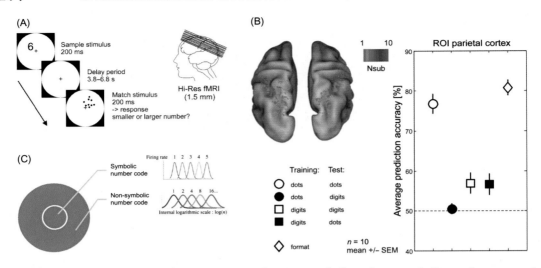

FIGURE 17.3 **Neural evidence for a convergence between symbolic and non-symbolic number representations**. (A) Example of stimuli in a high-resolution fMRI experiment where subjects performed a delayed comparison task with Arabic digits and dot patterns and a cartoon showing the scanned region [26]. (B) Regions active during the comparison task and the across-subject overlap of voxels (color coding indicating the number of subjects activating the corresponding voxel). Pairwise discrimination of mean-corrected activation patterns for different numerosities was significant for training and testing on data from dot pattern stimuli, but not for training on data from dot pattern stimuli and testing on data from digits. Training and testing on data from digits was significantly above chance but less accurate than for dot patterns, as was generalization from digits to dot patterns. Discrimination of the stimulus format (symbolic *vs* non-symbolic) for the same number was also significant and highly accurate. (C) Cartoon of a possible scenario accounting for the asymmetric pattern of generalization reported in (B) [26]. A subset of parietal neurons initially coding for approximate number undergo a process of tuning sharpening during the acquisition of symbolic number such that numerical quantity accessed by symbolic numbers is coded in a more precise, quasi-categorical fashion, consistent with the simulation by Verguts and Fias [17].

trained on parietal cortex activation to predict which Arabic is presented to subjects at any given trial, also correctly classified the numerosity of dot patterns, but not *vice versa* [26] (see Fig. 17.3). This data is consistent with the idea that the parietal quantity code accessed by symbolic numbers is more precise than the one for non-symbolic quantity even if it maintains some degree of fuzziness and compression (see Box 17.2).

The Relation Between the Developmental Trajectory of the ANS and the Initial Stages of Symbolic Number Acquisition

One puzzling feature of lexical acquisition in the number domain is that it is a very slow process. After they understand that the number words refer to numerical quantities (around two years of age), and before they discover the counting principles (around four years of age), children learn to map numbers 1 to 4 to the corresponding cardinalities one after the other, and it may take them up to six months to move onto the next number [65,66]. Some suggested that the cause underlying this difficulty is the need to reconcile two mutually incompatible systems: the ANS, providing approximate representations of number, and

BOX 17.2

REFINING THE APPROXIMATE NUMBER CODE: NEURAL MECHANISMS

One crucial step towards the construction of a representation of exact numbers is achieved when children understand the counting principles, thanks to which they can perform exact quantification on sets of any cardinality, thus overcoming the low resolution of ANS acuity. The mechanisms underlying this major achievement are still unexplored and thus remain largely unknown. One possibility is that one key aspect would involve a quick re-tuning of the coding schemes of a subset of parietal ANS neurons, such that through interaction with a precise symbolic system, where any number n is distinguished categorically from its neighbors $n - 1$ and $n + 1$, the tuning curves of a subset of numerosity detector neurons would become sharper, and the number representations would segregate into categorically quasi-distinct domains for the entire number range. This proposal, also modeled by means of a neuronal network simulation [17], is consistent with a recent neuroimaging study reporting that, while MVPA algorithms (classification algorithm based on the distributed pattern of activation over a voxels within a given brain region) trained to discriminate symbolic numbers on the basis of the activity of a distributed set of parietal cortex voxels, could accurately predict the corresponding non-symbolic numerical quantities, the contrary was not possible. This suggests that in the IPS (intraparietal sulcus) intermingled populations coding for numerical quantities show different coding schemes: broader for non-symbolic number, and sharper, but with preserved analog response properties, for numerical symbols. The emergence of such new coding schemes is possibly mediated by feedback "tuning sharpening" projections from categorical coding neurons in the frontal cortex [87,96,97], as suggested by higher frontal cortex activation reported in children compared to adults during both symbolic and non-symbolic comparison tasks [98–100]. The changes of parietal quantity coding schemes and the changes in their coupling with inferior frontal cortex activity should be visible using fine neuroimaging techniques during development.

the OTS, limited in capacity to three to four items, supporting operations on individual objects and providing an indirect notion of exact number [2,51,52]. Others hold that lexical acquisition is built upon the OTS without any contribution from the ANS, and attribute the seriality of this process to the fact that children have to learn the successor function (see Glossary), which comes from learning the count list by rote first, which is itself a serial process [2,52] (see Box 17.3). An alternative view, which I propose here, would be that two features of the ANS alone may account for the lexical acquisition process before understanding the counting principles: first, the ANS is not restricted to large numbers, but it extends to all numerosities [67–70]; and second, by virtue of its weberian code and its increase in precision during the life span, it comes to represent small numbers with extremely high precision by the first years of life. A representation of (exact) number N, which is a necessary condition

---

BOX 17.3

THE BOOTSTRAPPING ACCOUNT OF CAREY AND COLLEAGUES

Carey and colleagues suggest that children acquire the meaning of the first number words (one to four) by constructing and storing in long-term memory a mental model of a set of individuals for each number, along with a procedure that determines that the number words can be applied to any set that can be put in one-to-one correspondence with this model [2]. For example, a mental model for the number word "two" has the form of {j k}, and a new set of two elements (e.g., of two apples) is associated to its corresponding number ("two") by one-to-one correspondences between individual objects of the external set (each apple) and individual objects of the internal model ({j k}). While it is currently unstated in the theory whether the one-to-one correspondence is itself a parallel or a serial process, the emerging representation is clearly not intrinsically numerical, but rather, it is a "model of individuals" [52]. Once the child has constructed these models, the number words associated with them are then aligned with the ordered number words in the numerical sequence, which the child initially learns by route. This

happens via a mechanism called "bootstrapping". Bootstrapping is a mechanism by which so called "place-holder structures" are combined with pre-constructed concepts. In the case of numbers, the place-holder structure is held to be the counting list (initially acquired as a meaningless sequence of sounds), while the pre-constructed concepts are the small number representations, issuing from the OTS, stored in long-term memory together with the one-to-one correspondence rule. When children notice the correspondence between the first number words that refer to long-term memory representations of sets, and the first number-words in the numerical sequence they try and align those two independent representations. The alignment between order on the number list and order in a series of sets related by *additional individual*, children make the induction: for any word in the count list that refers to set with cardinality n, the next word in the list refers to set with cardinality $n + 1$, thus they are able to attribute meaning to any new number word.

---

for lexical acquisition of numbers, emerges only if children can consistently discriminate the set of N from the numerically adjacent sets (N − 1 and N + 1). Thus, children should be able to accurately understand the numeral "three" only when they can reliably distinguish a set of three from a set of two and a set of four (that is, when they become sensitive to a 3:4 ratio), which occurs, according to the fit to the existing available data, after the third year of life (see Fig. 17.1). Indeed, children become "3-knowers" at about this age [52,66]. The present proposal further predicts that it should be fairly difficult to teach new number words to children if their ANS does not allow a precise discrimination of the corresponding quantities, a prediction that was also recently confirmed [71]. A final testable prediction also follows: ANS acuity should tightly correlate with the inter-individual variability of lexical acquisition of number during the first years of life.

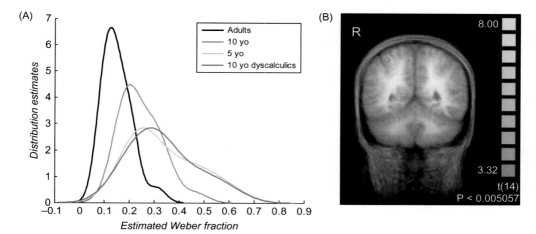

FIGURE 17.4   **ANS impairments in dyscalculia.** (A) Estimated Weber fraction distribution in four populations (using the same dots comparison task): normally developing adults ($n = 20$), kindergarteners ($n = 26$), 10-year-old children ($n = 26$) and 10-year-old, age- and IQ-matched children with developmental dyscalculia ($n = 23$) [22]. Dyscalculic ANS acuity is lower than age- and IQ-matched controls, and identical to that of children who are five years younger. (B) Right-parietal regions showing decreased ratio effect in non-symbolic number comparison in dyscalculic children compared with age- and IQ-matched controls [78].

The ANS and Developmental Dyscalculia

A strong prediction from the hypothesis that the ANS is a start-up system in symbolic number processing is that ANS impairment should engender difficulties in symbolic number acquisition. Thus, children with dyscalculia, a specific learning disability that affects the acquisition of knowledge about numbers and arithmetic [72], should show impairments in the ANS. This prediction received recent support [22,73,74] (see, however, [75,76] for failure in detecting ANS impairments in dyscalculics and [62] for no relationship between non-symbolic number discrimination and individual differences in children's mathematical achievement). In one study, a cohort of dyscalculic children aged about 10 was tested, diagnosed with a standardized battery probing knowledge of symbolic numbers and calculation. The performance of this group was compared to a group of age- and IQ-matched normally developing children as well as a group of kindergarteners [22]. Dyscalculics' ANS acuity (derived from performance in a dot comparison test) was severely impaired compared to their age-matched controls' and showed a five-year delay (see Fig. 17.4). Moreover, the size of the ANS impairment predicted symbolic number comparison impairments, consistent with another recent study reporting both non-symbolic and symbolic number comparison deficits in dyscalculic children [77]. Consistently, dyscalculia is associated with decreased mid-parietal activation during both quantity comparison tasks [78] and symbolic calculation [79], as well as anatomical alterations in mid-parietal cortex (reduced gray matter, abnormal gyrification and sulcal depth) compared to control, non-dyscalculic subjects [79,80].

Despite the importance of these results, however, because of their correlational nature, it is at present impossible to firmly establish the direction of the causal links between

---

BOX 17.4

QUESTIONS FOR FUTURE RESEARCH

- Does ANS acuity increase smoothly over development or are there any developmental discontinuities? If so, what are they related to?
- What is the direction of the causal relation between the ANS and mathematical achievement? Is ANS acuity as measured early in life a reliable and specific predictor of later mathematical achievement?
- Does the refinement of the ANS during the life span reflect maturation or is it

driven by the training with symbolic numbers?
- Do early impairments in the OTS engender developmental dyscalculia?
- What are the neural underpinnings of the OTS in adults and children?
- Currently there is only evidence that the neural code for approximate representations becomes less noisy, but there is no evidence that it becomes exact. How does the brain support representations of exact numbers?

---

dyscalculia, ANS impairments, and altered parietal function and structure. ANS impairments, together with the related parietal dysfunctions might be both the cause and the consequence of lack of learning to manipulate symbolic numbers, inasmuch as in the dyslexia literature lack of phonological awareness as well as altered activation in posterior perisilvian areas are seen both as a putative cause of the reading impairment, but also as a consequence of lack of learning to read [81].

In sum, while several strands of behavioral and neuroimaging evidence point toward an important and long-lasting role of the ANS in symbolic numerical thinking, the ultimate proof of its foundational role in the acquisition of symbolic numbers will only be provided by longitudinal investigations. At present, the only existing longitudinal study reporting a specific correlation between ANS acuity and mathematical achievement relates the ANS acuity of children at 14 years old to their mathematical proficiency earlier on (in 5 years old) [21]. Clearly, however, in light of the previously discussed issues of circular causality, it would be important to know if ANS acuity as measured early in life, and crucially before the acquisition of symbolic numbers, can reliably predict subsequent success in arithmetical tasks (see Box 17.4).

EVIDENCE FOR A FOUNDATIONAL ROLE OF THE OTS IN SYMBOLIC NUMBER PROCESSING

Some theories of the acquisition of symbolic numbers propose that the OTS is foundational because it provides the notion of exact number and allows endorsing the successor (+1) relations between adjacent numbers [2,50–52] (see Box 17.3). Indeed, it is often claimed that the ANS cannot provide semantic foundation to the representations of symbolic natural numbers because it lacks these two properties [50].

Traces of OTS Signatures in Symbolic Number Processing

The most important computational constraint of the OTS is that it is limited to small sets. Evidence for an important role of the OTS in symbolic number processing has been that the first number words are acquired initially for the small cardinalities, 1–4, and only after the discovery of the counting principles, to larger sets [65,66]. When the counting principles are acquired, however, traces of the OTS in symbolic number processing seem to disappear: to date there have been no reports of abrupt differences in behavioral or neural signatures of processing small (1–4) *vs* larger symbolic numbers in tasks such as comparison, naming, or arithmetic. Instead, distance and magnitude effects, reflecting a continuous approximate and compressed scaling of numbers, typically characterize symbolic number processing (see above). Further, there is no neuroimaging evidence in either children or adults showing activation specific to symbolic numbers that reflects a discontinuity around 3–4 in regions previously tentatively associated with the OTS, such as posterior parietal, occipital, or right temporo-parietal cortex. Instead, a progressive recruitment of mid- and inferior parietal cortex, partially overlapping with the cerebral circuits of the ANS, especially of the left hemisphere, together with a progressive reduced activation in frontal regions seems to support the progressive mastering of symbolic numbers during development (see [82] for a recent review). Data from neuropsychological studies is not more encouraging: acquired dyscalculia is not systematically, and not even frequently, associated with disorders of multiple object tracking. As discussed above, multiple object tracking deficits (simultanagnosia) typically occur after bilateral lesions in the posterior occipito-parietal cortex [45,46], and are not typically associated with calculation or number representation disorders.

The Relation Between the Developmental Trajectory of The OTS and the Initial Stages of Symbolic Number Acquisition

The capacity limit of the OTS develops quickly over the first year of life: on average, infants have an adult-like multiple object tracking capacity limit of three to four items already at 12 months [36–38]. This means that by the first year of life children already possess three or four "attentional pointers" that could be used to track up to four objects in parallel and thus to discriminate sets of one to three or four items. Thus, if lexical acquisition in young children were to build upon the OTS, as suggested [2], then children should be able to attach the words "one", "two", "three", and maybe "four" to the corresponding sets at once and with little effort. Instead, as reviewed, lexical acquisition for the first numbers is slow and strictly serial [65,66]. Accounts that the seriality of number acquisition is caused by the seriality of the acquisition of verbal counting [2,52] are rather unconvincing because the numerical sequence is acquired much earlier than numerical meaning, such that children understanding only the meaning of number "one" already know how to recite the number sequence of numbers up to eight or nine [52]. Moreover, in younger children and infants, there is evidence that the OTS can be detrimental in numerical tasks. As reviewed above, objects are represented in the OTS as distinct individuals, with a given set of physical features, such as identity, color, surface area, contour length, etc., and it was shown that for small sets falling within the limits of the OTS (<4) when certain such features (such as surface area or contour length) are pitted against number, infants sometimes automatically attend to those and thus fail to respond to number (see [51] for a review). It is extremely difficult to understand how a system that often interferes with numerical tasks might be relevant for learning yet more complex numerical representations.

OTS and Developmental Dyscalculia

In contrast to evidence for impairments in the ANS in dyscalculia, there seems to be no evidence to date for impaired OTS. Such evidence could take the form of impairments in subitizing, the adult measure of OTS capacity, in visuo-spatial short term memory capacity, also highly correlated with subitizing across subjects in adults (Piazza *et al.*, unpublished data), or in the multiple object tracking task, where subjects are asked to track the position of multiple objects moving along independent trajectories on the display. However, impairments in subitizing have not been convincingly reported in dyscalculia. On the contrary, dyscalculia seems to be associated with slowed serial counting for sets of more than four items [83,84]. As for visuo-spatial short term memory, the studies that report impairments in dyscalculia are plentiful, but they typically use tasks (such as the Corsi test) (e.g., [85,86]) that do not assess pure visuo-spatial span, but rather more complex abilities such as sequential order processing and complex visuo-motor co-ordination, allowing no strict conclusions on whether dyscalculics have a reduced OTS. In sum, current data do not strongly support a foundational role of OTS in symbolic number acquisition.

CONCLUDING REMARKS

Humans come to life with strong intuitions on approximate numerical quantities and their relations. There is evidence to suggest that culture-based acquisition of symbols representing exact numerical quantities is grounded on these pre-existing intuitions, while there is little evidence for a foundational role of the parallel individuation system. Current neuroimaging data suggest that representations of exact numbers emerge through important modifications of the pre-existing parietal coding schemes for approximate numerical quantity. Under investigation at the moment is the role of language and of visuo-spatial operations such as serial pointing and serial individuation, instantiating the one-to-one correspondence principle in counting, maybe initially mediated by frontal cortex regions acting as a "tuning sharpener" [87] of the core parietal approximate number code.

However, despite the current evidence suggesting the ANS rather than the OTS as being foundational in the construction of symbolic numerical thinking, there is a strong need for behavioral and neuroimaging data that would clarify the nature of the cognitive and neural changes occurring during the crucial period when children acquire the first symbolic numbers and learn the counting principles. Longitudinal studies mapping the exact status of knowledge before, during and after the crucial period between two and five years of age during which the natural number concepts are acquired would be of capital importance to understand the relative role of the early quantification systems, how they account for the speed and accuracy of cultural learning, and if and how they are in turn modified by cultural learning. This will be the starting point for new exciting discoveries on how humans, even though constrained by the limitations imposed by the functional architecture of their primate brains, manage to construct and combine a strikingly rich set of abstract representations.

GLOSSARY

Approximate Number System (ANS)

A system for representing the approximate number of items in sets, also sometimes referred to as 'analogue magnitude system'.

Cardinality

A property of sets indicating the number of elements in the set.

Object Tracking System (OTS)

A system for tracking multiple individuals, limited in capacity to 3 or 4 items, also sometimes referred to as 'parallel individuation system'.

Phonological Awareness

An individual's awareness of the phonological structure of words. It includes the ability to distinguish different units of speech, such as individual phonemes in syllables, syllables in words, and rhymes between words. Phonological skills are critical for the development of reading, as they are an important and reliable predictor of later reading ability [88,89].

Scalar Variability

A property of the response distribution in estimation tasks (including numerosity estimation), whereby the mean responses and standard deviation of the responses are proportional to each other as the quantity to be estimated varies, such that the coefficient of variation (CV = standard deviation/ mean) is constant across a wide range of quantities. Scalar variability is an instance of Weber's law [90].

Subitizing

The rapid, accurate, and confident judgment of the number of items in small collections "at a glance", without counting. Subitizing is thought to emerge from the ability to allocate attention over multiple individual items in parallel (i.e. the OTS system) [34,91].

Successor Function

A rule establishing the existence of a minimal quantity, ONE, which corresponds to the minimal distance between two successive numbers.

Weber's Fraction

The smallest variation to a quantity that can be readily perceived. When performing numerosity discrimination threshold experiments, the first analysis is often aimed at establishing whether or not Weber's law holds for that set of discriminations. If it does, the next step is to determine what the Weber fraction is. The Weber fraction can be straightforwardly derived from the accuracy performance as the difference between the two closest discriminable numerosities normalized by their size, and can sometimes also be expressed as a percentage. Better fits of numerosity response functions can sometimes be obtained by modeling the task with more refined psychophysical functions including some free parameters accounting for response biases which, in particular conditions, may influence performance [23,92,93]. The measure derived by this method has been labeled "internal Weber fraction" to differentiate it from the "behavioral Weber fraction". Irrespective of the method used to estimate the Weber fraction, different studies find broadly convergent results that an average adult can reliably discriminate sets with a numerical ratio of 7:8 (a Weber fraction of approx. 0.15) [22,23,64,91,92].

Weber's Law

A psychophysical law describing the relationship between the physical and the perceived magnitude of a stimulus. It states that the threshold of discrimination (also referred to as the "smallest noticeable difference") between two stimuli increases linearly with stimulus intensity. Weber's law (as first demonstrated by Gustav Fechner [14]) can be accounted for by postulating a logarithmic relation between the physical stimulus and its internal representation. $Dp = K^* \Delta S/S$, where Dp = smallest noticeable difference; dS = physical difference; S = stimulus intensity.

References

[1] E. Spelke, K. Kinzler, Core knowledge, Dev. Sci. 10 (2007) 89–96.
[2] S. Carey, The Origin of Concepts, Oxford University Press
[3] S. Dehaene, L. Cohen, Cultural recycling of cortical maps, Neuron 56 (2007) 384–398.
[4] E. Brannon, J. Roitman, Nonverbal representations of time and number in animals and human infants, in: W.H. Meck, (Ed.), Functional and Neural Mechanisms of Interval Timing, CRC, (2003) pp. 143–182.
[5] K. Jordan, et al., Monkeys match the number of voices they hear to the number of faces they see, Curr. Biol. 15 (2005) 1034–1038.
[6] K. Jordan, et al., Monkeys match and tally quantities across senses, Cognition 108 (2008) 617–625.
[7] K. McComb, et al., Roaring and numerical assessment in contests between groups of female lions, *Panthera leo*, Anim. Behav. 47 (1994) 379–387.
[8] M. Wilson, et al., Chimpanzees and the mathematics of battle, Proc. R. Soc. Lond., B, Biol. Sci. 269 (2002) 1107–1112.
[9] J. Krebs, N. Davies, An Introduction to Behavioural Ecology, Wiley–Blackwell
[10] B. Lyon, Egg recognition and counting reduce costs of avian conspecific brood parasitism, Nature 422 (2003) 495–499.
[11] J. Cantlon, E. Brannon, Basic math in monkeys and college students, PLoS Biol. 5 (2007) e328.
[12] J. Flombaum, et al., Rhesus monkeys (*Macaca mulatta*) spontaneously compute addition operations over large numbers, Cognition 97 (2005) 315–325.
[13] V. Izard, et al., Newborn infants perceive abstract numbers, Proc. Natl. Acad. Sci. USA. 106 (2009) 10382–10385.
[14] G.T. Fechner, Elemente der Psychophysik, Breitkopf & Hartel
[15] C.R. Gallistel, R. Gelman, Preverbal and verbal counting and computation, Cognition 44 (1992) 43–74.
[16] S. Dehaene, The neural basis of the Weber–Fechner law: a logarithmic mental number line, Trends Cog. Sci. 7 (2003) 145–147.
[17] T. Verguts, W. Fias, Representation of number in animals and humans: a neural model, J. Cog. Neurosci. 16 (2004) 1493–1504.
[18] M. Zorzi, B. Butterworth, A computational model of number comparison, in: M. Hahn, (Ed.), Proceedings of the Twenty-First Annual Conference of the Cognitive Science Society, Erlbaum, (1999) pp. 772–777.
[19] M. Piazza, et al., Tuning curves for approximate numerosity in the human intraparietal sulcus, Neuron 44 (2004) 547–555.
[20] M.E. Libertus, E.M. Brannon, Stable individual differences in number discrimination in infancy, Dev. Sci. (2010). Volume, DOI: 10.1111/j.1467-7687.2009.00948.x

[21] J. Halberda, et al., Individual differences in non-verbal number acuity correlate with maths achievement, Nature 455 (2008) 665–668.

[22] M. Piazza, et al., Developmental trajectory of number acuity reveals a severe impairment in developmental dyscalculia, Cognition 116 (2010) 33–41.

[23] J. Halberda, L. Feigenson, Developmental change in the acuity of the "Number Sense": the approximate number system in 3-, 4-, 5-, and 6-year-olds and adults, Dev. Psychol. 44 (2008) 1457–1465.

[24] J. Lipton, E. Spelke, Origins of number sense: large number discrimination in human infants, Psychol. Sci. 14 (2003) 396–401.

[25] F. Xu, E.S. Spelke, Large number discrimination in 6-month-old infants, Cognition 74 (2000) B1–B11.

[26] E. Eger, et al., Deciphering cortical number coding from human brain activity patterns, Curr. Biol. 19 (2009) 1608–1615.

[27] A. Knops, et al., Recruitment of an area involved in eye movements during mental arithmetic, Science 324 (2009) 1583–1585.

[28] V. Dormal, et al., Mode-dependent and mode-independent representations of numerosity in the right intraparietal sulcus, Neuroimage 52 (2010) 1677–1686.

[29] M. Piazza, V. Izard, How humans count: numerosity and the parietal cortex, Neuroscientist 15 (2009) 261–273.

[30] S. Dehaene, Origins of mathematical intuitions, Ann. N.Y. Acad. Sci. 1156 (2009) 232–259.

[31] G. Alvarez, P. Cavanagh, The capacity of visual short-term memory is set both by visual information load and by number of objects, Psychol. Sci. 15 (2004) 106–111.

[32] B. Scholl, Objects and attention: the state of the art, Cognition 80 (2001) 1–46.

[33] Z. Pylyshyn, Visual indexes, preconceptual objects, and situated vision, Cognition 80 (2001) 127–158.

[34] S.K. Revkin, et al., Does subitizing reflect numerical estimation?, Psychol. Sci. 19 (2008) 607–614.

[35] E. Vogel, M. Machizawa, Neural activity predicts individual differences in visual working memory capacity, Nature 428 (2004) 748–751.

[36] S. Ross-Sheehy, et al., The development of visual short-term memory capacity in infants, Child Dev. 74 (2003) 1807–1822.

[37] L. Oakes, et al., Rapid development of feature binding in visual short-term memory, Psychol. Sci. 17 (2006) 781–787.

[38] S. Rose, et al., Visual short-term memory in the first year of life: capacity and recency effects, Dev. Psychol. 37 (2001) 539–549.

[39] J. Todd, R. Marois, Capacity limit of visual short-term memory in human posterior parietal cortex, Nature 428 (2004) 751–754.

[40] Y. Xu, M.M. Chun, Dissociable neural mechanisms supporting visual short-term memory for objects, Nature 440 (2006) 91–95.

[41] M. Piazza, et al., Single-trial classification of parallel pre-attentive and serial attentive processes using functional magnetic resonance imaging, Proc. R. Soc. Lond., B, Biol. Sci. 270 (2003) 1237–1245.

[42] K. Sathian, et al., Neural evidence linking visual object enumeration and attention, J. Cogn. Neurosci. 11 (1999) 36–51.

[43] P. Vetter, et al., A candidate for the attentional bottleneck: set-size specific modulation of the right TPJ during attentive enumeration, J. Cog. Neurosci. (2010) 1–9.

[44] D. Ansari, et al., Linking visual attention and number processing in the brain: the role of the temporo-parietal junction in small and large symbolic and nonsymbolic number comparison, J. Cog. Neurosci. 19 (2007) 1845–1853.

[45] H.B. Coslett, E. Saffran, Simultanagnosia: to see but not two see, Brain 114 (1991) 1523–1545.

[46] M. Rizzo, S. Vecera, Psychoanatomical substrates of Balint's syndrome, Br. Med. J. 72 (2002) 162–178.

[47] S. Dehaene, L. Cohen, Dissociable mechanisms of subitizing and counting: neuropsychological evidence from simultanagnosic patients, J. Exp. Psychol. Hum. Percept. Perform. 20 (1994) 958–975.

[48] D. Hyde, E. Spelke, All numbers are not equal: an electrophysiological investigation of small and large number representations, J. Cog. Neurosci. 21 (2009) 1039–1053.

[49] S. Dehaene, J.P. Changeux, Development of elementary numerical abilities: a neuronal model, J. Cog. Neurosci. 5 (1993) 390–407.

[50] S. Carey, Cognitive foundations of arithmetic: evolution and ontogenesis, Mind Lang 16 (2001) 37–55.

[51] L. Feigenson, et al., Core systems of number, Trends Cogn. Sci. 8 (2004) 307–314.

[52] M. Le Corre, S. Carey, One, two, three, four, nothing more: an investigation of the conceptual sources of the verbal counting principles, Cognition 105 (2007) 395–438.

[53] L. Rips, et al., From numerical concepts to concepts of number, Behav. Brain Sci. 31 (2008) 623–642.

[54] C.K. Gilmore, et al., Symbolic arithmetic knowledge without instruction, Nature 447 (2007) 589–591.

[55] C.K. Gilmore, et al., Non-symbolic arithmetic abilities and mathematics achievement in the first year of formal schooling, Cognition 115 (2010) 394–406.

[56] I.D. Holloway, D. Ansari, Mapping numerical magnitudes onto symbols: the numerical distance effect and individual differences in children's mathematics achievement, J. Exp. Child Psychol. 103 (2009) 17–29.

[57] R.S. Moyer, T.K. Landauer, Time required for judgements of numerical inequality, Nature 215 (1967) 1519–1520.

[58] F. Van Opstal, et al., Dissecting the symbolic distance effect: comparison and priming effects in numerical and nonnumerical orders, Psychon. Bull. Rev. 15 (2008) 419–425.

[59] B. Reynvoet, et al., Semantic priming in number naming, Q. J. Exp. Psychol. A 55 (2002) 1127–1139.

[60] B. Reynvoet, et al., Children's representation of symbolic magnitude: the development of the priming distance effect, J. Exp. Child Psychol. 103 (2009) 480–489.

[61] M. Libertus, et al., Electrophysiological evidence for notation independence in numerical processing, Behav. Brain Funct. 3 (2007) 1.

[62] E. Temple, M.I. Posner, Brain mechanisms of quantity are similar in 5-year-olds and adults, Proc. Natl. Acad. Sci. USA. 95 (1998) 7836–7841.

[63] K. Notebaert, et al., The magnitude representation of small and large symbolic numbers in the left and right hemisphere: an event-related fMRI study, J. Cog. Neurosci. (In press).

[64] M. Piazza, et al., A magnitude code common to numerosities and number symbols in human intraparietal cortex, Neuron 53 (2007) 293–305.

[65] K. Wynn, Children's understanding of counting, Cognition 36 (1990) 155–193.

[66] K. Wynn, Children's acquisition of the number words and the counting system, Cogn. Psychol. 24 (1992) 220–251.

[67] K. vanMarle, K. Wynn, Infants' auditory enumeration: evidence for analog magnitudes in the small number range, Cognition 111 (2009) 302–316.

[68] J.F. Cantlon, E.M. Brannon, Shared system for ordering small and large numbers in monkeys and humans, Psychol. Sci. 17 (2006) 401–406.

[69] V. Izard, et al., Distinct cerebral pathways for object identity and number in human infants, PLoS Biol. 6 (2008) e11.

[70] J. Cantlon, et al., Spontaneous analog number representations in 3-year-old children, Dev. Sci. 13 (2010) 289–297.

[71] Y. Huang, et al., When is four far more than three? Psychol. Sci. 21 (2010) 600–606.

[72] B. Butterworth, Developmental dyscalculia, in: J.I.D. Campbell, (Ed.), Handbook of Mathematical Cognition, Psychology Press, (2005) pp. 455–467.

[73] M. Mazzocco, et al., Impaired acuity of the approximate number system underlies mathematical learning disability. Child Dev. (In press).

[74] C. Mussolin, et al., Symbolic and nonsymbolic number comparison in children with and without dyscalculia, Cognition 115 (2010) 10–25.

[75] L. Rousselle, M.P. Noel, Basic numerical skills in children with mathematics learning disabilities: a comparison of symbolic vs non-symbolic number magnitude processing, Cognition 102 (2007) 361–395.

[76] T. Iuculano, et al., Core information processing deficits in developmental dyscalculia and low numeracy, Dev. Sci. 11 (2008) 669–680.

[77] C. Mussolin, et al., Symbolic and nonsymbolic number comparison in children with and without dyscalculia, Cognition 115 (2010) 10–25.

[78] G.R. Price, et al., Impaired parietal magnitude processing in developmental dyscalculia, Curr. Biol. 17 (2007) R1042–1043.

[79] N. Molko, et al., Functional and structural alterations of the intraparietal sulcus in a developmental dyscalculia of genetic origin, Neuron 40 (2003) 847–858.

[80] E.B. Isaacs, et al., Calculation difficulties in children of very low birthweight: a neural correlate, Brain 124 (2001) 1701–1707.

[81] A. Castles, M. Coltheart, Is there a causal link from phonological awareness to success in learning to read? Cognition 91 (2004) 77–111.

[82] D. Ansari, et al., Effects of development and enculturation on number representation in the brain, Nat. Rev. Neurosci. 9 (2008) 278–291.

[83] K. Landerl, et al., Developmental dyscalculia and basic numerical capacities: a study of 8–9-year-old students, Cognition 93 (2004) 99–125.

[84] E. Maloney, et al., Mathematics anxiety affects counting but not subitizing during visual enumeration, Cognition 114 (2009) 293–297.

[85] R. Bull, et al., Exploring the roles of the visual–spatial sketch pad and central executive in children's arithmetical skills: views from cognition and developmental neuropsychology, Dev. Neuropsychol. 15 (1999) 421–442.

[86] J. McLean, G. Hitch, Working memory impairments in children with specific arithmetic learning difficulties, J. Exp. Child Psychol. 74 (1999) 240–260.

[87] D. Freedman, et al., Categorical representation of visual stimuli in the primate prefrontal cortex, Science 291 (2001) 312–316.

[88] J. Ziegler, U. Goswami, Reading acquisition, developmental dyslexia, and skilled reading across languages: a psycholinguistic grain size theory, Psych. Bull. 131 (2005) 3–29.

[89] L. Bradley, P.E. Bryant, Categorizing sounds and learning to read—a causal connection, Nature 301 (1983) 419–421.

[90] V. Izard, S. Dehaene, Calibrating the mental number line, Cognition 106 (2008) 1221–1247.

[91] D. Burr, et al., Subitizing but not estimation of numerosity requires attentional resources, J. Vis. 10 (2010).

[92] P. Pica, et al., Exact and approximate arithmetic in an Amazonian indigene group, Science 306 (2004) 499–503.

[93] S. Dehaene, Symbols and quantities in parietal cortex: elements of a mathematical theory of number representation and manipulation, in: Attention and Performance, Press HU ed., vol. 22, 2007, pp. 527–574.

[94] C.R. Gallistel, R. Gelman, The preverbal counting process, in: W. Kessen, et al. (Ed.), Thoughts Memories and Emotions: Essays in Honor of George Mandler, Lawrence Erlbaum Associates, (1991) pp. 65–81.

[95] S. Cordes, E.M. Brannon, Two systems or one? Infants discriminate small from large numerosities, Dev. Psychol. (In press).

[96] E. Meyers, et al., Dynamic population coding of category information in inferior temporal and prefrontal cortex, J. Neurophysiol. 100 (2008) 1407.

[97] I. Diester, A. Nieder, Semantic associations between signs and numerical categories in the prefrontal cortex, PLoS Biol. 5 (2007) e294.

[98] J. Cantlon, et al., The neural development of an abstract concept of number, J. Cog. Neurosci. 21 (2009) 2217–2229.

[99] D. Ansari, B. Dhital, Age-related changes in the activation of the intraparietal sulcus during nonsymbolic magnitude processing: an event-related functional magnetic resonance imaging study, J. Cog. Neurosci. 18 (2006) 1820–1828.

[100] D. Ansari, et al., Neural correlates of symbolic number processing in children and adults, Neuroreport 16 (2005) 1769–1773.

Natural Number and Natural Geometry

Elizabeth S. Spelke

Harvard University, Cambridge, USA

Summary

How does the human brain support abstract concepts such as *seven* or *square*? Studies of non-human animals, of human infants, and of children and adults in diverse cultures suggest these concepts arise from a set of cognitive systems that are phylogenetically ancient, innate, and universal across humans: systems of *core knowledge*. Two of these systems—for tracking small numbers of objects and for assessing, comparing and combining the approximate cardinal values of sets—capture the primary information in the system of positive integers. Two other systems—for representing the shapes of small-scale forms and the distances and directions of surfaces in the large-scale navigable layout—capture the primary information in the system of Euclidean plane geometry. As children learn language and other symbol systems, they begin to combine their core numerical and geometrical representations productively, in uniquely human ways. These combinations may give rise to the first truly abstract concepts at the foundations of mathematics.

For millenia, philosophers and scientists have pondered the existence, nature and origins of abstract numerical and geometrical concepts, because these concepts have striking features. First, the integers, and the figures of the Euclidean plane, are so intuitive to human adults that the systems underlying them are called "natural number" and, by some, "natural geometry" [1]. Second, these two systems are extremely useful: it is hard to find any important human cultural achievement—from money to measurement, to the arts, sciences, and mathematics—that does not depend on them. Third, these conceptual systems are simple: five postulates, together with some general axioms of logic, suffice to define all the objects of Euclidean geometry, and an even smaller set of postulates defines the positive integers. It is perhaps not surprising, therefore, that explorations of the origins of abstract concepts, from Plato [2] and Kant [3] to Piaget [4] and Carey [5], often use number or geometry as case studies.

Space, Time and Number in the Brain.
DOI: 10.1016/B978-0-12-385948-8.00018-9

© 2011 Elsevier Inc. All rights reserved.

Although natural number and natural geometry are important, intuitive, and formally simple, they are also highly puzzling from the standpoint of psychology and neuroscience. One puzzle concerns the sources of these concepts. Most concepts, like *crow* and *cell phone*, appear to be shaped by experience, but it is far from obvious how experience could produce these abstract concepts. All our perceptions have finite resolution, yet the objects of Euclidean geometry are points so small they have no extent, and lines so thin they have no thickness. All our actions, moreover, have finite extent and duration, yet we conceive of lines as infinitely long and of integers as arrayed in an endless sequence. A second puzzle concerns the application of these concepts. Most concepts apply to some things but not others: *cow* applies to cows and *brown* to a property of brown things. In contrast, concepts of number and geometry apply to everything: anything that we can conceive of at all can be characterized with numerical or spatial terms (*seven samurai, seas or sins; a distant village, era, or cousin*).

Where do these concepts come from? Despite the efforts of the world's greatest thinkers and experimenters, from Socrates to Helmholtz, this question has not been answered [6]. I believe, however, that it can be addressed by research that takes four comparative approaches. First, comparisons across species tracing continuity and change in the evolution of spatial and numerical abilities. Second, comparisons over human development can trace both the origins of these abilities and their changes with growth and education. Third, comparisons across cultures, or across individual humans with different degrees of access to the products of their culture, can elucidate universal and variable aspects of these abilities. Fourth, comparisons across levels of analysis, from cognition and action to brain systems, neurons and genes, can probe the systems on which our spatial and numerical concepts depend.

These strands of research provide converging evidence for at least four cognitive systems that are sources of our numerical and geometrical intuitions: a system for comparing and combining sets based on their cardinal values, a system for selecting and tracking small numbers of numerically distinct individuals, a system for representing the shape of the large-scale layout so as to determine one's own position, and a system for distinguishing the shapes of small-scale objects and visual forms so as to identify objects of particular kinds. Each of these systems has a long evolutionary history; none is unique to humans. Each system emerges early in development, largely independently of any specific experiences with the entities to which it applies. Above all, each of the systems has genuine numerical or spatial content on which we draw when we learn and perform symbolic mathematics. Because they are innate systems with mathematical content, I will call them *core systems of number and geometry*.

This chapter begins with a brief review of the evidence for the existence and properties of two of these core knowledge systems. Drawing on this evidence, I suggest that research has effectively addressed two of the more difficult problems in cognitive science: the problem of determining the content of non-linguistic representations, and the problem of determining the role of innate capacities in the development of those representations. Solutions to both problems hinge critically on the discovery that these systems are shared by humans and nonhuman animals. Thus, studies of educated humans shed light on animal minds, and studies of animals shed light on the development of human concepts.

This review will also elucidate two properties of these systems that distinguish them from truly abstract number and geometry: each system captures some but not all of the properties of natural number and Euclidean geometry, and each system applies to some but not all of the objects to which our abstract mathematical concepts apply. I conclude that no core system, by itself, accounts for our capacity to learn and use these fully abstract concepts. Finally, I offer

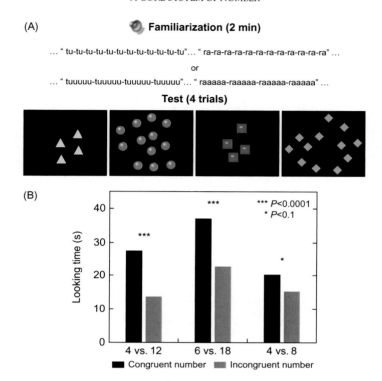

FIGURE 18.1 (A) Auditory and visual displays for an experiment on number representations by newborn infants, and (B) infants' looking times to the visual arrays that corresponded or differed in number from the accompanying auditory sequences ([7], reprinted with permission from PNAS).

two suggestions concerning the latter capacity: children and adults build systems of abstract number and geometry by productively combining the outputs of these four systems, and this process depends, in some way, on the acquisition and use of natural language.

A CORE SYSTEM OF NUMBER

An experiment by Izard *et al.* [7] serves to introduce the first core system. Newborn infants in a hospital nursery were presented with a series of syllable trains varying in pitch and duration. Across the different trains, the particular repeating syllable changed but the number of syllables per train was constant: four for half the infants and 12 for the others. After 2 min, a visual array of either four or 12 objects appeared on a large video screen (Fig. 18.1A). To ensure that no non-numerical variables connected these sounds to either array, the trains of four and 12 syllables were equated in extensive variables (train duration, total amount of sound) and differed in intensive variables (syllable frequency, duration of individual syllables), whereas the arrays of visible objects were equated in intensive variables (item size and density) and differed in extensive variables (array size, total amount of filled area on the screen). Across trials, the number of objects alternated between four and 12 while the syllable trains continued, and infants' looking time at each array was recorded, guided by findings that infants tend to look longer at visual arrays that correspond to an ongoing sound sequence (e.g., [8]). The newborn infants looked longer at the numerically corresponding visual arrays, detecting the numerical relationship between the auditory temporal sequences and visual spatial arrays (Fig. 18.1B, left).

Many experiments, conducted over the last decade, support the conclusion that prelinguistic infants are sensitive to number in spatial arrays (e.g., [9–11]) and temporal sequences (e.g., [12,13]). Evidence for these abilities comes from experiments using a variety of measures including preferential looking (e.g., Brannon, Chapter 14 of this volume), habituation of looking time (e.g., [9]), anticipatory head turning (e.g., [12]), exploratory reaching (e.g., [14]), and the neuroimaging measures of electroencephalography (e.g., [15,16]) and near infrared spectroscopy (e.g., [17]). Most important, this research reveals five important, non-obvious *signatures* of infants' numerical representations.

First, infants' ability to discriminate one numerical value from another depends on the ratio of the two values. In Izard *et al.*'s studies, newborn infants reliably discriminated between numbers that differed by a ratio of 3 (12 *vs* 4, 18 *vs* 6) but performed markedly less well when numbers differed by a ratio of 2 (8 *vs* 4; Fig. 18.1B). Over the first year, the critical ratio drops to 2 at six months and to 1.5 at 9 to 10 months (e.g., [12,18]). Second, at any given age, infants show the same ratio limit for different types of arrays: an infant who can just discriminate arrays of 8 *vs* 16 dots also will just discriminate sequences of 8 *vs* 16 sounds or actions [12,13]. Third, infants do not only discriminate numbers but can order them [9] and add two successively presented numbers and compare their sum to a third number [10]. Comparison and addition accuracy appear to be subject to the same critical ratio limit as discrimination. Fourth, numerical discrimination is impaired or abolished when arrays are presented under conditions that favor the attentive selection and tracking of individual objects. Although six-month-old infants can discriminate arrays of 4 *vs* 8 dots or sounds, even older infants tend to fail this discrimination when presented with objects that appear individually and move sequentially out of view ([19], Feigenson, Chapter 2 of this volume). Moreover, when infants are presented with arrays containing just a few simultaneously presented objects, each of which can be tracked in parallel, they tend to focus attention on the objects and ignore the cardinal value of the set [20–22].[1] Finally, infants spontaneously relate changes in number to changes in a different quantitative variable, line length. For example, infants who are habituated to arrays of dots that progressively increase (or decrease) in number will generalize habituation to arrays consisting of a line that progressively increases (or decreases) in length [27].

These five signatures provide clues to the nature and limits of infants' numerical representations. In particular, the ratio signature suggests that infants represent number

---

[1] These findings have sometimes been taken to suggest that infants cannot represent the approximate cardinal values of small numerical magnitudes, but more recent evidence refutes that suggestion (e.g., [23,24], see Brannon, Chapter 14 of this volume). Approximate numerical representations extend to the smallest numbers, but they are inhibited by processes of attentive object tracking, both in infants and in adults ([16,25], Burr, Chapter 3 and Cavanagh, Chapter 12 of this volume). When stimulus variations block object-directed attention or present objects that are usually perceived in large collections, representations of small cardinal values emerge [14,26].

imprecisely, and the evidence for a common ratio limit across diverse types of arrays and operations suggests that the source of the limit is to be found in the numerical system itself, which functions both to compare numerosities and to combine them in accord with the operations of arithmetic. For these reasons, this system has been called the *Approximate Number System*, or ANS: a term I will use hereafter. Infants' failures to enumerate the objects to which they are attending suggest that their ANS does not make explicit the identity or properties of the individual entities that it enumerates. Indeed, representations of individual entities may block the operation of this system: infants can see the forest and the trees, but they may not readily see both at once. Finally, the linkage between representations of number and length suggest that this system of numerical representation is one part of a more general sensitivity to magnitude (Lourenco, Chapter 15 of this volume).

The five signatures also provide a means to track this system of representation over the time-scales of evolution and human development, across different cultures and tasks, and into the human and animal brain. Experiments reveal all five signatures in nonhuman primates, providing evidence that the ANS is not unique to humans (see Brannon, Chapter 14 of this volume). Studies of children and adults in North America and Europe reveal the same five signatures, provided that the participants are tested under conditions that prevent verbal counting or other symbolic forms of enumeration. Thus, the system persists over human development and education, although its precision increases with growth and learning (see [28]). Studies of adults in remote cultures, lacking formal education, again reveal these signatures, indicating that the system is maintained over the lifespan without support from instruction in mathematics. Finally, studies of human and animal brains at the levels of cortical regions and single neurons reveal these systems as well (see Chapters 8 and 17 of this volume), opening the door to detailed studies of the neural coding of abstract number.

Armed with these findings, I believe it is now possible to address a vexed question: how can one determine the *content* of a mental representation as it is found in the mind of an infant, an animal, or a member of a culturally remote community? The research described above provides evidence that infants discriminate, compare, and combine arrays that educated adults would describe with numbers and arithmetic, but this evidence does not suffice to ensure that the arrays evoke number representations or arithmetic operations in infants. For example, consider infants' perception not of number but of surface lightness. Research on visual development provides evidence that infants, like adults, perceive edges by detecting abrupt luminance changes across visual arrays. Psychophysicists use mathematics to describe the mechanisms that detect these changes. We would not conclude, however, that infants who see contrast borders form representations of number: they perceive edges, not numbers. The fact that we can use mathematics to describe infants' or animals' responses to arrays of dots or sequences of sounds does not in itself imply that infants or animals represent number, because mathematics is a powerful tool for characterizing all the mental representations formed by any creature. How can psychologists determine if representations of these arrays have numerical content?

The research reviewed above suggests an answer to this question. Tests of the signatures of the system found in infants and animals reveal that the ANS is shared in large part by older children and adults. School children and adults, however, also have *symbolic* systems for representing number: including number words, Arabic notation, number lines, and

BOX 18.1

RELATIONSHIPS BETWEEN NON-SYMBOLIC AND SYMBOLIC NUMERICAL COGNITION

When preschool children first master number words and counting, they draw spontaneously on the ANS to solve new symbolic problems. Asked to add two symbolic numbers and to compare the results to a third number that differs from the sum (Box 18.1 Fig. 1, bottom left), children who have been taught no symbolic arithmetic perform above chance, as they do when they are presented instead with numbers instantiated non-symbolically, as arrays of dots (Box 18.1 Fig. 1, top left). Moreover, children's performance

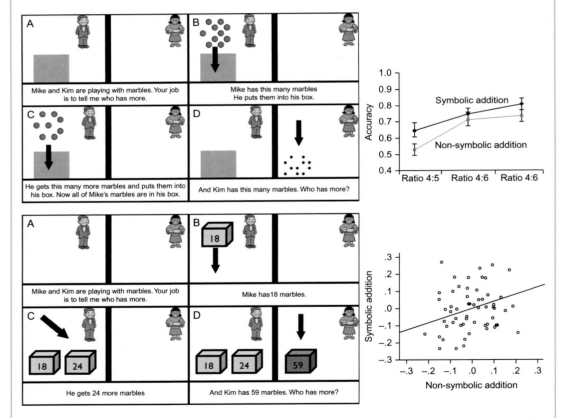

BOX 18.1 FIGURE 1 Example problems from tests of non-symbolic and symbolic addition (left). The accuracy of five-year-old children was affected by ratio on both tasks (top right), and performance on the two tasks was correlated (bottom right). Gilmore et al., 2007, 2010, and in review, reprinted with permission from Nature, and reprinted from Cognition, 115/3, Gilmore, C. K., McCarthy, S. E., & Spelke, E. S., Non-symbolic arithmetic abilities and mathematics achievement in the first year of formal schooling, 394–406, 2010, with permission from Elsevier

BOX 18.1 *(cont'd)*

shows critical signatures of their performance with non-symbolic numbers, such as the ratio limit ([29]; Box 18.1 Fig. 1, top right). The children who perform these problems best also perform better on non-symbolic problems, controlling for IQ and literacy ([31]; Box 18.1 Fig. 1, bottom right). Similarly, when young children, or adults lacking formal education, are introduced to a number line and are asked to place symbolic numbers on the line, their placements reveal the compressed pattern observed with non-symbolic numerical arrays [32,33]. Thus the ANS provides usable information that guides children's performance on symbolic number tasks.

When school children learn mathematics, moreover, individual differences in their non-symbolic numerical performance correlate with individual differences in school mathematics achievement. In adolescents, the precision of the ANS retrodicts symbolic mathematics performance at seven years of age, controlling for IQ and performance in other school subjects [34]. Studies of adults with varying levels of schooling suggest that non-symbolic numerical representations are activated, exercised, and sharpened during learning and performance of symbolic mathematics (Piazza, Chapter 17 in this volume). Moreover, children who perform better on a non-symbolic addition task at the start of schooling go on to higher achievement in mathematics at the end of the first

school year, controlling for IQ and literacy [30]. Symbolic and non-symbolic numerical representations therefore appear to have bidirectional effects on each other, although these effects are not shown on all measures of non-symbolic performance [35,36], and definitive claims about causal relationships must await the findings of training experiments.

Further evidence for a relation between ANS representations and symbolic numerical abilities comes from studies in neuropsychology and cognitive neuroscience. Adults activate the same brain areas when they compare or operate on non-symbolic and symbolic numbers (see [28]; Piazza, Chapter 17 in this volume). When non-symbolic numerical abilities are impaired by brain injury or transcranial magnetic stimulation, adults show corresponding impairments on symbolic numerical tasks [37,38]. Most important, activation to dot arrays of a given number produces adaptation of neural responses to symbolic arrays and the reverse [39], and fine-grained cortical responses to particular numbers of dots can be predicted from cortical responses to the corresponding symbolic numbers [40].

All these findings provide evidence that ANS representations have numerical content for adults and children. Because these ANS representations are shared by infants and animals, it follows that infants and animals have representations with some numerical content as well.

other symbolic devices. Thus, we can ask whether the ANS found in infants or animals has numerical content by investigating whether, and how, ANS representations relate to the symbolic numerical representations that are unique to human children and adults. Three types of findings provide evidence for a close relationship between the ANS and symbolic numerical abilities (Box 18.1). These findings of course do not imply that infants or animals have the full array of numerical abilities found in educated adults. Nevertheless, they

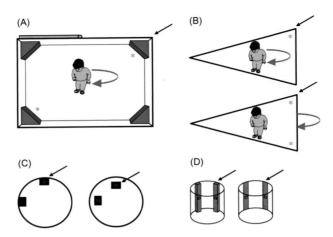

FIGURE 18.2   Displays and findings from studies of children's search (A) in a rectangular room (after [42]), (B) in an isosceles triangular room after disorientation of the child (top) or the room (bottom; after [44]), (C) in a circular room with two columns against the wall (left) or offset from it (right; after [43], or (D) in a circular room in which the columns (left) were replaced by flat stripes (right; after [43]). Arrows indicate the location of a hidden object, and asterisks indicate the location(s) at which children searched for the object. Rooms are depicted from above (A–C) or from the side (D).

provide evidence that the system by which infants and animals discriminate, compare, and combine arrays of discrete dots or sounds contains numerically relevant information.

In summary, research provides evidence for a core system of number. The system is present in newborn infants and in other animals [41], and therefore is not learned through experience counting, communicating about, or even manipulating sets of objects. The system, moreover, is a foundation for learning of symbolic mathematics. Nevertheless, the system has two striking limits. First, it is imprecise and therefore fails to support representations such as *exactly seven*. Second, the system fails to operate under conditions in which objects are presented individually and can be attended to and tracked over time and occlusion. For both reasons, the ANS fails to represent explicitly the individual entities that comprise the set whose approximate cardinal value it registers, and it fails to capture the fundamental operation of *adding one individual* to a set.

A CORE SYSTEM OF GEOMETRY

Geometry is the measurement of the earth. True to this meaning, the first core system of geometry is a system by which navigating humans and animals compute their own positions, and those of significant objects, by measuring properties of the surrounding terrain. An experiment by Lee and Spelke [42] serves to introduce this system. Children (aged three to four years) were brought into a closed rectangular room with four corner panels (Fig. 18.2A). Because the room was uniformly colored and contained no distinctive, asymmetrically placed objects, only the relative lengths of the walls broke its four-fold symmetry, and no information distinguished any direction from its diagonal opposite. While children watched, a sticker was hidden at one corner, and then children turned with eyes closed until they were disoriented. Finally children were allowed to open their eyes and search for the sticker. Children used the shape of the room to confine their search to two corners: the correct location and the opposite location with the same distance and directional relationships (e.g., the corner to the *left* of one of the two *more distant* walls). This finding provides evidence that children were sensitive to these properties of the shape of their surroundings.[2]

Although full disorientation rarely occurs during human navigation, experiments using reorientation tasks are valuable, because they reveal the information about the environment that navigators encode and rely on automatically (since children do not expect to be disoriented). As a consequence, a rich array of experiments has investigated children's reorientation in diverse environments. Reorientation by room geometry is highly robust across age (from infancy to adulthood), across variations in room size and shape, and across variations in the nature and presence of landmarks (see [43], for review). As in the case of core number representations, however, the most interesting findings from studies of children's reorientation concern not the existence of geometry-guided navigation but the signature limits on this capacity. These limits again provide clues to the nature of the representations that guide children's navigation, and they allow investigators to track these representations across species, ages, cultures, tasks, and brain systems.

The first signature concerns the task-specificity of geometry-guided navigation: the system serves to locate the child in relation to her surroundings, but it does not directly specify the relative locations of movable objects. Elegant experiments by Lourenco and Huttenlocher [44] (see also [45,46]) reveal this limit. Children searched for an object hidden in one of the three corners of a triangular enclosure. In one condition, the child was disoriented while the enclosure remained stationary (Fig. 18.2B, top). In a second condition, the child remained oriented, with eyes closed, while the enclosure was moved around her (Fig. 18.2B, bottom). Both conditions ended with the same perceptible environment and behavioral instruction, but they presented different cognitive problems: determining one's own position in a stable environment or relocating a displaced object. As in past research, children used the distances and directions of the triangular walls to reorient themselves, but they used only distance, not direction, to locate the displaced object in the rotated room. Searching for a displaced object is not simply more difficult, however: when an object is hidden at a distinctive landmark, children are better able to use the landmark when they are oriented and it moves than when they are disoriented and it is stable [46]. Children use the distances and directions of surfaces to specify their own location but not as direct landmarks to the locations of hidden objects.

A second signature of this core geometry system concerns the kind of layout information that it accepts: children reorient by the distances and directions of extended surfaces but not by the distances and directions of freestanding objects, even large ones. A recent study by Lee and Spelke [43] (see also [47,48]) illustrates this limit. In a series of experiments, children were

---

[2]One question that is frequently raised in studies of spatial representation concerns the coordinate system within which information is represented: do navigating children represent the shape of their surroundings allocentrically (for example, as a rectangular room with two long and two short walls) or egocentrically (for example, as an array of surfaces standing at particular distances and directions from their current station point)? Although a great deal has been learned about the representations that guide navigation in children and animals, this question has proved to be very difficult to answer in this domain, as it is in the domain of visual form analysis discussed below. For this reason, I do not address questions concerning spatial reference frames and coordinate systems in this chapter.

disoriented in a cylindrical environment with two large, stable columns that contrasted with the walls of the cylinder in brightness and color, positioned so that they both stood on one side of the room, separated by 90 degrees. When the columns stood flush against the cylindrical wall of the room (Fig. 18.2C, left), children used them to reorient themselves and locate a hidden object, both when that object was hidden directly at one of the columns and when it was hidden elsewhere. When the columns were offset slightly from the walls, however, children failed to use their positions to locate the hidden object. This failure did not stem from a failure to attend to or remember the relation of the object to the columns: if the object was hidden directly at one of the two columns, children searched only at the columns, showing that they appreciated their relevance to the task (Fig. 18.2C, right). Children failed, however, to confine their search to the column with the correct directional relationship to the child: e.g., the freestanding column *on the left*. Columns only specified the child's position when they were placed flush against the walls, and therefore contributed to the shape of the room.

A third signature concerns the dimensionality of the information that children use to track their own positions: children reorient by the distances and directions of extended 3D surfaces but not by the distances and directions of extended 2D patterns. Another experiment by Lee and Spelke [43] reveals this limit (see also [48–50]). Children were tested in the same cylindrical environment as in the above studies. Instead of viewing two 3D columns against the wall (Fig. 18.2D, left), however, children were presented with two 2D patches on the walls (Fig. 18.2D, right): patches of the same angular size as the columns, made of the same material and contrasting dramatically from the surrounding walls in brightness, texture and color. When an object was hidden at one of these patches, children confined their search to the two patches, showing again that they detected them and appreciated their relevance for the task. As in the case of freestanding objects, however, children searched equally at the correct patch (e.g., the patch on the right) and the incorrect patch (on the left). Although the patches were clearly detectable, they did not alter the shape of the cylindrical environment so as to break its symmetry. Accordingly, the geometric navigation system did not analyze their distance and directional relationships to specify the position of the child (Box 18.2).

BOX 18.2

REORIENTATION DEPENDS ON 3D BUT NOT 2D GEOMETRY

Research by Lourenco and Huttenlocher highlights the obliviousness of navigating children to 2D geometrical forms that could specify their own position [51,52]. Children were disoriented in a square room whose opposing walls displayed distinctive 2D patterns (for example, crosses *vs* discs: see Box 18.2 Fig. 1A–C). The patterns differed only in shape, but children did not reorient by this geometric information. In contrast, children confined their search to the two directionally consistent corners whenever the opposite walls were covered with forms of the same shape but of differing size and density (Box 18.2 Fig. 1D). Children therefore reoriented by a contrast between large and small discs, but not by a contrast between discs and crosses or between discs and a blank wall.

What accounts for this pattern? When equidistant surfaces are covered by forms differing in size and density, the surface with larger forms appears closer to the

BOX 18.2   *(cont'd)*

viewer. Depth perception based on *relative size* begins in infancy [54], and it could lead children to perceive the square room as slightly rectangular, triggering the reorientation system. This interpretation leads to two predictions. First, children should reorient in uniformly colored environments that are only very slightly rectangular (because the effect of relative size on depth is subtle). Second, relative size should interact predictably with other depth cues to enhance or diminish children's reorientation. Lee *et al.* [55] confirmed both these predictions. In an unpatterned room, children successfully reoriented by a subtly rectangular shape (sides differing in an 8:9 ratio). When large and small discs were added to these walls, children reoriented successfully when larger discs adorned the closer walls, but not when they adorned the more distant walls (Box 18.2 Fig. 1E). Flat geometrical patterns therefore serve as a depth cue, allowing children to reorient by a subtle, perceived difference in surface distance. Such patterns do not serve as independent information guiding children's reorientation, however, for children fail to reorient by them when the depth effect is cancelled.

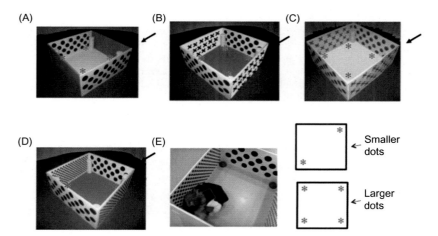

BOX 18. 2 FIGURE 1   Displays and findings from studies of the effects, on children's reorientation, of (A) the presence of a pattern, (B) the shapes of the pattern elements, (C) the shapes and colors of the pattern elements, or (D) the size and density of the pattern elements (Huttenlocher & Lourenco, 2007, and Lourenco et al., 2009, reprinted with permission from John Wiley and Sons, reprinted from Journal of Experimental Child Psychology, 104, Lourenco, S., Addy, D., & Huttenlocher, J., Location representation in enclosed spaces: What types of information afford young children an advantage? 313–325, 2009, with permission from Elsevier, and reprinted with permission from S. Lourenco, 2010). Rooms are shown from the side, arrows indicate the location of the hidden object, and asterisks indicate the locations at which children searched. In (E), pattern elements of different size and density were placed on the walls of a slightly elongated rectangle; children's performance (depicted from above) depended on the pairings of patterns to wall lengths (after [53]).

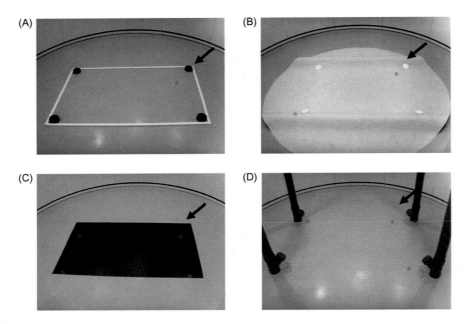

FIGURE 18.3   Displays and findings from studies of reorientation by subtle perturbations to the 3D layout on the ground surface (A and B), by a salient 2D figure on the ground surface (C), or by freestanding columns connected by a frame that was offset from the ground and constrained children's motion (D). Rooms are shown from the side; arrows indicate the location of the hidden object, and asterisks indicate the locations at which children searched (after [55]).

A fourth signature of the geometric navigation system concerns the primacy of the ground surface and its borders as information for one's own position: children reorient effectively not only in enclosed environments with a distinctive shape, but in environments where the only distinctive shape is provided by a tiny rectangular frame or arrangement of bumps on the floor (Fig. 18.3A and B). In contrast, children fail to reorient by salient 2D contrast borders or by large freestanding columns connected by a raised barrier that similarly constrains their motion but does not contact the ground (Fig. 18.3C and D) [57]. The system's high sensitivity to subtle perturbations of the ground surface, coupled with its insensitivity to much larger vertical landmarks, provides evidence against a popular theory whereby reorientation depends on processes for matching brightness contrast borders in 2D panoramic images of the layout [56–58] (the experiments described in Box 18.2 provide further evidence against this theory). Image-matching processes contribute to a wealth of navigation processes in animals (e.g., [59]) and they may aid in landmark guidance in humans [60], but they do not account for the process by which children locate themselves within the larger spatial layout.

There are other features of this system, related to its automaticity and robustness over variations in attention (see [61,62]) and motion [43], but I will focus on only one final signature: this system is sensitive to two fundamental properties of Euclidean geometry—*distance* and *direction*—but not to a third Euclidean property, *angle*. Children's insensitivity

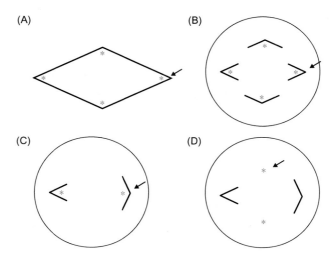

FIGURE 18.4 Displays and findings from studies of reorientation by length and by angle in (A) a connected rhomboid environment (after [63]), (B) a circular environment containing a fragmented rhombus with no informative aspect ratio, or (C and D) a circular environment containing two angles differing in size and four hiding containers (not shown) in a symmetrical arrangement (after [64]). Displays are depicted from above; arrows indicate the location of the hidden object and asterisks indicate the locations where children searched. In (C), the object was hidden at one of the two containers nested within the angles, and children divided their search between those two containers; in (D), the object was hidden at one of the two containers displaced from the angles, and children divided their search between those two containers.

to the angles at which walls meet at corners was first shown by Hupbach and Nadel [63], who reported that 2 to 3-year-old children failed to reorient by the distinctive shape of a rhomboid environment consisting of four walls that were equal in length but met at unequal angles (Fig. 18.4A). In a recent replication and extension of this research, we found that such children were strikingly insensitive to angle when the four angles of a rhombus were presented in an array with no informative aspect ratio (Fig. 18.4B), and they remained insensitive to angle when tested in the simplest environments [64]. In one experiment, two corners of markedly different angle (an obtuse angle of 120 degrees and an acute angle of 60 degrees) were placed opposite one another in a cylindrical room, each adjacent to one of four hiding containers (Fig. 18.4C and D). When an object was hidden in the container directly in front of the obtuse-angled corner, disoriented children searched only the two containers in front of corners, showing that they noticed the corners and appreciated their relevance as landmarks. Nevertheless, the children searched those two containers equally: they didn't use the angular difference between the corners to reorient themselves or to specify the object's unique location.

As in the case of the core number system, these five signatures allow investigators to test for this system of geometry in other animals, in human adults in diverse cultures and circumstances, in specific systems in the brain, and even into the genes. For brevity, I will discuss only the first and the last two of these tests. Studies of reorientation began with the classic studies of Cheng and Gallistel [65] and Cheng [66], conducted on rats. Reorientation

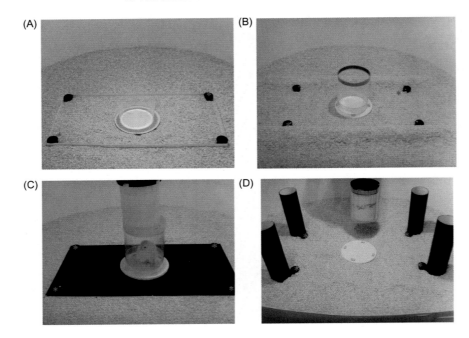

FIGURE 18.5 Displays and findings from studies of reorientation in chicks. Displays are depicted from the side; arrows indicate the location of the hidden object, and asterisks indicate the locations at which chicks searched. Chicks viewed the hiding of the object while confined in a transparent cylinder at the center of the room (depicted in A); for disorientation, a second cylinder with opaque walls was inserted in the first and chicks were turned (depicted in B). Then the opaque cylinder was lifted (C) and the cylinder was removed to allow the chick to search (D; after [68]).

by the shape of the environment has now been shown in a wide range of nonhuman animals, from primates to birds and even to ants [67] (see [61] for review). The literature is vast and complex, and studies that involve training give divergent findings, likely due to effects of training on attention to landmarks. Moreover, not all of the signatures have been tested in all animal species. Where untrained animals have been tested, however, they show the same signatures of reorientation found in children. Like children, for example, ants use 2D geometric patterns as beacons but reorient only by the 3D shape of the environment [67]. Moreover, newly hatched chicks reorient by the same patterns of subtle geometric information as children, and they too use 2D patterns and large freestanding objects as beacons but fail to reorient by them [68] (Fig. 18.5). Mice show the same reorientation performance as children in square rooms containing patterning information evoking the relative size depth cue [69]. Rats are strikingly insensitive to angle when tested in rooms whose shape is perturbed so as to change angle information while holding length relations constant [70].

In research using neurophysiological methods, the same signatures have been found in the brains of navigating animals, in areas whose activity specifies the animal's location, heading, or motion (see Burgess, Chapter 5 in this volume). The firing patterns of place cells in the hippocampus, and of grid cells and boundary cells in the nearby entorhinal cortex, are systematically affected by the distance and direction of the walls of the chamber [71,72], but markedly

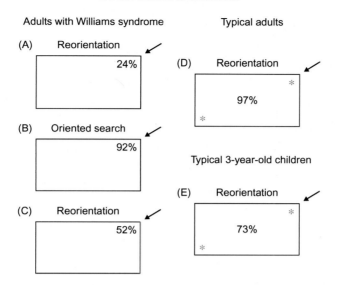

FIGURE 18.6 Displays and findings from studies of adults with WS who (A) were disoriented in a rectangular room with no landmarks, (B) remained oriented with eyes closed for a similar delay in the same room, or (C) were disoriented in a rectangular room with a single colored wall. For comparison, (D) and (E) show the performance of typical adults and young children in the same environment and test as (A; after [76]). Displays are depicted from above; arrows indicate the location of the hidden object. In A–C, numbers give the percentage search at each of the correct locations; in D and E, numbers give the percentage of search at either of the two geometrically correct locations (indicated by asterisks).

unaffected by the positions of freestanding objects [72] or the orientations of walls and angles of corners [73]. New research using neuroimaging methods provides indirect evidence for place and grid cells in humans as well, activated when humans learn object locations in a virtual environment in relation to extended surface boundaries ([74]; Burgess, Chapter 5 in this volume). Hippocampal activity associated with learning an environmental location in relation to an extended surface in the virtual layout is markedly impervious to effects of attention and interference, in contrast to activity in other brain structures associated with learning a location in relation to a freestanding landmark object [75]. These studies show a remarkable convergence across humans and rodents, and across behavioral and neurophysiological methods, in the core mechanisms for encoding the shape of the surrounding surface layout.

Finally, an exciting new line of research hints that the core system of geometry may have a specific genetic basis. Lakusta, Dessalegn and Landau studied adults with Williams Syndrome (WS), a developmental disability stemming from a genetic deletion that produces a variety of structural and cognitive abnormalities including an especially impaired capacity for spatial reasoning [76]. WS adults perform a wide variety of spatial tasks at roughly the level of typical three-year-old children, but the reorientation task shows a different pattern. Lakusta et al. [76] tested the reorientation performance of adults with WS in a homogeneously colored, rectangular room and found complete failure: in contrast to all the studies reviewed above, WS adults searched the four corners of the room equally (Fig. 18.6A). Their performance did not stem from a failure to remember the location of the hidden object, because they performed well after a delay over which they remained oriented (Fig. 18.6B). Their performance also did not stem from any debilitating effects of the disorientation procedure, because they performed fairly well when tested, after disorientation, in a rectangular room with one distinctively colored wall (Fig. 18.6C). The reorientation performance of the adults with WS contrasted both with that of typical adults (Fig. 18.6D) and with that of typically developing children (Fig. 18.6E). Indeed, the experiments revealed a striking double dissociation: whereas young children successfully navigated in accord with the shape of the environment and failed to navigate in accord with the colored wall, WS adults did the reverse. WS therefore seems to produce a specific deficit in the core system for navigating by layout geometry. Because WS is caused by a genetic deletion, and mouse models of WS have been developed [77], future experiments on mice can probe the mechanisms by which this cognitive system develops or goes awry.

These new findings raise a second vexed question in cognitive science: what are the effects of experience in a geometrically structured world, and of intrinsic, genetically specified developmental processes, on the emergence of this system of geometry? Questions concerning the innateness of knowledge systems are as thorny as questions concerning the content of those systems. In the case of human navigation by layout geometry, the debate has been particularly difficult to resolve, because children don't begin to navigate independently until the end of the first year. Children's system of geometry-guided navigation is shared by other animals, however, so studies of animals can probe its developmental foundations. Studies of controlled-reared chicks by Chiandetti and Vallortigara reveal that the system develops independently of any experience in a geometrically structured surface layout. Chicks reared in a geometrically uninformative, cylindrical environment reorient by the distances and directions of extended surfaces as consistently as do chicks reared in rectangular or asymmetrical environments [78], even on their first exposure to those surfaces (Vallortigara, Chapter 13 in this volume). The system for locating the self in relation to the distinctive shape of the surface layout therefore develops independently of any experience with layouts of distinctive shapes.

Research probing the innate foundations of human cognition is sometimes criticized as leading to an impasse: when a capacity is found to be innate, it is argued, there is no further research for developmental and comparative psychologists to do. Research on core geometry provides an illuminating counterexample to this argument. Since Plato, thinkers have wondered about the effects of experience on the development of knowledge of geometry: would a lifetime spent navigating in environments that systematically violate Euclidean relationships change our geometrical intuitions? With the controlled rearing methods of Vallortigara and others, these questions can be addressed, and the literature on effects of controlled rearing on navigation already is yielding intriguing findings. In particular, Brown *et al.* [79] and Twyman *et al.* [80] have investigated effects, on navigating fish and mice, of rearing in a geometrically structured environment with one or more salient landmarks. Like Chiandetti and Vallortigara [78], Brown *et al.* [79] find that reorientation in accord with the distances and directions of surfaces is independent of experience in a geometrically structured environment (Twyman *et al.* did not test for this effect). In contrast, experiments in both labs reveal that navigation by landmarks is affected by rearing experience: animals reared with a distinctively colored wall in a stable position are more likely to use that wall to guide their navigation. Research is therefore beginning to chart both the foundations and the malleability of cognitive mechanisms guiding navigation.

In summary, research provides evidence for a core system of geometry that emerges in human children soon after they begin to locomote independently, that is common to a broad range of animals, and that can develop independently of any prior experiences with the geometrical relationships that it analyzes. Like the core system of number, however, this system is limited. Although human adults use Euclidean geometry to characterize the shapes of freestanding objects and 2D forms arrayed at any orientation, this core system only applies to extended surfaces and privileges surfaces that border the ground over which we navigate. Whereas Euclidean geometry can be used for many purposes, this core system only serves to specify the position and heading of the navigator with respect to the surrounding environment. And whereas Euclidean transformations (rigid displacements) preserve distance, angle and direction, this core system is blind to angle and preserves only information about surface distances and directions. Core geometry for navigation cannot be the sole source of our Euclidean geometrical intuitions.

MORE CORE SYSTEMS

If the above two systems are not the sole sources of natural number and Euclidean geometry, what other sources do we draw on? Research on human cognitive development, animal cognition, cognition across cultures, and cognitive neuroscience provides evidence for two more core systems of number and geometry. The second number system, whose nature and limits are described by Feigenson (Chapter 2 in this volume), serves to represent sets of up to three to four numerically distinct individuals, as well as the operation of adding one individual to a set. The second geometry system, whose nature and limits are described by Izard (Chapter 19 in this volume), serves to represent the shapes of 2D visual forms and moveable objects, capturing the relations of length and angle that are invariant over changes in size.

Each of these systems is activated under conditions complementary to the conditions that activate the two core systems described above. Whereas core representations of numerical magnitudes are inhibited under conditions in which a small number of objects are attentively tracked, these are just the conditions that elicit activity in the second number system. And whereas core representations of layout geometry do not include the shapes of 2D patterns or freestanding objects, these are just the arrays that activate the system of visual form analysis. Moreover, each of these systems captures information that the other system lacks. In the case of number, the first core system captures cardinal information across a broad range of values, but only does so imprecisely, whereas the second core number system captures the exact number of individuals in an array, but only when those numbers are small. In the case of geometry, the core system for navigation represents distance and direction but not angle, whereas the system for form analysis represents distance and angle but not the directional information that distinguishes a form from its mirror image (Izard, Chapter 19 in this volume).

The contrasting properties of the two core systems of number and geometry are summarized in Fig. 18.7. This summary suggests that more powerful and abstract mathematical concepts could arise if the representations from the core systems could be productively combined. If children could systematically combine representations of sets and their cardinal

Core systems of number and geometry

(A)	2 vs. 3	4 vs. 8
Comparing sets by cardinal values	--	√
Tracking individuals, adding one	√	--

(B)	Distance	Angle	Direction
Navigating in 3D layouts	√	--	√
Recognizing 2D forms	√	√	--

FIGURE 18.7   Contrasting properties of, and limits on, the core systems of number and geometry. Checks indicate successful performance, and dashes indicate failures of performance, by (A) six-month-old infants whose numerical sensitivity is assessed with large or small numbers of objects, and (B) preschool children whose geometrical sensitivity is assessed with large-scale layouts or small-scale forms.

values with representations of numerically distinct individuals, formed by successive addition of one, they could overcome both the ratio limit on the representation of cardinal values and the set size limit on the representation of individuals, representing sets of any size with exact cardinal values. Similarly, if children could systematically combine the geometric properties they extract from large-scale navigable layouts and from small-scale forms, they could overcome the limits on the domains of application of these systems and increase the power of their geometrical analyses. By combining these systems, children might navigate by angle as well as distance by viewing the extended surface layout through the lens of visual form analysis, as painters do. Moreover, children might distinguish forms and objects from their mirror images by viewing those forms and objects through the lens of geometry-guided navigation, using real or mental rotation to view objects from changing perspectives. In the next two sections, I turn to evidence bearing on these possibilities.

CONSTRUCTING NATURAL NUMBER

Children appear to overcome the limits of the core number systems when they begin to use number words in natural language expressions and counting. For most children, counting begins to be mastered at about two years of age, when children learn the first 10 or so words of the counting list. Initially, these words have little numerical meaning beyond the fact that they are elicited by the presence of a collection of objects (a display that is likely to activate representations of approximate cardinal values) and they are accompanied by gestures of pointing to each object in turn (an activity that likely depends on attentive object tracking). At some point in the third year, most children learn that *one* designates a single

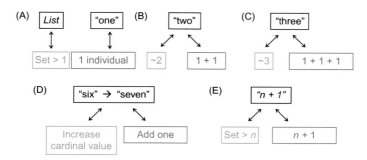

FIGURE 18.8 Successive steps in children's learning of counting (after [5,81,82]), and a proposed account of these steps as the progressive combination of information from the two core systems of number.

object and that all the other number words designate a plurality of objects. Over the next year, children learn that *two* designates exactly two objects, and that *three* designates exactly three objects. Some children also learn that *four* designates exactly four objects, but children then abandon this pattern of piecemeal learning and make two related inductions: every word in the counting list designates a set of individuals with a unique cardinal value, and each cardinal value can be constructed through progressive addition of one. Figure 18.8 suggests how children might learn this mapping by connecting each word in the counting list to representations from the two core number systems.

For most children, the language of number words and verbal counting appears to provide the critical system of symbols for combining the two core systems, and some evidence suggests that language may be necessary for this construction (Box 18.3). Once natural number concepts are constructed, however, does language continue to play a role in their use? Intuition suggests that language plays no role in mature mathematical reasoning (see [89]). Contrary to this intuition, however, three sources of evidence suggest that language serves throughout life as the medium by which representations from the two distinct core systems of number are combined (Box 18.4). I believe the role played by language is small (consistent with the intuitions of mathematicians), but crucial. All of the information supporting our numerical intuitions derives from the two core number systems, and these systems are fully independent of language. Nevertheless, the language of number words and quantified expressions may serve to link this information together. Absent language, human infants and other animals may have all the information they need to represent the natural numbers, but they may lack the means to assemble that information into a set of workable concepts.

CONSTRUCTING NATURAL GEOMETRY

Although the development of natural number has been subjected to intense investigation since the pioneering studies of Piaget [94] and Gelman and Gallistel [95], the development of Euclidean geometry has received less attention. Some experiments nevertheless provide clues to its development. Like counting, full Euclidean geometry develops in humans with or without formal education. Also like counting, its development requires a protracted process.

BOX 18.3

IS LANGUAGE NECESSARY FOR THE CONSTRUCTION OF NATURAL NUMBER?

The counting list learned by most children is composed of words with the grammatical properties of quantifiers [83], but the relation of language to number is debated. Is language merely a convenient source of symbols for combining information from the two number systems so as to enumerate entities exactly, or is it necessary for the construction of natural number concepts?

Children and adults in remote cultures, whose languages lack words for most numbers, tend to preserve approximate, but not exact, numerical equivalence when matching numbers larger than three [84,85] (cf. [86,87]). The interpretation of these studies is debated, however, in part because of the difficulty of disentangling effects of language and culture on cognitive capacities and predispositions.

Deaf adults who live in a numerate culture, but who have little or no exposure to a deaf community and, therefore, speak no conventional language, provide a different test of the role of language in the development of natural number and counting. Spaepen *et al.* [88] studied four adults living in remote areas of Nicaragua, who communicate with their hearing families and friends through a gestural system called *homesign* [88]. These homesigners received no formal education, but they hold jobs and use and exchange money, possibly both by recognizing the distinctive appearances of different bills and coins and by recognizing Arabic notation to some degree. When the homesigners communicate about number, they do not count or make tally marks. Although they use their fingers to convey numerical information, they do so with only approximate accuracy. Finally, they perform non-symbolic numerical matching tasks with approximate but not exact accuracy. These findings suggest a special role for language in the construction of natural number, but they leave many questions open. First, it is not clear which of the many aspects of language that are available to hearing people and to deaf speakers of sign language, but not to homesigners, are critical for the development of natural number concepts. Moreover, it is not clear whether language is necessary for the construction of natural number concepts or whether other symbolic systems, also not available to these homesigners, could support this construction.

Evidence for the spontaneous emergence of Euclidean geometry comes from three experiments performed on the Munduruku, who lack both formal education and experience with symbolic maps. First, Munduruku adults and older children were asked to navigate to a specific location in a simplified 3D layout (a triangular arrangement of containers) when the location was indicated by means of a Euclidean, 2D map (three small forms in the shape of a similar triangle, oriented variably with respect to the environment: Fig. 18.9A). Over a set of trials that varied the shape of the triangle, the Munduruku used distance, angular and sense relationships to specify the 3D location [98]. In further tests, moreover, the Munduruku used information on the map indicating landmark objects as well: their performance was enhanced when the location indicated on the map was a form with a distinctive color and shape that

---

BOX 18.4

LANGUAGE AND NUMERICAL REASONING IN EDUCATED ADULTS

Evidence for a role of language in mature numerical reasoning comes from experiments that compare educated adults' performance of approximate symbolic arithmetic (which could be supported by the ANS alone) to their performance of exact symbolic arithmetic (which goes beyond the limits of the ANS). First, educated adults who suffer language impairments often show impairments in exact numerical reasoning, despite preserved approximate numerical abilities [37]. Second, bilingual adults who are taught new number facts in one of their languages show a cost if they must produce exact number facts in the untrained language, relative to performance in the trained language [90,91]. Third, adults who perform exact, but not approximate, mental arithmetic respond more slowly when the numbers they must add require more time to pronounce, even though the numbers are presented in Arabic notation, not as words [92]. If language merely scaffolded the acquisition of natural number concepts and abilities, and then was replaceable by other symbol systems, one would not expect adults to translate Arabic symbols into words for purposes of exact computation.

Despite this evidence, it is clear that non-linguistic symbols contribute to numerical reasoning: arithmetic is far easier to perform with Arabic than with Roman numerals, and devices such as the abacus can greatly speed its execution [93]. The role of language in mature natural number concepts therefore continues to be debated.

---

conformed to the color and shape of a landmark in the 3D array. As in non-symbolic navigation tasks, representations of landmarks and representations of layout geometry were found to be distinct and possibly mutually inhibitory: Munduruku showed higher sensitivity to the geometric information in maps when landmark information was absent [96].

Second, Izard *et al.* [99] presented Munduruku adults and children with a computer-animated depiction of a large-scale spatial layout consisting of two locations, described as villages, on a textured surface that was either flat or curved. They were shown the directions of two paths leaving from each location; one was described as leading straight to the other visible village and the other was described as leading straight to a third, unseen village. Then participants were asked to determine both the location of the third village and the angle at which the two paths converged at that location. Across trials, the distance between the two visible villages and the angles of the paths varied. When the surface was planar, the Munduruku used both the distance between the villages and the angles formed by the paths that left them to specify the distance and angle of the third, unseen apex of the triangle. In particular, they produced angles whose size followed from the principle that the three angles of a planar triangle will sum to 180 degrees, in accord with Euclidean geometry, whereas the three angles of a triangle on a sphere will sum to a larger value [99] (see Izard, Chapter 19 in this volume).

Munduruku adults

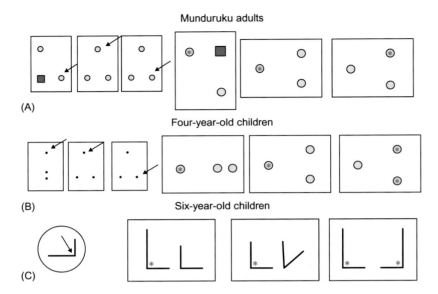

(A)

Four-year-old children

(B)

Six-year-old children

(C)

FIGURE 18.9 Geometric map tasks performed (A) by Munduruku adults and older children (after [96]), (B) by four-year-old U.S. children (after [97]), and (C) by six-year-old US children (after [98]). Arrows designate the target positions indicated on the maps (left); asterisks indicate the positions in the 3D arrays chosen by the participants (right). Across trials, the target location and the map orientation varied relative to the array. Maps were presented as participants faced away from the test arrays, so that a map and the array that it depicted were not simultaneously visible.

The third task presented the Munduruku with a series of questions about the behavior of abstract, dimensionless points and one-dimensional lines on a planar or spherical surface. For this task, the visual displays were zoomed in so as to remove all perceptual differences between the planar and spherical surfaces: all questions about the behavior of points and lines on the plane *vs* the sphere therefore were accompanied by identical displays. The intuitions of the Munduruku about points and lines accorded well with the principles of Euclidean geometry when they were asked to consider the points and lines as lying on the planar surface. When they were presented with two non-parallel, short line segments, for example, they judged that two segments, if extended, would cross on only one side; when given an single line segment and a point that was displaced from the line on which the segment lay, they judged that a line could be placed through the point such that it never crossed another line [99] (Izard, Chapter 19 in this volume). The Munduruku also modulated their judgments to some degree, but not fully, when asked to imagine the extensions of straight lines on the sphere: they judged that lines would cross on both sides of two visible segments, but they continued erroneously to judge that a line could be placed through a point such that it never crossed a second line. All these findings provide evidence that Euclidean geometry develops, by middle childhood, even in a culture lacking formal education, rulers, or maps.

Studies of younger children suggest, nevertheless, that Euclidean geometry develops gradually over childhood. Shusterman *et al.* [97] presented versions of the Munduruku map

Navigation by geometric maps

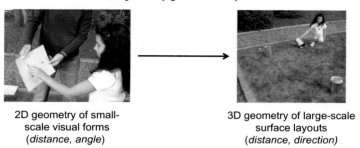

2D geometry of small-
scale visual forms
(*distance, angle*)

3D geometry of large-scale
surface layouts
(*distance, direction*)

FIGURE 18.10   Navigation by geometric maps in relation to the two core systems of geometry.

task to four-year-old children in the US (Fig. 18.9B). Like the Munduruku, children performed well when the target location was distinctive in color and shape, and they proved more sensitive to geometry when no distinctive landmarks were presented (see also [100]). Analyses of performance across the different shapes suggested, however, that children were not sensitive to all the geometric relationships detected by the Munduruku adults and older children. When the map consisted of three collinear but unequally spaced points, children reliably used the relative distances of the points on the map to distinguish among the similarly spaced 3D objects. Children performed no better, however, when angle was added to distance information (in a triangular map), and they failed altogether to use sense information to distinguish the two similar corners of an isosceles triangle. At four years, children may be sensitive only to distance in purely geometric maps. Further experiments suggest a regular developmental progression in map understanding. At six years, children navigate by both distance and angle information in maps [98] (Fig. 18.9C), but they still fail to navigate by sense information, as adults do [96].

Studies using the tests developed for the Munduruku, provide further evidence that six-year-old US children have only limited command of Euclidean geometry [99]. On the triangle completion test with virtual villages on a flat surface, children's placement of the third corner of the triangle was reasonably accurate, but their estimation of the angle at which the two paths met at that corner was not: children's estimates were appropriately influenced by the distance between the two visible villages but not by the angles of the paths leading from them. On the intuitions task, moreover, six-year-old children performed poorly, and they failed to distinguish the properties of points and lines arrayed on planar or curved surfaces. Although Euclidean geometry develops in the absence of education or experience with maps, that development appears to be a long, protracted process that may begin with a focus on distance: the Euclidean property that is shared by the two core systems of geometry.

When children use a map, they display an ability to combine geometric information from two different systems: the core system for navigation that analyzes geometric information in the 3D layout in which they must place or find an object, and the core system for form analysis that analyzes information in the 2D image that serves as the map (Fig. 18.10). What allows children to make this link? Prior experience with maps evidently is not necessary, since it is unlikely that the Munduruku, or most of the young children in these studies, had ever used a map before. Both Munduruku adults and US children, however, can use language to specify spatial locations. In all the above studies, the experimenter used object names and spatial terms to connect each form on the map to an object in the 3D layout (e.g., "Big Bird wants to sit in this chair [pointing to a dot on the map]. Can you put him in his favorite chair [pointing in the direction of the 3D array]?"). The act of using the same spatial expression to refer both to a 2D point and to a 3D position may have served to link these representations for children [101].

It is possible, therefore, that the spatial expressions of natural language initially serve to connect geometric information in 2D forms to geometric information in 3D navigable arrays. If that suggestion is correct, then there is a parallel between the construction of natural number and natural geometry: both would depend first on language, and then on other symbol systems (Arabic notation, number lines, maps). Far more research is needed, however, to explore the process by which children integrate information from the two core systems of geometry, and to test the roles of language and of other symbol systems in that process. I end by considering one line of research exploring a small corner of this terrain: studies of the role of spatial language in integrating representations of the shape of the layout with representations of the positions of landmarks.

These experiments focused on children's reorientation in a rectangular environment with one landmark that broke the rectangle's symmetry: a single distinctively colored wall. Although young children can use a colored wall to directly mark the location of a hidden object, they typically fail to use such a wall to guide their reorientation [44,48,50,51,57]. Young children use wall colors as beacons, and wall lengths and directions to specify their own position and heading, but they fail to combine these sources of information. Studies of older children reveal a change, however, at about the age when children begin to master spatial expressions involving the terms *left* and *right*. At about six years, children begin to reorient in accord with the lengths, directions *and* colors of walls. The development of this ability coincides with the acquisition of spatial language [102] and is enhanced by spatial language training [103], but these findings do not reveal the role that language plays. Does language serve as a medium for combining information about the spatial layout with information about landmark objects?

Recent studies of adult speakers of Nicaraguan Sign Language (NSL) shed light on this question [104]. NSL is a new sign language that began to emerge in the 1970s, developed by children attending a new school for the deaf. It is now the primary language spoken by the school's graduates. Importantly, the first cohort of graduates entered the school with a variable array of homesign gestural systems, and the common language on which they converged lacks many of the grammatical devices of fully developed signed or spoken languages. These first-cohort speakers have no consistent means for expressing or interpreting spatial relationships such as *left of X* [105]. The second cohort of graduates entered the school at a later point in the development of NSL, and their language is richer and more lawful. Second-cohort speakers are more consistent in their use of expressions for left–right relationships, and they communicate these relationships more effectively [108]. Except for these language differences, however, members of the two cohorts are similar: all are adults who live in the same culture and communicate regularly with one another. They provide, therefore, an excellent population for studying whether differences in their spatial language lead to differences in performance on non-linguistic navigation tasks.

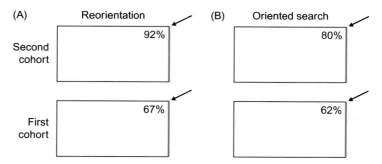

FIGURE 18.11 The performance of first- and second-cohort speakers of Nicaraguan sign language on (A) a test of reorientation in a rectangular environment with one colored wall, and (B) a test of oriented search for an object in a rectangular box with one colored side, following rotation of the box (after [104]). Arrows indicate the location of the hidden object: numbers indicate the percentage of first searches at the correct hiding location.

To address this question, Pyers *et al.* [103] presented first- and second-cohort NSL speakers with two spatial tasks: a reorientation task in a rectangular room with a single colored wall, and an oriented search task in which an object was hidden in a rectangular box with a single colored side that was then rotated on a table (Fig. 18.11). After completing both tasks, participants were asked to describe where the object was hidden, and their spatial expressions were coded. There were three principal findings. First, second-cohort signers performed markedly better than first-cohort signers on both spatial tasks, although performance was well above chance (25%) for each group. Second, across the entire sample, use of the colored wall for reorientation correlated with one specific aspect of spatial language: the consistency of signing of expressions involving the relations *left* and *right*. Third, across the sample, use of the colored side of the box to locate the hidden object correlated with a different aspect of spatial language: the consistency of the positioning of the colored wall within the signing space. Importantly, neither language variable consistently predicted performance on the opposite task. Thus, these correlations do not reflect individual differences in the overall proficiency of language or spatial cognition. They testify to more specific relationships between spatial language and spatial representation.

How might spatial expressions such as *left of the tree* serve to combine geometric and landmark information automatically and productively? These combinations may depend on three attainments achieved by speakers of any natural language [106]. First, speakers have learned a lexicon of words referring to entities in diverse cognitive domains including objects (*box, wall*), properties (*red*), numbers (*three*), and spatial relationships (*left, longer*). Second, speakers have induced a set of rules for combining these words to form expressions, and those rules are conditioned only by the grammatical properties of the words that they serve to combine, not by their content domains. Although *red* and *long* refer to properties in different cognitive domains, both are adjectives, and so for any grammatical expression that includes one (*left of the long wall*), there is a possible grammatical expression that includes the other (*left of the red wall*). Third, speakers who have learned the words and rules of a language can infer the meaning of an expression in the language the first time that they hear it, because the meanings of expressions follow from the meanings of their words and the rules for combining them. If one learns a new color term (say, *chromium*) and already

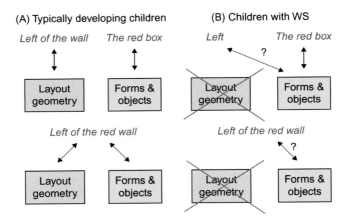

FIGURE 18.12 Schematic and simplified depiction of the possible learning (top) and use (bottom) of language to combine representations of layout geometry and landmark objects in (A) typical development and (B) Williams Syndrome.

knows the meaning of phrases like *the red tray*, one needs no further learning to know the meaning of phrases like *the chromium tray* [107].

With these three properties, language could serve as the medium in which information about object properties, and information about the shape of the surrounding layout, could be productively combined. With a cognitive system for representing objects, children can learn terms like *red* and *triangle* by mapping words and expressions to object representations. And with a separate cognitive system for representing distances and directions in the navigable environment, children can learn terms like *long* and *left* by mapping words and expressions to representations of the extended surface layout. The combinatorial machinery of natural language could then derive the meanings of expressions that combine these terms, and thereby serve as a medium in which information from these diverse representations is productively combined (Fig. 18.12A). On this account, as in the case of natural number, the information that guides adults' navigation resides entirely in core systems for representing objects and the surface layout; language serves only to link information from these distinct systems together.

Perhaps, however, language plays a different role. When children learn an expression like *left of the blue wall*, they may gain a means for encoding properties of the environment that bypasses core representations altogether.[3] Lakusta, Dessalegn and Landau's studies of adults with Williams Syndrome shed light on this possibility. Recall that WS adults appear to lack altogether the core system of geometry for navigation: after disorientation, they show no ability to distinguish among the corners of a rectangular room by representing the distances and directions of its walls. In contrast, however, WS adults have relatively proficient language, including some spatial language, and considerable abilities to use the distinctive color of a wall to specify the location of a hidden object. If language serves to

---

[3] I am grateful to Susan Carey for this suggestion (see also [5]).

bypass geometric representations, then these two abilities should be related to one another as they are for Nicaraguan signers: WS adults with more consistent spatial language should be more consistent in their search to the left or right of a colored wall. Contrary to this prediction, WS adults show no relation between the consistency of their spatial language and the consistency of their reorientation performance in a room with one colored wall. These findings support the view that language serves to combine core representations. In the absence of a core representation of layout geometry, spatial language cannot play this role (Fig. 18.12B), and it does not enhance navigation.

CONCLUSION AND PROSPECTS

Abstract concepts in general, and the concepts of natural number and geometry in particular, present a longstanding puzzle to the brain and cognitive sciences. Nevertheless, a rich array of studies in cognitive development, animal cognition, cognitive psychology, comparative cultural psychology, and cognitive neuroscience is providing clues that may lead to its solution. Four cognitive systems found in infants, animals, and human adults across widely varying cultures give rise to representations with true numerical or geometrical content. The systems develop on the basis of little or no experience in numerically or geometrically structured environments, and therefore are innate. Abstract concepts of natural number and Euclidean geometry build on these systems of core knowledge.

Nevertheless, each of these four systems is limited in its domain of application (none is fully abstract) and in the information that it makes available (none has the power of the system of integers or of Euclidean geometry). The limits on the two core number systems, and on the two core geometry systems, are complementary: richer systems of number and geometry could be constructed if representations from the different core systems could be productively combined. Research suggests that children begin to make these combinations in the preschool years. Thus, the most intuitive, abstract geometrical and numerical concepts that we possess as adults may not be given to us as infants; they may develop as children come to combine their core representations productively.

The processes that give rise to fundamental human conceptual integrations are only beginning to be explored. Some of the research reviewed in this chapter suggests that natural language plays a pivotal role in the development of abstract numerical and geometric concepts, and does so by serving as the primary medium for combining information productively across distinct systems of core knowledge. These suggestions raise many questions, however, concerning the aspects of language that play this role, and the ways in which language interfaces with non-linguistic conceptual representations. Research is also needed to probe whether other symbolic devices can substitute for language and serve to combine core representations productively. Finally, research into other abstract concepts, in domains such as morality, politics or economics, is needed to explore whether core systems and productive combinatorial abilities produce a broad range of abstract concepts or apply more narrowly to the concepts of mathematics. By addressing such questions, research in cognitive science promises to elucidate the mechanisms by which humans go beyond the core knowledge systems that we share with other animals and construct truly abstract knowledge systems that are unique in the living world.

References

[1] R. Descartes, The Optics, In P.J. Olscamp (Ed. and Trans.), Discourse on Method, Optics, Geometry and Meteorology. Hackett, Indianapolis, IN: (1637/2001).

[2] Plato, Meno (B. Jowett, trans.). Bobbs-Merrill, Indianapolis, IN: (ca. 380 B. C./1949).

[3] I. Kant, Critique of Pure Reason, Cambridge University Press, Cambridge, 1781, 2006.

[4] J. Piaget, Biology and Knowledge, University of Chicago Press, Chicago, 1971.

[5] S. Carey, The Origin of Concepts, Oxford University Press, N.Y., 2009.

[6] G. Hatfield, The Natural and the Normative: Theories of Spatial Perception from Kant to Helmholtz: MIT Press, Cambridge, M. A., 1990.

[7] V. Izard, C. Sann, E.S. Spelke, A. Streri, Newborn infants perceive abstract numbers, Proc. Natl. Acad. Sci. U.S.A. 106 (25) (2009) 10382–10385.

[8] L.E. Bahrick, The development of perception in a multimodal environment, in: G. Bremner, A. Slater (Eds.), Theories of Infant Development, Blackwell, Oxford, 2004.

[9] E.M. Brannon, The development of ordinal numerical knowledge in infancy, Cognition 83 (2002) 223–240.

[10] K. McCrink, K. Wynn, Large-number addition and subtraction by 9-month-old infants, Psychol. Sci. 15 (2004) 776–781.

[11] F. Xu, E.S. Spelke, Large number discrimination in 6-month-old infants, Cognition 74 (2000) B1–B11.

[12] J.S. Lipton, E.S. Spelke, Origins of number sense: large number discrimination in human infants, Psychol. Sci. 14 (2003) 396–401.

[13] J.N. Wood, E.S. Spelke, Infants' enumeration of actions: numerical discrimination and its signature limits, Dev. Sci. 8 (2) (2005) 173–181.

[14] K. vanMarle, K. Wynn, Tracking and quantifying objects and non-cohesive substances. Dev. Sci. (in press).

[15] M.E. Libertus, L.B. Pruitt, M.G. Woldorff, E.M. Brannon, Induced alpha-band oscillations reflect ratio-dependent number discrimination in the infant brain, J. Cogn. Neurosci. 21 (2009) 2398–2406.

[16] D.C. Hyde, E.S. Spelke, Neural signatures of number processing in human infants: evidence for two core systems underlying numerical cognition. Dev. Sci. 14(2) (2011) 360–371.

[17] D.C. Hyde, D.A. Boas, C. Blair, S. Carey, Near-Infrared Spectroscopy shows right parietal specialization for number in pre-verbal infants. NeuroImage. 53(2) (2010) 647–652.

[18] F. Xu, R. Arriaga, Number discrimination in 10-month-old infants, Br. J. Dev. Psychol. 25 (2007) 103–108.

[19] L. Feigenson, S. Carey, M. Hauser, The representations underlying infants' choice of more: object files versus analog magnitudes, Psychol. Sci. 13 (2) (2002) 150–156.

[20] M.W. Clearfield, K.S. Mix, Number versus contour length in infants' discrimination of small visual sets, Psychol. Sci. 10 (1999) 408–411.

[21] L. Feigenson, S. Carey, E.S. Spelke, Infants' discrimination of number vs. continuous extent, Cognit. Psychol. 44 (2002) 33–66.

[22] F. Xu, Numerosity discrimination in infants: evidence for two systems of representation, Cognition 89 (2003) B15–B25.

[23] S. Cordes, E.M. Brannon, Crossing the divide: infants discriminate small from large numerosities. To appear in Dev. Psychol. 45(6) (2009) 1583–1594.

[24] K. vanMarle, K. Wynn, Infants' auditory enumeration: evidence for analog magnitudes in the small number range, Cognition 111 (2009) 302–316.

[25] D.C. Hyde, E.S. Spelke, All numbers are not equal: an electrophysiological investigation of small and large number representations, J. Cogn. Neurosci. 21 (6) (2009) 1039–1053.

[26] D.C. Hyde, J.N. Wood, Spatial attention determines the nature of non-verbal numerical cognition. J. Cogn. Neurosci. (in press).

[27] M.D. de Hevia, E.S. Spelke, Number–space mapping in human infants, Psychol. Sci. 21 (5) (2010) 653–660.

[28] S. Dehaene, Origins of mathematical intuitions: the case of arithmetic, Ann. N. Y. Acad. Sci. 1156 (2009) 232–259.

[29] C.K. Gilmore, S.E. McCarthy, E.S. Spelke, Symbolic arithmetic knowledge without instruction, Nature 447 (2007) 589–592.

[30] C.K. Gilmore, S.E. McCarthy, E.S. Spelke, Non-symbolic arithmetic abilities and mathematics achievement in the first year of formal schooling, Cognition 115 (3) (2010) 394–406.

[31] C.K. Gilmore, S.E. McCarthy, E.S. Spelke, Relationships between symbolic and non-symbolic arithmetic in 5-year-old children (in review).

[32] R.S. Siegler, J.E. Opfer, The development of numerical estimation: evidence for multiple representations of numerical quantity, Psychol. Sci. 14 (2003) 237–243.

[33] S. Dehaene, V. Izard, E.S. Spelke, P. Pica, Log or linear? Distinct intuitions of the number scale in Western and Amazonian cultures, Science 320 (5880) (2008) 1217–1220.

[34] J. Halberda, M.M. Mazzocco, L. Feigenson, Individual differences in non-verbal number acuity correlate with maths achievement, Nature 455 (2008) 665–668.

[35] I.D. Holloway, D. Ansari, Mapping numerical magnitudes onto symbols: the numerical distance effect and individual differences in children's mathematics achievement, J. Exp. Child Psychol. 103 (2009) 17–29.

[36] T. Iuculano, J. Tang, C.W.B. Hall, B. Butterworth, Core information processing deficits in developmental dyscalculia and low numeracy, Dev. Sci. 11 (2008) 669–680.

[37] C. Lemer, S. Dehaene, E. Spelke, L. Cohen, Approximate quantities and exact number words: dissociable systems, Neuropsychologia 41 (2003) 1942–1958.

[38] M. Cappelletti, H. Barth, F. Fregni, E.S. Spelke, A. Pascual-Leone, rTMS over the intraparietal sulcus disrupts numerosity processing, Exp. Brain Res. 179 (2007) 631–642.

[39] M. Piazza, P. Pinel, D. Le Bihan, S. Dehaene, A magnitude code common to numerosities and number symbols in human intraparietal cortex, Neuron 53 (2) (2007) 293–305.

[40] E. Eger, V. Michel, B. Thirion, A. Amadon, S. Dehaene, A. Kleinschmidt, Deciphering cortical number coding from human brain activity patterns, Curr. Biol. 19 (2009) 1608–1615.

[41] C.R. Gallistel, The Organization of Learning, MIT Press, Cambridge, M.A., 1990.

[42] S.A. Lee, E.S. Spelke, Children's use of geometry for reorientation, Dev. Sci. 11 (2008) 743–749.

[43] S.A. Lee, E.S. Spelke, A modular geometric mechanism for reorientation in children, Cognit. Psychol. 61(2) (2010) 152–176.

[44] S.F. Lourenco, J. Huttenlocher, How do young children determine location? Evidence from disorientation tasks, Cognition 100 (2006) 511–529.

[45] J. Huttenlocher, C.C. Presson, The coding and transformation of spatial information, Cognit. Psychol. 11 (1979) 375–394.

[46] L. Hermer, E.S. Spelke, Modularity and development: the case of spatial reorientation, Cognition 61 (1996) 195–232.

[47] A.R. Lew, K.A. Foster, J.G. Bremner, Disorientation inhibits landmark use in 12–18-month-old infants, Infant Behav. Dev. 29 (2006) 334–341.

[48] R.F. Wang, L. Hermer, E.S. Spelke, Mechanisms of reorientation and object localization by children: a comparison with rats, Behav. Neurosci. 113 (1999) 475–485.

[49] S.A. Lee, S. Shusterman, E.S. Spelke, Reorientation and landmark-guided search by young children: evidence for two systems, Psychol. Sci. 17 (2006) 577–582.

[50] S. Gouteux, E.S. Spelke, Children's use of geometry and landmarks to reorient in an open space, Cognition 81 (2001) 119–148.

[51] J. Huttenlocher, S.F. Lourenco, Coding location in enclosed spaces: is geometry the principle?, Dev. Sci. 10 (2007) 741–746.

[52] S. Lourenco, D. Addy, J. Huttenlocher, Location representation in enclosed spaces: what types of information afford young children an advantage?, J. Exp. Child Psychol. 104 (2009) 313–325.

[53] S.A. Lee, N. Winkler-Rhoades, E.S. Spelke, Children's reorientation depends on the perceived shape of the spatial layout (in preparation).

[54] A. Yonas, C.E. Granrud, L. Pettersen, Infants' sensitivity to relative size information for distance, Dev. Psychol. 21 (1) (1985) 161–167.

[55] S.A. Lee, E.S. Spelke, Young children reorient by computing layout geometry, not by matching images of the environment. Psychon. Bull. Rev. 18(1) (2011) 192–198.

[56] K. Cheng, Whither geometry? Troubles of the geometric module, Trends Cogn. Sci. 12 (2008) 355–361.

[57] W. Sturzl, A. Cheung, K. Cheng, J. Zeil, The information content of panoramic images I: the rotational errors and the similarity of views in rectangular experimental arenas, J. Exp. Psychol. Anim. Behav. Process. 34 (2008) 1–14.

[58] D. Sheynikhovich, R. Chavarriaga, T. Strösslin, A. Arleo, W. Gerstner, Is there a geometric module for spatial orientation? Insights from a rodent navigation model, Psychol. Rev. 116 (2009) 540–566.

[59] B.A. Cartwright, T.S. Collett, How honey bees use landmarks to guide their return to a food source, Nature 295 (1982) 560–564.

[60] R.F. Wang, E.S. Spelke, Human spatial representation: insights from animals, Trends Cogn. Sci. 6 (9) (2002) 376–382.

[61] K. Cheng, N.S. Newcombe, Is there a geometric module for spatial reorientation? Squaring theory and evidence, Psychon. Bull. Rev. 12 (2005) 1–23.

[62] C.F. Doeller, N. Burgess, Distinct error-correcting and incidental learning of location relative to landmarks and boundaries, Proc. Natl. Acad. Sci. U.S.A. 105 (2008) 5909–5914.

[63] A. Hupbach, L. Nadel, Reorientation in a rhombic environment: no evidence for an encapsulated geometric module, Cogn. Dev. 20 (2005) 279–302.

[64] S.A. Lee, E.S. Spelke, Navigation as a source of geometric knowledge: young children's use of distance, direction, and angle in a disoriented search task (in review).

[65] K. Cheng, C.R. Gallistel, Testing the geometric power of an animal's spatial representation, in: H.L. Roitblat, T.G. Bever, H.S. Terrace, (Eds.), Animal Cognition: Proceedings of the Harry Frank Guggenheim Conference, Erlbaum, Hillsdale, NJ, 1984.

[66] K. Cheng, A purely geometric module in the rats' spatial representation, Cognition 23 (1986) 149–178.

[67] A. Wystrach, G. Beugnon, Ants learn geometry and features, Curr. Biol. 19 (2009) 61–66.

[68] S.A. Lee, E.S. Spelke, G. Vallortigara, Spontaneous reorientation behavior in chicks: Evidence against image-matching processes underlying reorientation (in preparation).

[69] A.D. Twyman, N.S. Newcombe, T.G. Gould, Of mice (*Mus musculus*) and toddlers (*Homo sapiens*): evidence for species-general spatial reorientation, J. Comp. Psychol. 123 (2009) 342–345.

[70] J.M. Pearce, J. Ward-Robinson, M. Good, C. Fussell, A. Aydin, Influence of a beacon on spatial learning based on the shape of the test environment, J. Exp. Psychol. Anim. Behav. Process. 27 (2001) 329–344.

[71] J. O'Keefe, N. Burgess, Geometric determinants of the place fields of hippocampal neurons, Nature 381 (1996) 425–428.

[72] C. Lever, T. Wills, F. Cacucci, N. Burgess, J. O'Keefe, Long-term plasticity in hippocampal place-cell representation of environmental geometry, Nature 416 (2002) 90–94.

[73] T. Solstad, C.N. Boccara, E. Kropff, M. Moser, E.I. Moser, Representation of geometric borders in the entorhinal cortex, Science 322 (2008) 1865–1868.

[74] C.F. Doeller, C. Barry, S. Burgess, Evidence for grid cells in a human memory network, Nature 463 (2010) 657–661.

[75] C.F. Doeller, J.A. King, N. Burgess, Parallel striatal and hippocampal systems for landmarks and boundaries in spatial memory, Proc. Natl. Acad. Sci. U.S.A. 105 (2008) 5915–5920.

[76] L. Lakusta, B. Dessalegn, B. Landau, Impaired geometric reorientation caused by genetic defect, Proc. Natl. Acad. Sci. U.S.A. 107 (2010) 2813–2817.

[77] L.R. Osborne, Animal models of Williams syndrome, Am. J. Med. Genet. 154C (2010) 209–219.

[78] C. Chiandetti, G. Vallortigara, Is there an innate geometric module? Effects of experience with angular geometric cues on spatial re-orientation based on the shape of the environment, Anim. Cogn. 11 (2008) 139–146.

[79] A.A. Brown, M.L. Spetch, P.L. Hurd, Growing in circles: rearing environment alters spatial navigation in fish, Psychol. Sci. 18 (2007) 569–573.

[80] A. Twyman, N. Newcombe, T. Gould, Malleability in the development of spatial reorientation (in review).

[81] K. Wynn, Children's understanding of counting, Cognition 36 (1990) 155–193.

[82] J.S. Lipton, E.S. Spelke, Preschool children master the logic of number word meanings, Cognition 98 (3) (2006) B57–B66.

[83] P. Bloom, K. Wynn, Linguistic cues in the acquisition of number words, J. Child Lang. 24 (3) (1997) 511–533.

[84] P. Gordon, Numerical cognition without words: evidence from Amazonia, Science 306 (2004) 496–499.

[85] P. Pica, C. Lemer, V. Izard, S. Dehaene, Exact and approximate arithmetic in an Amazonian Indigene group, Science 306 (5695) (2004) 499–503.

[86] M.C. Frank, D.L. Everett, E. Fedorenko, E. Gibson, Number as a cognitive technology: evidence from Pirahã language and cognition, Cognition 108 (2008) 819–824.

[87] B. Butterworth, R. Reeve, F. Reynolds, D. Lloyd, Numerical thought with and without words: evidence for indigenous Australian children, Proc. Natl. Acad. Sci. U.S.A. 105 (2008) 13179–13184.

[88] E. Spaepen, M. Coppola, E.S. Spelke, S. Carey, S. Goldin-Meadow, Number without a language model 108(8) (2011) 3163–3168.

[89] J. Hadamard, An Essay on the Psychology of Invention in the Mathematical Field, Princeton University Press, Princeton, 1945.

[90] S. Dehaene, E.S. Spelke, P. Pinel, R. Stanescu, S. Tsivkin, Sources of mathematical thinking: behavioral and brain-imaging evidence, Science 284 (1999) 970–974.

[91] E.S. Spelke, S. Tsivkin, Language and number: a bilingual training study, Cognition 78 (2001) 45–88.

[92] Lemer, C. (2004). Unpublished doctoral thesis.

[93] M.C. Frank, D. Barner, Mental abacus represents large exact numerosities using pre-existing visual resources (in review).

[94] J. Piaget, The Child's Conception of Number, Routledge and Kegan Paul, London, 1952.

[95] R. Gelman, C.R. Gallistel, The Child's Understanding of Number: Harvard University Press, Cambridge, MA, 1978.

[96] S. Dehaene, V. Izard, P. Pica, E.S. Spelke, Core knowledge of geometry in an Amazonian indigene group, Science 311 (2006) 381–384.

[97] A. Shusterman, S.A. Lee, E.S. Spelke, Young children's spontaneous use of geometry in maps, Dev. Sci. 11 (2008) F1–F7.

[98] E.S. Spelke, C.K. Gilmore, S. McCarthy, Kindergarten children's sensitivity to geometry in maps. Dev. Sci. (in press).

[99] V. Izard, P. Pica, E.S. Spelke, S. Dehaene, Euclidean intuitions of geometry in an Amazonian indigene group (in review).

[100] J.S. DeLoache, D.V. Kolstad, K.N. Anderson, Physical similarity and young children's understanding of scale models, Child Dev. 62 (1991) 111–126.

[101] N. Winkler-Rhoades, S. Carey, E.S. Spelke, Two-year-old children spontaneously read abstract, purely geometric maps (in preparation).

[102] L. Hermer-Vasquez, A. Moffet, P. Munkholm, Language, space, and the development of cognitive flexibility in humans: the case of two spatial memory tasks, Cognition 79 (2001) 263–299.

[103] A. Shusterman, E.S. Spelke, Language and the development of spatial reasoning, in: P. Carruthers, S. Laurence, S. Stich, (Eds.), The Innate Mind: Structure and Contents, Oxford University Press, New York, NY, 2005, pp. 89–106.

[104] J. E. Pyers, A. Shusterman, A. Senghas, E.S. Spelke, K. Emmorey, Evidence from an emerging sign language reveals that language supports spatial cognition. Proc. Natl. Acad. Sci. U.S.A. 107(27) (2010) 12116–12120.

[105] A. Senghas, S. Kita, A. Özyurek, Children creating core properties of language: evidence from an emerging sign language in Nicaragua, Science 305 (2004) 1779–1782.

[106] E.S. Spelke, What makes us smart? Core knowledge and natural language, in: D. Gentner, S. Goldin-Meadow (Eds.), Language in Mind: Advances in the Investigation of Language and Thought, MIT Press, Cambridge, MA, 2003.

[107] S. Carey, E. Bartlett, Acquiring a single new word, Proc. Stanford Child Lang. Conf. 15 (1978) 17–29.

Geometry as a Universal Mental Construction

Véronique Izard[*][†], *Pierre Pica*[‡],
Stanislas Dehaene[§][¶][**][††], *Danielle Hinchey*[***],
Elizabeth Spelke[***]

[*]Laboratoire Psychologie de la Perception, Université Paris Descartes, Paris,
France; [†]CNRS UMR 8158, Paris, France; [‡]UMR 7023 "Formal Structure of
Language", CNRS and Université Paris 8, Paris, France; [§]INSERM, Cognitive
Neuroimaging Unit, Gif-sur-Yvette, France; [¶]CEA, I2BM, NeuroSpin,
Gif-sur-Yvette, France; [**]Université Paris-Sud, Orsay, France; [††]Collège de
France, Paris, France; [***]Department of Psychology, Harvard University,
Cambridge, USA

Summary

Geometry, etymologically the "science of measuring the Earth", is a mathematical formalization of space. Just as formal concepts of number may be rooted in an evolutionary ancient system for perceiving numerical quantity, the fathers of geometry may have been inspired by their perception of space. Is the spatial content of formal Euclidean geometry universally present in the way humans perceive space, or is Euclidean geometry a mental construction, specific to those who have received appropriate instruction? The spatial content of the formal theories of geometry may depart from spatial perception for two reasons: first, because in geometry, only some of the features of spatial figures are theoretically relevant; and second, because some geometric concepts go beyond any possible perceptual experience. Focusing in turn on these two aspects of geometry, we will present several lines of research on US adults and children from the age of three years, and participants from an Amazonian culture, the Mundurucu. Almost all the aspects of geometry tested proved to be shared between these two cultures. Nevertheless, some aspects involve a process of mental construction where explicit instruction seem to play a role in the US, but that can still take place in the absence of instruction in geometry.

Space, Time and Number in the Brain.
DOI: 10.1016/B978-0-12-385948-8.00019-0

© 2011 Elsevier Inc. All rights reserved.

The axioms of geometry introduced by Euclid circa 300 B.C. [1] define concepts with spatial content, such that any theorem or demonstration of Euclidean geometry can be realized in the construction of a figure. Just as intuitions about numerosity may have inspired the early mathematicians to develop mathematical theories of number and arithmetic, Euclid may have appealed to universal intuitions of space when constructing his theory of geometry. In the current chapter, we investigate this proposition by assessing how much of the spatial content of Euclidean geometry is present in our spontaneous intuitions about space.

There are two major aspects of the spatial content of Euclidean geometry that may depart from our perception of space. First, in geometry, only some of the features of spatial figures are theoretically relevant. For example, Euclid introduces axioms pertaining to angles, where he points to the right angle as a special figure; but he does not introduce definitions related to orientation, such as a definition of horizontal or vertical lines. In this sense, geometric representations may be more specific than spatial representations: to qualify as "geometric", spatial representations must instantiate invariance by the properties that are not theoretically relevant to formal geometry. Second, some of the concepts of geometry transcend spatial perception by their very definition. Hence, Euclid's axioms introduce ideal concepts whose extension in space is either infinitely small or large, extending beyond the limits of our perception. For example, for Euclid a line is an object so infinitely thin that it has no width, while at the same time its extension in the length direction may be infinite.

In the following, we will focus in turn on those two aspects of geometry and raise the questions of their universality and development. A first possibility would be that all humans have access to the spatial content of Euclidean geometry, either because we all come to learn

---

BOX 19.1

TWO DISSOCIATED SYSTEMS OF CORE KNOWLEDGE FOR GEOMETRY

A large part of the research effort in geometry has focused on navigation tasks, following the classic behavioral and neurophysiological research of Tolman [33] and O'Keefe and Nadel [34], respectively, and invigorated by Cheng's seminal discovery that animals use the geometry of their surroundings to establish their orientation [35]. The system encoding space for reorientation is truly geometric in the sense that it encodes information about the shape of the environment, and ignores featural information such as colors, or landmark objects [36] (but see [37] for a different view). However, the system of geometry-informed navigation fails to reach abstraction in two points. First, it fails to encode some geometric information,

namely angle [31,38,39]. Second, it also fails to recognize geometry in 2D displays, a main domain of Euclidean geometry [31,40]. Nevertheless, sensitivity to 2D shapes is present even in infants [41], which leads us to postulate the existence of a second cognitive system of geometric content, dedicated to small, manipulable objects and 2D displays [31]. As reviewed in the present chapter, this system is sensitive to angle and length, while it ignores distinctions of sense: it is thus complementary to the geometry-informed navigation system, which encodes length and sense, but not angle. Children may need to learn to combine the information given by these two systems to create an integrated representation of Euclidean geometry.

it on the basis of an experience of space that is general enough to be universal, or because Euclidean geometry expresses core aspects of our perception of space (Box 19.1). On the contrary, geometric concepts may only be available to those who have received relevant instruction, or invested considerable energy in their mental construction. To address these issues, the present chapter will present several lines of evidence involving children of different ages, and people from an Amazonian culture, the Mundurucu.

UNIVERSAL GEOMETRIC INTUITIONS

In a first study, we probed a variety of geometric intuitions in a people from the Amazon, the Mundurucu [2]. The participants had no instruction in geometry, and their language does not have terms for basic Euclidean concepts such as parallelism or right angle. In one test, participants had to detect an image that was "different" or "weird" in slides of six images. Five of these images illustrated a geometric property (e.g., parallelism), while the remaining one lacked this property (non-parallel lines) (Fig. 19.1A). Care was taken to introduce maximal variation on irrelevant aspects of the images. For instance, in the previous example, the distractor pair of lines varied in terms of the distance between the two lines, the length of each line, and their orientation. This variation created several options for the participants, who may have relied either on geometry or on other aspects of the shapes to elect their answer. Nevertheless, across a variety of trials targeting different geometric properties, adult and children Mundurucu used principally the abstract geometric properties of the figures and performed well above chance. Furthermore, their performance across trials correlated tightly with the performance of adult and children control participants from the US (Fig. 19.1B). Despite dramatic differences in geometric education between these two groups, the trials that were harder for the Munducuru were also harder for the US participants. This test therefore reveals a signature of geometric intuitions, by establishing a hierarchy of saliency between the different geometric and non-geometric properties of images. This signature is impervious to instruction in geometry, and potentially universal across cultures. More recently, we also found evidence for continuity through development in a study including 448 participants from the US, ranging in age from three to 51 years: the same correlations were observed across all age groups [3] (Fig. 19.1C).

However, because the test spans a large range of geometric properties, and each trial is unique, it cannot suffice to infer the content of our geometric intuitions. In particular, the correlational findings suggest that participants relied mostly on geometry in processing shapes, but also used non-geometric cues when choosing an outlying figure. In an attempt to better characterize the geometric content of our spatial intuitions, the following sections will present new experimental tests controlling more closely the type of spatial variations introduced in the images (geometric and non-geometric). These tests will focus on features that are particularly diagnostic of the concepts of Euclidean geometry: global size, length proportions, angle, sense, and orientation.

PERCEPTION OF ABSTRACT GEOMETRIC FEATURES

Under the framework of transformational geometry (Box 19.2), Euclidean geometry can be conceived as a list of embedded theories, which differ by the type of features they make

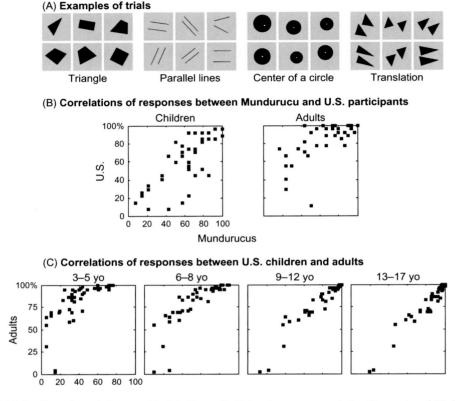

FIGURE 19.1 **Generic test of geometric intuitions.** Participants were presented with a series of 45 slides such as those in (A), each illustrating a distinct geometric property. In each slide, five of the images share a geometric property which the last image lacks. The participants were asked to pick the image that was "different", or "weird and ugly". The test was first administered to 14 children and 30 adults from the Mundurucu population, as well as control groups of 26 children and 28 adults in the US. The responses across trials were highly correlated between these two populations, in each age group (B). Later, the test was also administered to 448 participants from the US aged three to 51 years, and revealed the same correlation across age groups (C). A and B adapted from [2]; C adapted from [3].

explicit. Briefly, in all versions of Euclidean theory, angle and length proportions are defining features of figures, while position or orientation are not; the status of sense and global size is variable. From a psychologist's point of view, the framework of transformational geometry defines a research program: to look at the perception of some abstract geometric feature despite variations of other aspects of the displays, such as orientation, position, or global size [4]. If people are sensitive to geometry in the sense of one of the Euclidean theories, the defining features of this geometry should be easy to perceive, even with concomitant variations of non-defining features, and hard to ignore when their variation is made

BOX 19.2

TRANSFORMATIONAL GEOMETRY

In Klein's transformational geometry framework, any geometric theory (such as Euclidean geometry) can entirely be defined by the set of its invariant transformations, i.e. transformations that do not affect the theorems of that theory [42]. For example, if a geometry theory is invariant by translation, then for that geometry two figures that are identical, except that they are placed in different positions in space, are considered equivalent: exactly the same list of theorems can be proven of either of these two figures. (Of course, the relationships between these two figures could be the object of other theorems, such as theorems describing how the sides of these two figures are parallel to each other: such theorems are concerned with the global figure formed of the two translated versions, and therefore do not consider the two subfigures equivalent. In other words, invariant transformations must be thought as irrelevant when applied to the whole figure, not only a subpart.)

The transformational framework allows us to think of geometric theories as embedded within each other, with increasing levels of invariance: as long as a subset of the parent geometry's invariant transformations set verifies certain combination properties, this subset defines a valid theory of geometry. For example, in 2D geometry, Euclid's axioms create a high level of invariance, with four types of invariant transformations: translation (position in space), rotation (orientation), symmetry (sense), and homothecy (global size) (see Box 19.2 Fig. 1). This list of invariant transformations leaves angle and length proportions as essential properties of a figure. By comparison, in the geometry created by solid movement of objects, which is embedded within Euclid's full theory, only translations and rotations are included in the set of invariant transformations: besides angle and length proportions, sense and global size are also defining features of figures in this geometry. Embedded between these two geometries, one can also define a Euclidean geometry that is sensitive to angle, length proportions, and global size while being agnostic to sense: we will refer to this system of geometry as "the geometry of non-oriented solid movements".

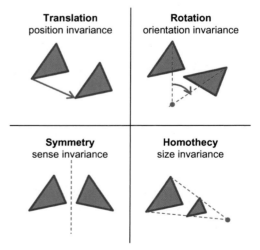

BOX 19.2 FIG. 1 Illustration of the four types of invariant transformations for Euclidean geometry.

irrelevant to a task. On the contrary, the properties that are irrelevant to Euclidean geometry, such as orientation and position, should be easy to ignore.[1]

To our knowledge, the question has rarely been addressed in this form in the literature (see [8–11] for a few exceptions). However, evidence from infants [12–14], young children [15,16], adults [7–11,17,18], and single-unit recordings [19] (see a review of mirror image confusions in [20]) seem to indicate that length (both relative and absolute) and angle have a privileged status in form perception. In contrast, the perception of sense requires an additional step of mentally aligning the objects, as in the classical experiments of mental rotation [7]. This would argue that the intuitive basis for geometry is a non-oriented Euclidean geometry. However, all the evidence summarized above comes from a variety of tasks, displays, measures, and population, thus making direct comparisons difficult.

We designed a new test focusing specifically and systematically on the defining features of some or all of the Euclidean geometries: angle, size, and sense [3]. As in the original intruder test [2], participants were presented with six figures for each trial, and instructed to find the figure that was "very different". Each figure was shaped like an L, except that the orientation of the figure, its size, its sense (akin to an L or the mirror image of an L), and the angle between the two branches could vary. On "pure trials", one of the figures differed from the others in terms of size, angle, or sense, while all other parameters were kept constant, except for the global orientation and position of the figure (Fig. 19.2A). On "interference trials", a second dimension was allowed to vary progressively across figures, but not in a way that defined a unique deviant: for example, when size was the interfering dimension, each of the six figures was presented in a different size. The test was administered to 104 participants from three to 34 years of age. In all the groups tested, angle and size deviants were detected better than the sense deviants (Fig. 19.2B). Even the youngest children (mean age 3.91 years) were able to use angle and size, but only adults relied on sense in their search for the deviant figure. Furthermore, in "interference" trials, introducing irrelevant variations of size or angle impaired the detection of the deviant, while participants were not disturbed by irrelevant variations of sense (Fig. 19.2C). In fact, when an irrelevant variation of size or angle was present, participants sometimes used this dimension to make their choice, electing for example the largest or the smallest shape.

More recently, we observed the same pattern of performance in a group of 25 Mundurucu participants: on the "pure" trials, adults and children detected the size and angle deviants successfully while failing to detect the sense deviants. Similarly, "interference trials" revealed that they were sensitive to irrelevant variations of size and angle, but not sense.

Our results on sense may seem surprising, given that even preschoolers can succeed at mental rotation tasks, when they are given explicit instruction or when the stimuli are embedded in an ecological Tetris game task [21,22]. In adults, the detection of sense variations is specific in that it requires the use of mental rotation, whereas metric differences can be perceived

---

[1] In terms of mechanisms, for any of the relevant features, organisms could opt for either of two computational solutions: the first solution would be to extract that feature directly, abstracting away non-relevant aspects in the figure. It has been proposed that this kind of solution is used for encoding numerosity [5], and reflects the organization of the visual system at large [6]. Another solution would be to impose a mental transformation and realign the displays, to then apply direct pattern matching between the realigned displays. This solution is used, for example, to detect sense deviations in classic mental rotation tasks [7].

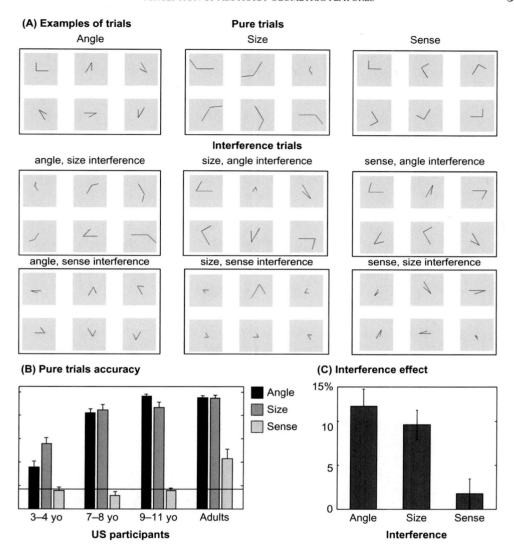

FIGURE 19.2 **Test on the perception of angle, size and sense**. Participants (US children and adults: $n = 104$; Mundurucu children and adults: $n = 25$) were presented with 27 to 162 slides of six images and asked to pick the image that seemed "different" or "weird and ugly". Trials were of two types. In the "pure" trials (A), the deviant was defined by a single difference in either angle, size, or sense, while the non-deviant figures differed only in orientation. In the "interference" trials, variations were introduced in a second dimension, but not in a way to define a clear deviant. (B) Responses were more accurate to the angle and size pure trials than to the sense pure trials. (C) Also, an interference of angle or size reduced the level of accuracy in the responses, compared to corresponding pure trials without this inference. On the contrary, trials on angle and size were not affected by an irrelevant variation of sense. Adapted from [3].

directly, without a need to mentally realign shapes [23]. The context of a Tetris game can facilitate the recruitment of motor resources for children: they can manipulate the shapes with a joystick to fit them in a hole pictured at the bottom of the screen. Our task made it less natural for participants to engage motor resources, because the shapes did not present any motor affordance, and also because the sense trials were interleaved with other trials where mental rotation was not needed. Together, these task features could explain the failure of the youngest participants. More crucially, the judgment we asked from our participants differed from the same/different judgments involved in mental rotation tasks: our instructions (to find a "very different" shape amongst shapes that were "all a little bit different") boiled down to asking participants what type of differences they found relevant to shape classification. The refusal of the children to use mental rotation reveals that sense differences do not appear an important factor of shape classification to their eyes: children did try hard to solve the sense trials, but instead of using mental rotation and checking for sense deviants, they looked at subtle differences in the pixelization, or sometimes chose randomly with evident frustration. These results suggest that adults entertain a more integrated concept of shape, rooted in a variety of cognitive mechanisms, whereas the concept of the children is only linked to shape perception systems. Before the integration of motor resources into the concept of shape, sense does not appear to be an important, defining aspect of shapes, at least in a context where shapes are allowed to vary in orientation.

Together, these results indicate that when classifying shapes, sensitivity to angle and size is universal, while sensitivity to sense is not. When comparing to Euclidean geometry systems, the intuitive geometry implied by the participants' classification of shapes picks the invariants of the non-oriented geometry of solid objects, maybe because these invariants are the most useful in object identification and classification.[2]

NORMATIVE GEOMETRIC CONCEPTS

We now turn to a second aspect of geometric knowledge, namely the ability to grasp concepts that go beyond any perceptual experience. As a first window into these concepts, we consider first the angle categories. Much as discrete integers are crystallized from a continuous representation of numerosity [24], educated adults crystallize angles into sharp categories of acute, right, and obtuse angles; parallel lines may be viewed as a kind of remarkable angle too. Although it is not necessary to possess a rich conceptual structure to be able to form categories, such absolute, sharp angle categorization is a prerequisite to reasoning about non-perceivable, normative properties, such as the fact that in some special cases, lines may never cross.

We studied children's judgment of categorizations by presenting 141 participants from the US (aged three to 34 years) with displays such as those of Fig. 19.3 [25]. In none of the trials did angle define a clear deviant, unless participants elected to use the angle categories of Euclidean geometry. Indeed, all adults picked the right angles, the parallel lines or the perpendicular lines as deviant in those displays. However, in children, parallelism and right angles were dissociated: all the groups chose the parallel lines as being special, while

---

[2] Nevertheless, the role of metric properties in object identification has been debated: perhaps, the identification of shapes is computed only on the basis of structural or "non-accidental" properties [27,28].

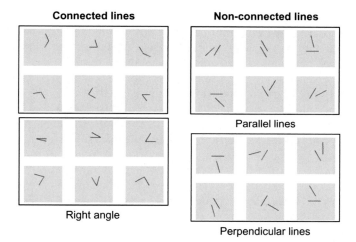

FIGURE 19.3 **Test on angle categories**. In this new version of the intruder task, variations in angle do not define a clear deviant unless the participants are sensitive to exact angle categories. Stimuli with connected lines probed the sensitivity to right angle, while stimuli with non-connected lines tested parallel and perpendicular lines.

only children aged seven years and over picked the right angle and perpendicular lines. Furthermore, in a short post-test we asked the children to draw a right angle, parallel lines and perpendicular lines in order to assess their knowledge of the relevant lexical terms: in accord with the general performance at the categorization task, the knowledge of the lexical terms "right angle" or "perpendicular lines" facilitated the detection of these figures in children, while the knowledge of the term for "parallel lines" had no effect on the detection of parallels. These results indicate that different normative categories develop along different trajectories, with a category for parallelism possibly present from start, while the category of right angle gets constructed once the child has acquired the relevant lexicon.

Because some Mundurucu do not receive any instruction in geometry, testing them helps to probe the universality of the right angle category. If specific instruction or an appropriate lexicon is necessary, Mundurucu should not pick a right angle as being special amongst a range of angles; however, if the lexicon just acts as a mere catalyst in the US children, the Mundurucu may direct their choices towards the right angles. Although the previous test has not yet been administered to Mundurucu participants, an examination of a subtest of the trials in the previous experiment (trials on sense with angle interference) could address this question (Fig. 19.2A): indeed, since Mundurucu were not sensitive to sense, these trials must have appeared as a test of angle categories to the participants. Examination of the responses in those particular trials revealed that the Mundurucu did choose the right angles more often than chance. This result raises the possibility that right angle may be a universal category of angle, even though instruction on the relevant lexicon appears to play a role in the acquisition of this category in young US children.

In further research, it would be interesting to evaluate the role of experience in the categorization of right angles by separating different subgroups of Mundurucu participants, living either in carpentered villages (where right angles are prominent) or in very rural areas. On the other hand, the performance of the Mundurucu suggests that the role played by instruction in US children may be limited in scope. It is possible that the acquisition of geometric vocabulary helps children forming a category of right angle, without implying any sensitivity to the geometric properties of this figure: perhaps children considered right angles to be special only because they have a name. In this case, the effect of elementary instruction would be initially superficial but may still have enduring effects on the development of geometry, by directing the attention of the child towards categories relevant to Euclidean geometry and therefore facilitating later conceptual learning.

In general, although sharp categories can provide a window onto normative concepts, being able to categorize parallel lines or right angles does not require an elaborate conceptual apparatus and could even be derived from experience. Thus, we attempted to design one last test probing the most abstract geometric concepts directly [26]. Participants were introduced to an ideal shape, either an infinite plane or a sphere. The experimenter narrated the properties of the shape ("it is very, very flat and goes on forever and ever" or "it is very round, like a ball"), straight, infinite lines, as well as dots (Fig. 19.4A). Following this introduction phase, participants were given a list of questions pertaining to the properties of straight lines. Impressively, Mundurucu adults and children performed extremely accurately at the test, especially on the plane. Most of them agreed that a new straight line may always be placed in such way that "it would never cross" a first straight line. They also correctly modulated their responses to adapt them to the planar and spherical environments tested. Beyond categorization, this last test argues for elaborate, non-perceivable concepts being universal.

These concepts may either be part of an innate "core knowledge", or may have been acquired by interactions with the environment. In order to separate these hypotheses, we tested five- and six-year-old US children on the same questionnaire task. Although the young children performed above chance in the plane test, they were much less accurate compared to the other groups; in particular, they responded at chance when asked about parallelism. Moreover, they failed to adapt their responses to the spherical context. These results indicate that the concepts of Euclidean geometry are only partially in place at the age of five or six years; while being universal, Euclidean geometry nevertheless appears to result from a mental construction.

The finding on parallelism has important implications for our interpretation of the results of the previous task. Contrary to adults, the categorization of parallel lines by young children does not rely on a rich conceptual theory of geometry, but probably on perceptual properties of parallel lines, such as the fact that the distance between them is constant, the fact that the two parallel segments look identical, or the fact that parallelism represents a singular point in angle values. Indeed, parallel lines may be regarded as a case where there is no angle to compute, therefore different from all other configurations; or the parallel lines may be perceived as related by an angle of 0°/180°, which is at the same time both a global minimum and a global maximum for non-oriented angles. This singularity might be extracted on the basis of accumulated perceptual experience. Again, as in the case of the category of right angle, the perceptual categorization of parallel lines is compatible with the concepts of geometry. Even if it is not rooted in a rich conceptual understanding of geometry, it could provide a stepping stone to conceptual development.

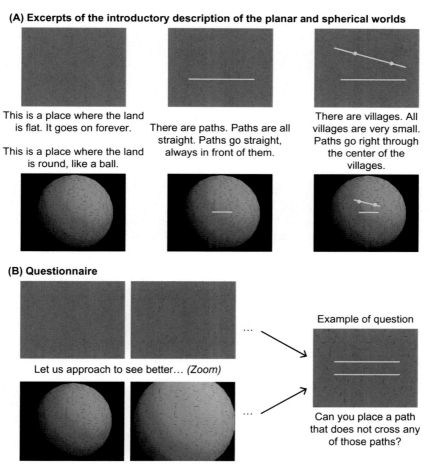

(A) Excerpts of the introductory description of the planar and spherical worlds

This is a place where the land is flat. It goes on forever.

This is a place where the land is round, like a ball.

There are paths. Paths are all straight. Paths go straight, always in front of them.

There are villages. All villages are very small. Paths go right through the center of the villages.

(B) Questionnaire

Let us approach to see better... *(Zoom)*

Example of question

Can you place a path that does not cross any of those paths?

FIGURE 19.4 **Test of Euclidean reasoning**. (A) Participants were first introduced to one of two ideal worlds, shaped either as a plane or a sphere. The experimenter narrated the properties of this world, and introduced the existence of very small villages (points), and paths that never turned or ended (straight lines). Following this introduction, participants were asked a series of 21 illustrated questions pertaining to the properties of points and lines in these worlds (B). Crucially, the sketches presented in the two subsets were identical: a zooming animation created the impression of coming so close to the sphere that it appeared flat.

CONCLUSION

Our research provides evidence that the basic principles of Euclidean geometry are reflected in intuitions of space that develop progressively throughout childhood, but still appear universal. From early childhood, the perception of shapes provides an intuitive ground corresponding to the geometry of non-oriented solid objects: preschoolers are sensitive to angle and length, can abstract differences of orientation and position, but they also abstract away sense relations. These early intuitions are enriched over development in three ways. First, in their classification of shapes, adults recruit a special process to detect sense: mental rotation. Second, mental continua are progressively carved out into discrete categories that give prominence to particular figures. Third, children become able to reason about elaborate non-perceptible concepts. Although the acquisition of the relevant geometric lexicon seems to play a role in the formation of some discrete geometric categories for US children, this role may be reduced to that of a category-maker and catalyst. Indeed, in a population that did not receive any education or share any relevant lexicon in geometry, a brief description of ideal shapes sufficed to elicit elaborate thoughts about the fundamental ideal concepts of Euclidean geometry, such as infinite lines or parallelism.

How could geometry be universal, and at the same time develop progressively? A first possibility would be that geometric knowledge is derived from a type of spatial experience that is so general that every human would encounter it. For example, all humans may come to compute some geometric features of shapes such as angle, or length, because they are especially relevant to object identification and classification [15], or to action. This view raises the question of the development of ideal geometric concepts, which by definition can never be experienced directly, and would need to be derived from incomplete or approximate experience. For example, the Euclidean concept of a line with no width would need to be derived from experience with very thin lines; or the concept of parallelism for infinite straight lines would need to be derived from experience with lines that do not cross locally—still a far cry from the property that parallel lines will *never* cross. Assuming this derivation to be impossible, Kant famously argued for knowledge of space (as well as geometry) being available *a priori* to experience [29,30].

Another possibility would be for geometry to be grounded on "core knowledge" [31], i.e. representations of abstract content that were selected by evolution, and provide useful guidelines to interpret the environment and learn. Representations of ideal straight lines or planes may be present in the architecture of the perceptual system to serve as anchors for perception, a strategy that has proven useful to reduce processing loads and increase reliability in artificial vision [32]. Under this hypothesis, during childhood these implicit anchors would need to be progressively reformatted into explicit representations, to be able to enter thought processes and be manipulated directly—a process that may be time consuming, but potentially accessible to every human being.

In conclusion, we have provided evidence that geometric knowledge appears universal, based on two cultures that are maximally different in terms of education and lifestyle. Ultimately, however, claims of universality can never be verified directly, and would be better informed by looking at the factors that favor the acquisition of geometric knowledge. Geometric concepts may emerge spontaneously on the basis of a universal experience with space, or reflect intrinsic properties of the human mind. Precisely what type of experience is relevant, and what limits younger children in their conception of geometry awaits further research.

GLOSSARY

Universal

Present in all normally developing human beings, irrespective of their environment, level of education, etc. Some properties may even be universal beyond the human species, but in the present article we will only consider claims pertaining to humans.

Innate

Determined by genetic or epigenetic mechanisms, rather than learned from the environment. Some innate features may not be present at birth, as for example the beard in human males. Claims of innateness are hardly accessible to experimentation, contrary to claims of universality.

Intuition

A form of knowledge that is accessible to explicit report, although its justification is not. In the present experiments, participants were often able to pick the correct response without being able to explain why they took such choice.

Sense

The geometric property that distinguishes two figures that are mirror images of each other. More generally, given a trajectory in a geometric space, a value of sense can be attributed to this trajectory depending on whether it bears more often to the left or to the right.

Acknowledgments

The authors thank the members of the "Development Perception-Action" team at the Laboratoire Psychologie de la Perception, the members of E. Spelke's laboratory, two anonymous reviewers and T.R. Virgil for useful discussions and comments on earlier versions of the paper. The work with the Mundurucu is part of a larger project on the nature of quantification. It is based on psychological experiments and linguistics studies conducted in the Mundurucu territory (Pará, Brazil) under the direction of Pierre Pica, in accordance with the Consehlo de Desenvolvimento Cientifico et Tecnologicico and the Fundacão do Indio (Funaï; Processo 2857/04). This work benefited greatly from advice from Lucia Braga (SARAH Network of Neurorehabilitation Hospitals, Brasilia), Andre Ramos (Coordenação Geral de Educação, Funaï), and C. Romeiro (Nucleo de Documentação e Pesquisa, Funaï); M. Karu, and C. Tawe assisted in the data collection. Most of the US children were tested by Danielle Hinchey, Amy Heberle, and Annie Douglas at the Boston Museum of Science, as part of a program coordinated by Marta Biarnes (Boston Museum Science). Supported by INSERM (Stanislas Dehaene), the Département des Sciences Humaines et Sociales of CNRS (Pierre Pica), NIH (Elizabeth Spelke), NSF (Elizabeth Spelke), and the McDonnell Foundation (Stanislas Dehaene).

References

[1] T.L. Heath, The Thirteen Books of Euclid's Elements, Dover Publications.
[2] S. Dehaene, Core knowledge of geometry in an Amazonian indigene group, Science 311 (2006) 381–384.
[3] V. Izard, E.S. Spelke, Development of sensitivity to geometry in visual forms, Hum. Evol. 23 (2009) 213–248.
[4] C.R. Gallistel, The Organisation of Learning, MIT Press.
[5] M. Piazza, V. Izard, How humans count: numerosity and the parietal cortex, Neuroscientist 15 (2009) 261–273.
[6] K. Grill-Spector, R. Malach, The human visual cortex, Annu. Rev. Neurosci. 27 (2004) 649–677.
[7] R.N. Shepard, J. Metzler, Mental rotation of three-dimensional objects, Science 171 (1971) 701–703.

[8] J.F. Norman, J.T. Todd, V.J. Perotti, J.S. Tittle, The visual perception of three-dimensional length, J. Exp. Psychol., Hum. Percept. Perform. 22 (1996) 173–186.

[9] D. Regan, Evidence for a neural mechanism that encodes angles, Vision Res. 36 (1996) 323–330.

[10] S. Chen, D.M. Levi, Angle judgment: is the whole the sum of its parts?, Vision Res. 36 (1996) 1721–1735.

[11] G.J. Kennedy, Global shape versus local feature: an angle illusion, Vision Res. 48 (2008) 1281–1289.

[12] S.F. Lourenco, J. Huttenlocher, The representation of geometric cues in infancy, Infancy 13 (2008) 103–127.

[13] A. Slater, Size constancy at birth: newborn infants' responses to retinal and real size, J. Exp. Child Psychol. 49 (1990) 314–322.

[14] A. Slater, Form perception at birth: Cohen and Younger (1984) Revisited, J. Exp. Child Psychol. 51 (1991) 395–406.

[15] E.J. Gibson, A developmental study of the discrimination of letter-like forms, J. Comp. Physiol. Psychol. 55 (1962) 897–906.

[16] A. Shusterman, Young children's spontaneous use of geometry in maps, Dev. Sci. 11 (2008) F1–7.

[17] I. Biederman, E.E. Cooper, Evidence for complete translational and reflectional invariance in visual object priming, Perception 20 (1991) 585–593.

[18] E. Gregory, M. McCloskey, Mirror-image confusions: implications for representation and processing of object orientation, Cognition 116 (2010) 110–129.

[19] J.E. Rollenhagen, C.R. Olson, Mirror-image confusion in single neurons of the macaque inferotemporal cortex, Science 287 (2000) 1506–1508.

[20] S. Dehaene, Reading in the Brain: The Science and Evolution of a Human Invention, Penguin Viking

[21] A. Frick, Motor processes in children's mental rotation, J. Cogn. Dev. 10 (2009) 18–40.

[22] A. Frick, N. Newcombe, Measuring mental rotation in 4-year-olds using a nonverbal touch screen paradigm, in: VI Biennal Meeting of the Congitive Development Society, 2009.

[23] J. Vanrie, Multiple routes to object matching from different viewpoints: mental rotation versus invariant features, Perception 30 (2001) 1047–1056.

[24] S. Dehaene, The Number Sense, Oxford University Press, Penguin Press

[25] V. Izard, D. Hinchey, E.S. Spelke, The development of angle categories, (in preparation).

[26] V. Izard, P. Pica, E.S. Spelke, S. Dehaene, Flexible intuitions of Euclidean geometry in an Amazonian indigene group, (under revision).

[27] I. Biederman, Recognition-by-components: a theory of human image understanding, Psychol. Rev. 94 (1987) 115–147.

[28] I. Biederman, Representation of shape in individuals from a culture with minimal exposure to regular, simple artifacts: sensitivity to nonaccidental versus metric properties, Psychol. Sci. 20 (2009) 1437–1442.

[29] L. Shabel, Reflections on Kant's concept (and Intuition) of space, Stud. Hist. Philos. Sci. 34 (2003).

[30] G. Hatfield, The Natural and the Normative: Theories of Spatial Perception from Kant to Helmholtz, The MIT Press

[31] E.S. Spelke, Beyond core knowledge: natural geometry, Cogn. Sci. 34 (2010) 863–884.

[32] A.P. Gee, Discovering Higher Level Structure in Visual SLAM, Institute of Electrical and Electronics Engineers

[33] E.C. Tolman, Cognitive maps in rats and men, Psychol. Rev. 55 (1948) 189–208.

[34] J. O'Keefe, L. Nadel, The Hippocampus as a Cognitive Map, Clarendon Press, Oxford University Press

[35] K. Cheng, N.S. Newcombe, Is there a geometric module for spatial orientation? Squaring theory and evidence, Psychon. Bull. Rev. 12 (2005) 1–23.

[36] A. Shusterman, E.S. Spelke, Language and the development of spatial reasoning, in: P. Carruthers, et al. (Ed.), The Innate Mind: Structure and Contents, Oxford University Press, pp. 89–106.

[37] N.S. Newcombe, Is cognitive modularity necessary in an evolutionary account of development, in: L. Tommasi, et al. (Ed.), Cognitive Biology: Evolutionary and Developmental Perspectives on Mind, Brain and Behavior, The MIT Press, pp. 105–126.

[38] A. Hupbach, L. Nadel, Reorientation in a rhombic environment: no evidence for an encapsulated geometric module, Cogn. Dev. 20 (2005) 279–302.

[39] S.A. Lee, E.S. Spelke, Signature limits on children's spatial representations: young children navigate by distance and direction but not angle, J. Exp. Psychol., General (in review).

[40] S.A. Lee, E.S. Spelke, Children's use of geometry for reorientation, Dev. Sci. 11 (2008) 743–749.

[41] N.S. Newcombe, J. Huttenlocher, Making Space: The Development of Spatial Representation and Reasoning, The MIT Press

[42] F.C. Klein, A comparative review of recent researches in geometry, Bulletin of the New York Mathematical Society 2 (1893) 215–249.

How Languages
Construct Time

Lera Boroditsky

Department of Psychology, Stanford University, Stanford, USA

Summary

How do people construct their mental representations of time? I focus on work examining the role that spatial metaphors and basic spatial representations play in constructing representations of time across languages. The results reveal that the metaphors we use to talk about time have both immediate and long-term consequences for how we conceptualize and reason about this fundamental domain of experience. How people conceptualize time appears to depend on how the languages they speak tend to talk about time, the current linguistic context (what language is being spoken), and also on the particular metaphors being used to talk about time in the moment. Further, people who conceptualize space differently also conceptualize time differently suggesting that people co-opt representations of the physical world (e.g., space) in order to mentally represent more abstract or intangible entities (e.g., time). Taken all together these findings show that conceptions of even such fundamental domains as time differ dramatically across cultures and groups. The results reveal some of the mechanisms through which languages and cultures help construct our basic notions of time.

One of the great mysteries of the mind is how we are able to think about things we can never see or touch. How do we come to represent and reason about abstract domains like time, justice, or ideas? All of our experience of the world is physical, accomplished through sensory perception and motor action. And yet our internal mental lives go far beyond those things observable through physical experience; we invent sophisticated notions of number and time, we theorize about atoms and invisible forces, and we worry about love, justice, ideas, goals, and principles. The ability to cognitively transcend the physical is one of the very hallmarks of human intelligence. So how is it possible that physical organisms who collect photons through their eyes, respond to physical pressure in their ears, and bend their knees and flex their toes in just the right amount to defy gravity are able to invent and

© 2011 Elsevier Inc. All rights reserved.

reason about the unperceivable and abstract? The mystery of abstract thought has vexed scholars from Plato to Darwin.

One proposed solution to this mystery is that representations of the abstract might be constructed through analogical extensions from more experience-based domains (e.g., [3,5]). That is, in order to construct mental representations of abstract or intangible entities, we co-opt the representations we have developed for more tangible and concrete domains. In this paper I will focus on the domain of time and the role that representations of space play in constructing representations of time.

Time is a topic of central interest in our culture. The word "time" is the most frequent noun in the English language, with other temporal words like "day" and "year" also ranking in the top 10 [1,2]. Time is ubiquitous yet ephemeral. It forms the very fabric of our experience, and yet it is unperceivable: we cannot see, touch, or smell time. So how do we mentally represent and organize this fundamental domain of experience?

To represent time, people around the world rely on space. We spatialize time in cultural artifacts like graphs, time-lines, orthography, clocks, sundials, hourglasses, and calendars; we gesture temporal relations, and rely heavily on spatial words (e.g., forward, back, long, short) to talk about the order and duration of events (e.g., [3–5]). People's private mental representations of time also appear to be based in space; irrelevant spatial information readily affects people's judgments of temporal order and duration [6–11], and people seem to implicitly and automatically generate spatial representations when thinking about time [12–18].

However, the particular ways that time is spatialized differ across languages and cultures. Research done around the world has uncovered dramatic variability in representations of time across cultures and groups. Several aspects of linguistic, cultural, and personal experience appear to shape people's temporal reasoning:

1. The pattern of spatial metaphors that people use to talk about time [19–24];
2. The set of spatial representations and reference frames that are available for co-opting for thinking about time (either in the linguistic or cultural environment more generally, or in the immediate context more specifically) [6–10];
3. Organizational patterns in cultural artifacts (e.g., writing direction) [15,25–27];
4. Aspects of cultural or individual disposition, age and experience [28–30].

In the following sections, I focus on work revealing the role that spatial metaphors and basic spatial representations play in constructing representations of time across languages. Languages around the world rely on spatial terms to talk about time. In some cases, it is difficult or impossible to talk about time without invoking spatial language. However, languages differ in the spatial terms that are most commonly used to talk about time. For example, depending on the language we are speaking, we might talk about the future as if it lies ahead of us (in English), behind us (in Aymara), or below us (in Mandarin Chinese). Do such differences in metaphors matter for how people mentally organize the domain of time?

THE AXES OF TIME

One prominent example of how spatiotemporal metaphors shape temporal thinking comes from comparisons of English and Mandarin. Mandarin speakers are more likely to talk about time using vertical metaphors than are English speakers [31–33]. Are Mandarin speakers also more likely to think about time vertically than are English speakers?

To test this, Boroditsky [20] compared English and Mandarin speakers' representations of time. In the studies, English and Mandarin speakers made temporal judgments following horizontal or vertical spatial primes. Participants' response times to the target questions about time following either the horizontal or vertical primes were the measure of interest. The results revealed a behavioral pattern consistent with the linguistic observation: Mandarin speakers appeared more likely to think about time vertically than did English speakers. Beyond comparing English and Mandarin speakers, the studies also compared the results of Mandarin speakers who had learned English at different stages of life, and further compared the results of English speakers tested with and without training to talk about time vertically. In each case, more experience with talking about time vertically lead to more vertical representations of time.

Results using this paradigm have been challenged (see [34–36]), but more recent work using a variety of methods has confirmed these cross-linguistic differences [22,26,37,38]. For example, when native English and native Mandarin speakers were asked to spatially arrange temporal sequences shown in pictures, Mandarin speakers arranged the pictures in vertical arrays 30% of the time (18–39% depending on group), whereas English speakers never did so [26]. In a 3D variant of this task, Boroditsky [39] asked English and Mandarin speakers to arrange time by pointing in 3D space around them. Mandarin speakers (tested in Mandarin) arranged time on the vertical axis 43.6% of the time, whereas English speakers did so only 2.5% of the time. Further, the studies found that the more proficient the participants were in Mandarin, the more likely they were to arrange time vertically. Mandarin–English (ME) bilinguals who were tested in Mandarin were more likely to arrange time vertically when they were tested in Mandarin as opposed to in English.

Lai and Boroditsky [24] examined whether metaphor use plays a causal in-the-moment role in how people construct representations of time. The results revealed that Mandarin speakers are more likely to construct front–back representations of time when understanding front–back metaphors, and more likely to construct vertical representations of time when understanding vertical metaphors. It appears that Mandarin speakers flexibly reorganize time along the front–back or up–down axis depending on whether they are processing front–back or up–down metaphors for time.

Finally, several studies have used a non-linguistic implicit space–time association task to measure how English and Mandarin speakers spatialize time [22,23,38]. The studies consistently find differences between the two language groups along the vertical axis. Mandarin speakers show an implicit vertical pattern of space–time association consistent with vertical space–time metaphors in Mandarin, with earlier events above and later events below. English speakers do not show evidence of this vertical space–time association. The findings are consistent with other work showing that experience with speaking Mandarin [22], and processing vertical time metaphors in particular [20,24] helps create and maintain Mandarin speakers' representations of time on the vertical axis. These results reveal that people automatically instantiate spatial representations of time that are consistent with the set of spatiotemporal metaphors in their linguistic environment, even in nonlinguistic tasks.

MOTION IN TIME

Linguistic analyses have suggested that Mandarin relies more heavily on time-moving (as opposed to ego-moving) metaphors than does English. That is, in Mandarin, metaphors that suppose an observer moving along a stationary timeline are less likely than those that suppose a stationary observer and a moving time-line. Do these differences in metaphors predict differences in thinking about time between English and Mandarin speakers?

Lai and Boroditsky [24] measured the relative cognitive salience of ego-moving and time-moving conceptualizations in three groups with different histories of linguistic experience with time metaphors: English monolinguals, Mandarin monolinguals, and ME bilinguals. The results revealed that English and Mandarin monolinguals indeed tend to take different perspectives on time, with Mandarin speakers more likely to take the time-moving perspective (consistent with the linguistic analyses of metaphor use in the two languages). Further, ME bilinguals differ from both groups of monolinguals. When understanding time metaphors in English, ME bilinguals are more likely to adopt the time-moving perspective than are English monolinguals. Interestingly, when understanding time metaphors in Mandarin, ME bilinguals are less likely to adopt the time-moving perspective than are Mandarin monolinguals. That is, for bilinguals there are influences of both their first language on conceptualizing time in their second language, and of their second language on conceptualizing time in their first language.

REVERSING THE DIRECTION OF TIME

So far we have discussed whether time can be laid out on different axes, and whether it is perceived as moving or stationary. What about the direction of time within an axis? A number of studies have found striking reversals in the direction of time between cultural groups.

One factor that affects the perceived direction of time is writing direction. People who read text arranged from left to right, tend to lay out time as proceeding from left to right, and people who read text arranged from right to left (e.g., Arabic, Hebrew) arrange time from right to left. This reversal has been documented in picture arrangement tasks [15,25], in patterns of elicited gestures or points around the body [15], in implicit non-linguistic spatial association tasks [15] and in auditory tasks [27].

Patterns in spatio-temporal metaphors have also revealed striking reversals of the direction of time. For example, in languages like English and Spanish spatial metaphors put the past behind the observer (e.g., the worst is already behind us) and the future in front (e.g., the best is still ahead of us). In Aymara, this pattern is reversed and the future is said to be behind the observer while the past is in front [19]. This pattern in metaphors is reflected in patterns in spontaneous co-speech gesture. When talking about the past, the Aymara gesture in front of them, and when talking about the future, they gesture behind them, a striking reversal from the patterns observed with speakers of English or Spanish (e.g., [19]).

DURATION

Beyond event ordering, interesting cross-linguistic differences have been observed in a separate aspect of time: representations of duration. English speakers talk about duration more often in terms of linear distance (e.g., a long time), whereas Greek speakers talk about duration more often in terms of amount (e.g., *poli ora*, tr. "much time"). To determine whether this difference in language corresponds to a difference in thinking, Casasanto *et al.* [40] compared Greek and English speakers' ability to estimate duration in the presence of distracting information about distance or amount, using simple duration reproduction tasks with non-linguistic stimuli and responses. Participants' non-linguistic duration estimates varied as predicted by the space–time metaphors in their native languages: English speakers' duration estimates were more influenced by irrelevant distance information, and Greek speakers' by irrelevant amount information. Next, English speakers were trained to use Greek-like metaphors for duration (e.g., a week is more than a day), which resulted in Greek-like performance on a non-linguistic duration estimation task. These findings demonstrate that (a) people who talk about time differently also think about it differently, and (b) language not only reflects the structure of our non-linguistic mental representations, it can also shape those representations in fundamental ways that can be observed even in low-level perceptuo-motor tasks.

REPRESENTATIONS OF TIME IN ABSOLUTE SPACE

Because people tend to recruit spatial representations to think about time, representations of time also differ depending on what spatial representations are most cognitively available to co-opt for time (either in the immediate environment or in the culture more generally) [6,7,9,10,41].

One such demonstration comes from spatial representations of time in a remote Australian aboriginal community of Pormpuraaw. Unlike English, the Pormpuraaw languages do not routinely use relative spatial terms like left and right, and instead rely on absolute direction terms (e.g., North/South/East/West), saying things like "move your cup over to the NNW a little bit" or "the boy standing to the South of Mary is my brother"[42–45]. Members of such linguistic communities must always stay oriented, just in order to be able to speak the language properly. In Kuuk Thaayorre (one of the languages included in this study), to say hello, one says "where are you going?" an appropriate response being "a long way to the SSW." That is, if you do not know which way is which, you literally cannot get past hello. Previous work has documented that speakers of such languages do indeed stay oriented, show precision in spontaneous co-speech gesture, and exhibit remarkable skill in dead reckoning [46–50]. How might members of such speech communities think about time?

To find out, Boroditsky and Gaby [41] gave participants sets of pictures that showed some kind of temporal progression (e.g., a man aging, or a crocodile growing, or a banana being eaten) (see Fig. 20.1). Their job was to arrange the shuffled photos on the ground to

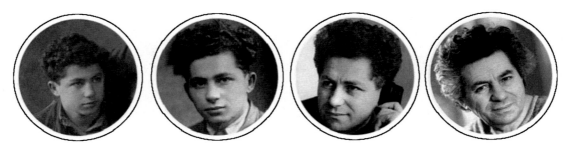

FIGURE 20.1   Example of a picture series participants were asked to arrange.

show the correct temporal order. Each participant was tested in two separate sittings, each time facing in a different cardinal direction. If you ask English speakers to do this, they will arrange the cards so that time proceeds from left to right. Hebrew speakers will tend to lay out the cards from right to left, showing that writing direction in a language plays a role. So what about folks like the Kuuk Thaayorre, who do not use words like "left" and "right"? What will they do?

The Kuuk Thaayorre did not arrange the cards more often from left to right than from right to left, nor more toward or away from the body. However, their arrangements were not random: there was a beautiful pattern, just a different one from that of English speakers. Instead of arranging time from left to right, they arranged it from east to west. That is, when they were seated facing south, the cards went left to right. When they faced north, the cards went from right to left. When they faced east, the cards came toward the body, and so on. This was true even though we never told any of our subjects which direction they faced. The Kuuk Thaayorre not only knew that already, but they also spontaneously used this spatial orientation to construct their representations of time.

This example illustrates that cross-cultural differences in thought can be more than a matter of style or preference. Pormpuraawans think about time in ways that other groups cannot (because they lack the necessary spatial knowledge). Many Americans simply could not lay out time in absolute coordinates even if they wanted to, because they lack the basic spatial knowledge necessary to do so (see [41]): two-thirds of the American sample could not reliably point to the compass directions even though they were tested outside on a sunny day in a familiar environment); and even those Americans who could have in principle done it, would be highly unlikely to spontaneously think to do it that way. This example reveals that speakers of different languages can arrive at qualitatively different ways of constructing even such fundamental domains of experience as space and time (in this case, representations that operate in entirely independent coordinate frames).

SUMMARY

Across the studies cited here, people in different cultures or groups have been shown to differ in whether they think of time as stationary or moving, limited or open-ended, as distance or quantity, horizontal or vertical, oriented from left to right, right to left, front to back,

back to front, or in cardinal space (e.g., East to West). The findings reviewed in the first four sections above demonstrate that the metaphors we use to talk about time (and other cultural factors) have both immediate and long-term consequences for how we conceptualize and reason about this fundamental domain of experience. How people conceptualize time appears to depend on how the languages they speak tend to talk about time, the current linguistic context (what language is being spoken), and also on the particular metaphors being used to talk about time in the moment. Further, the findings reviewed in the fifth section (*Representations of Time in Absolute Space*) demonstrate that people co-opt representations of the physical world (e.g., space) in order to mentally represent more abstract or intangible entities (e.g., time). It appears that differences in basic spatial representations may have far-reaching consequences in many other knowledge domains in the cognitive system. Taken all together these findings show that conceptions of even such fundamental domains as time differ dramatically across cultures and groups and reveal some of the mechanisms through which languages and cultures help construct our basic notions of time.

References

[1] H. Kucera, W.N. Francis, Computational Analysis of Present-day American English, Brown University press, Providence, 1967.

[2] M. Brysbaert, B. New, Moving beyond Kucera and Francis: a critical evaluation of current word frequency norms and the introduction of a new and improved word frequency measure for American English, Behav. Res. Meth. 41 (4) (2009) 977–990.

[3] H. Clark, Space, time, semantics, and the child, in: T.E. Moore, (Ed.), Cognitive Development and the Acquisition of Language, Academic Press, New York, 1973.

[4] E. Traugott, On the expression of spatiotemporal relations in language, in: J.H. Greenberg, (Ed.), Universals of Human Language. Vol. 3. Word Structure, Stanford University Press, Stanford, California, 1978, pp. 369–400.

[5] G. Lakoff, M. Johnson, Metaphors We Live By, University of Chicago Press, Chicago, 1980.

[6] L. Boroditsky, Metaphoric structuring: understanding time through spatial metaphors, Cognition 75 (1) (2000) 1–28.

[7] L. Boroditsky, M. Ramscar, The roles of body and mind in abstract thought, Psychol. Sci. 13 (2002) 185–189.

[8] L. Boroditsky, A. Gaby, Remembrances of times East: Absolute Spatial Representations of time in an Australian Aboriginal Community Psychol. Sci (2010) doi: 10.1177/095679610386621.

[9] T. Matlock, M. Ramscar, L. Boroditsky, The experiential link between spatial and temporal language, Cogn. Sci. 29 (2005) 655–664.

[10] R. Núñez, B. Motz, U. Teuscher, Time after time: the psychological reality of the Ego- and Time-Reference-Point distinction in metaphorical construals of time, Metaphor Symbol 21 (2006) 133–146.

[11] D. Casasanto, L. Boroditsky, Time in the mind: using metaphor to think about time, Cognition 106 (2008) 579–593.

[12] W. Gevers, B. Reynvoet, W. Fias, The mental representation of ordinal sequences is spatially organized, Cognition 87 (2003) B87–B95.

[13] M. Ishihara, P.E. Keller, Y. Rossetti, W. Prinz, Horizontal spatial representations of time: evidence for the STEARC effect, Cortex 44 (2008) 454–461.

[14] U.W. Weger, J. Pratt, Time flies like an arrow: space–time compatibility effects suggest the use of a mental time-line, Psychon. Bull. Rev. 15 (2) (2008) 426–430.

[15] O. Fuhrman, L. Boroditsky, Cross-cultural differences in mental representations of time: evidence from an implicit nonlinguistic task, Cogn. Sci. (2010), doi: 10.1111/j.1551-6709.2010.01105.x.

[16] A. Torralbo, J. Santiago, J. Lupianez, Flexible conceptual projection of time onto spatial frames of reference, Cogn. Sci. 30 (2006) 745–757.

[17] J. Santiago, J. Lupiáñez, E. Pérez, M.J. Funes, Time (also) flies from left to right, Psychon. Bull. Rev. 14 (3) (2007) 512–516.

[18] L.K. Miles, L.K. Nind, C.N. Macrae, Moving through time, Psychol. Sci. (2010), doi: 10.1177/0956797609359333.

[19] R.E. Núñez, E. Sweetser, With the future behind them: convergent evidence from aymara language and gesture in the crosslinguistic comparison of spatial construals of time, Cogn. Sci. 30 (3) (2006) 401–450.

[20] L. Boroditsky, Does language shape thought? English and Mandarin speakers' conceptions of time, Cogn. Psychol. 43 (1) (2001) 1–22.

[21] D. Casasanto, L. Boroditsky, W. Phillips, J. Greene, S. Goswami, I. Bocanegra-Thiel, et al., How deep are effects of language on thought? Time estimation in speakers of English, Indonesian, Greek, and Spanish, in: K. Forbus, D. Gentner, T. Regier, (Eds.), Proceedings of the 26th Annual Conference Cognitive Science Society, Lawrence Erlbaum Associates, Hillsdale, NJ, 2004, pp. 575–580.

[22] L. Boroditsky, O. Fuhrman, K. McCormick, Do English and Mandarin speakers think about time differently? Cognition (2010), doi:10.1016/j.cognition.2010.09.010.

[23] O. Fuhrman, D. Shu, S. Mao, E. Chen, H. Jiang, L. Boroditsky, How linguistic and cultural forces shape conceptions of time: English and Mandarin time in 3D. Cog. Sci. (in press).

[24] V. Lai, L. Boroditsky, The metaphorical construction of time: English and Mandarin from front to back, Cognitive Linguistics (2011), (forthcoming).

[25] B. Tversky, S. Kugelmass, A. Winter, Crosscultural and developmental-trends in graphic productions, Cogn. Psychol. 23 (1991) 515–557.

[26] T.T. Chan, B. Bergen, Writing direction influences spatial cognition, in: Proceedings of the Twenty-Seventh Annual Conference of the Cognitive Science Society, 2005.

[27] M. Ouellet, J. Santiago, Z. Israeli, S. Gabay, Is the future the right time? Exp. Psychol. (2010), doi: 10.1027/1618-3169/a000036.

[28] L.L. Carstensen, The influence of a sense of time on human development, Science 312 (2006) 1913–1915.

[29] A. Gonzalez, P.G. Zimbardo, Time in perspective, Psychol. Today (1985) 21–26.

[30] L. Ji, T. Guo, Z. Zhang, D. Messervey, Looking into the past: cultural differences in perception and representation of past information, J. Pers. Soc. Psychol. 96 (4) (2009) 761–769.

[31] L. Chun, A cognitive approach to UP metaphors in English and Chinese: what do they reveal about the English mind and the Chinese mind? Research Degree Progress Report for Hong Kong Polytechnic University, 1997, pp. 125–140.

[32] L. Chun, Conceptualizing the world through spatial metaphors: an analysis of UP/DOWN vs. SHANG/XIA metaphors: Proceeding of the 19th Annual Meeting of the Cognitive Science Society, Erlbaum, Mahwa, NJ, 1997.

[33] A. Scott, The vertical dimension and time in Mandarin, Aust. J. Linguist. 9 (1989) 295–314.

[34] D. January, E. Kako, Re-evaluating evidence for the linguistic relativity hypothesis: response to Boroditsky (2001), Cognition 104 (2) (2007) 417–426.

[35] J.Y. Chen, Do Chinese and English speakers think about time differently? failure of replicating Boroditsky (2001), Cognition 104 (2) (2007) 427–436.

[36] C.-S. Tse, J. Altarriba, Evidence against linguistic relativity in Chinese and English: a case study of spatial and temporal metaphors, J. Cogn. Cult. 8 (2008) 335–357.

[37] L. Liu, J. Zhang, The effects of spatial metaphorical representations of time on cognition, Foreign Lang. Teach. Res. 41 (4) (2009) 266–271.

[38] C.N. Macrae, L.K. Miles, The time traveler's life in: ESCON 2, Gothenberg, Sweden, 2010.

[39] L. Boroditsky, Do English and Mandarin speakers think differently about time? in: B.C. Love, K. McRae, V.M. Sloutsky (Eds.), Proceedings of the 30th Annual Conference of the Cognitive Science Society, Cognitive Science Society, Austin, TX, 2008, pp. 64–70.

[40] D. Casasanto, L. Boroditsky, W. Phillips, J. Greene, S. Goswami, I. Bocanegra-Thiel, et al., How deep are effects of language on thought? Time estimation in speakers of English, Indonesian, Greek, and Spanish, in: K. Forbus, D. Gentner, T. Regier, (Eds.), Proceedings of the 26th Annual Conference Cognitive Science Society, Lawrence Erlbaum Associates, Hillsdale, NJ, 2004, pp. 575–580.

[41] L. Boroditsky, A. Gaby, Remembrances of times East: Absolute Spatial Representations of time in an Australian Aboriginal community, Psychol. Sci. (2010), doi: 10.1177/0956797610386621.

[42] I. Smith, S. Johnson, Kugu Nganhcara, in: R.M.W. Dixon, B.J. Blake (Eds.), Handbook of Australian Languages, vol. 5, Oxford University Press, pp. 357–489.

[43] B. Sommer, The deixis of space in Oykangand, in: B. Merry (Ed.), Essays in Honour of Keith Val Sinclair, 1991, pp. 273–282, Capricornia 9.

[44] C. Kilham, M. Pamulkan, J. Pootchemunka, T. Wolmby, Dictionary and Source Book of the Wik-Mungkan Language, Summer Institute of Linguistics

[45] A. Gaby, A Grammar of Kuuk Thaayorre, University of Melbourne, 2006.

[46] S.C. Levinson, Frames of reference and Molyneux's question: cross-linguistic evidence, in: P. Bloom, et al. (Eds.), Language and Space, MIT Press, pp. 109–169.

[47] S.C. Levinson, Space in Language and Cognition: Explorations in Cognitive Diversity, Cambridge University Press, 2003.

[48] J.B. Haviland, Anchoring, iconicity, and orientation in Guugu Yimithirr pointing gestures, J. Linguist. Anthropol. 3 (1993) 3–45.

[49] A. Majid, M. Bowerman, S. Kita, D.B.M. Haun, S.C. Levinson, Can language restructure cognition? The case for space, Trends Cogn. Sci. 8 (3) (2004) 108–114.

[50] S.C. Levinson, D. Wilkins, Grammars of Space: Explorations in Cognitive Diversity, Cambridge University Press, 2006.

Improving Low-Income Children's Number Sense

Robert S. Siegler*, *Geetha B. Ramani†*

*Carnegie Mellon University, Department of Psychology, Pittsburgh, USA,
†Department of Human Development, University of Maryland,
College Park, USA

Summary

This article describes how a theoretical analysis and empirical findings regarding number sense led to the development of an educational intervention that produces large and rapid increases in low-income children's mathematical knowledge. Roughly an hour of playing a simple numerical board game based on the mental number line construct led to substantial gains in their knowledge of numerical magnitudes, counting, numeral identification, number line estimation, and arithmetic. The gains remained present two months after the last game-playing session. Both physical features of the game board and the way in which children interact with it proved important in the size of the gains. Reasons why such a brief intervention produces such substantial learning were discussed.

Throughout the developed world, the mathematical knowledge of children from low-income families lags behind that of children from wealthier families [1]. Even before children enter school, the differences are seen on a wide range of foundational tasks: counting from one, counting up or down from numbers other than one, recognizing written numerals, comparing numerical magnitudes, adding, and subtracting [2,3].

These early differences in numerical knowledge have lasting consequences. Kindergartners' mathematical knowledge is strongly predictive of their mathematics achievement in third grade, fifth grade, eighth grade, and even high school [4–6]. The long-term predictive relations of early mathematical knowledge are unusually strong, more than twice as strong as the relations in reading, attention control, and emotional self-regulation [4]. Moreover, absolute differences in

© 2011 Elsevier Inc. All rights reserved.

mathematical knowledge between children from richer and poorer backgrounds, already substantial in kindergarten, steadily widen over the course of schooling [7].

These differences in the mathematical knowledge of children from richer and poorer backgrounds reflect differences in environmental support for learning mathematics. Middle-income parents more frequently engage in mathematical activities with their children than do low-income parents [3,8], and children whose parents present them with more mathematical activities generally have greater mathematical knowledge [9]. A study of home, preschool and daycare environments indicated that most children from working-class backgrounds received mathematical input in 0 of the 180 segments observed [10].

One result of the minimal mathematical input they receive is that children from low-income families often enter school with poorly developed number sense. There is widespread agreement that acquiring number sense is an important part of mathematical development and an important goal of mathematics instruction (e.g., [11–13]). However, reaching this goal is harder than it sounds. One reason that improving number sense is difficult is that there is little agreement on what number sense is. This lack of an accepted definition has contributed to difficulties in knowing how to study number sense and how to help children acquire it.

A review of the literature [14] suggested one promising definition of number sense: "a process of translating between alternative quantitative representations." The translations can be between spatial and numerical representations (e.g., "About how many feet wide is this room?"), temporal and tactile representations (e.g., "tap your finger once every 10s"), luminance and pressure (e.g., "the brighter this light, the harder you should press on this pad"), and so on. This definition suggests three key questions for understanding number sense: How can we best think about number sense? How can we measure children's ability to approximate numerical magnitudes? and How can we help improve children's number sense, including their approximation of numerical magnitudes?

With regard to the first question, the core of number sense seems to us to be the presence of a linearly increasing mental number line. A wide range of theories of numerical cognition propose that knowledge of whole numbers is organized around a mental number line, in which number symbols (e.g., "7") are connected to nonverbal representations of quantity in an ordered, horizontally oriented array. The nonverbal representations of quantity appear to be largely spatial (e.g., [15]), though other sensory modalities also seem to be included in the representation [16]. Both behavioral and neural data support the mental number line construct. One body of evidence comes from studies of the SNARC Effect (spatial–numerical associations of response codes), the tendency of people in cultures with left-to-right orthographies to respond faster on the left to smaller numbers and on the right to larger numbers. For example people more quickly answer the question, "Which is bigger, seven or four?" when seven is chosen with a right side key press than with a left side key press [17]. A second source of evidence comes from brain-damaged patients with left-side neglect who displace upward (rightward on the number line) their bisections of numerical ranges (e.g., they estimate that the midpoint of the range 11–19 is 17), just as they do with physical lines [18]. A third set of evidence comes from brain imaging studies. The horizontal, intraparietal sulcus (HIPS), a brain area believed to be central to the mental number line, shows greater activation during comparison of numbers close in magnitude than during comparison of numbers further apart, presumably because finer magnitude discriminations require greater activation of relevant brain areas [19,20]. Fourth and especially important, the precision of

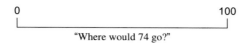

"Where would 74 go?"

FIGURE 21.1   A typical number line estimation task involves presenting lines with a number at each end (e.g., 0 and 100) and no other numbers or marks in between, and asking participants to locate a third number on the line (e.g., "Where does 74 go?"). Then a new number line is presented, and participants are asked to locate a different number on that line. The procedure continues until participants have estimated numbers from all parts of the numerical range. The mathematical function that best fits the relation between the presented numbers and the estimates of their locations provide evidence regarding representations of numerical magnitudes.

children's approximation of numerical magnitudes and their mental number line representations has been found to be quite highly correlated with their performance in arithmetic, memory for numbers, and overall mathematics achievement test scores [21,22]. Thus, our strategy for improving number sense in children from low-income backgrounds was to help them generate a mental number line that precisely and accurately related symbolically expressed numbers to nonverbal numerical representations.

With regard to the second question, estimation tasks, especially number line estimation tasks, have several advantages for measuring and investigating number sense. As shown in Fig. 21.1, the number line estimation task involves asking children to translate between numerical and spatial representations, for example, asking them to estimate the location of 74 on a number line with 0 at one end and 100 at the other. This task has several desirable characteristics. Number line estimation can be used with any real number—large or small, positive or negative, whole number or fraction. The task transparently reflects the ratio characteristics of the number system. Just as 80 is twice as large as 40, the estimated location of 80 should be twice as far from 0 as the estimated location of 40. It is non-routine; neither parents nor teachers typically instruct children in how to do number line estimation, so children's sense of the magnitudes of the numbers is reflected in their estimates.

Estimated values on the number line should increase linearly with a slope of 1 with the size of the number being estimated. Thus, the distance on the physical number line between 0 and the estimated location of 20 should be the same as the distance between the estimates of 20 and 40, 40 and 60, 60 and 80, and 80 and 100. The number line task allows several measures of the quality of children's estimates, including the percent absolute error (the absolute distance between the number that was presented and the number corresponding to the child's estimate on the number line), the slope of the best fitting linear function relating the number presented to the child's estimate on the number line, and whether the best-fitting function relating the number presented to the child's estimates is linear, logarithmic, or exponential.

Although the linear relation between the number presented and the estimate on the number line might seem obvious, children do not understand it for a surprisingly long time. Instead, children seem to progress through a rough three-step progression in which they first lack knowledge of even the ordinal properties of symbolically expressed numbers, then know the numbers' order but do not relate them in a linearly increasing fashion, and then represent the relation between numbers and their magnitudes as increasing linearly, as in the equation $y = x$. With regard to the first period, many three- and four-year-olds who count flawlessly from one to 10 do not even know the rank order of the numbers. For example, their percent correct on magnitude comparison tasks is close to chance, and they show knowledge of only the smallest

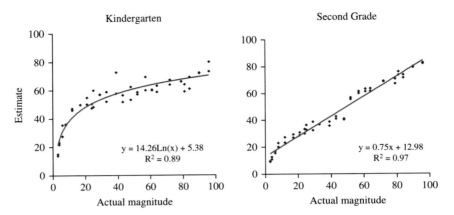

FIGURE 21.2   Kindergartners' logarithmic and second graders' linear estimation patterns [44].

numbers (e.g., 1 and 2) on other tasks [23]. Somewhat older children know the rank order of the numbers but still fail to understand that equal differences between two pairs of numbers mean that the magnitudes of the two pairs of numbers must be equally discrepant. Instead, these children use a logarithmic representation of numerical magnitudes, in which estimates of magnitudes at the low end of the scale are farther apart than estimates at the high end for any given difference between numbers. Thus, as shown in Fig. 21.2, most kindergartners, and about half of first graders, think that on a 0–100 number line, the magnitudes of 12 and 20 are much more discrepant than the magnitudes of 72 and 80. Not until second grade do the number line estimates of most children indicate understanding that these differences are equal, and not until fourth grade do most children show similar knowledge on 0–1000 number lines [21,24].

The number line estimation findings are far from isolated phenomena. Similar patterns of developmental changes have been found with other types of estimation, including numerosity estimation ("Here's a beaker with one dot and here's a beaker with 1000 dots. Put about N dots in this empty glass on the screen by holding down the mouse") and measurement estimation ("Here's a line 1 zip long and here's a line 1000 zips long; draw a line N zips long.") Most children either generate logarithmic estimation patterns on all three estimation tasks or generate linear estimation patterns on all three [21]. Perhaps most striking, the linearity of number line estimates of children in all grades through fourth grade correlate substantially with the children's mathematics achievement test scores [21,25,26].

Given that children can count from one to 10 at least a year before they show knowledge of the magnitudes of knowledge in this range, counting is clearly insufficient for generating accurate numerical magnitude representations. This raises the question of what other experiences might contribute. One common activity that might help children generate linear representations is playing linear, number board games—that is, board games with linearly arranged, consecutively numbered, equal-size spaces (e.g., *Chutes and Ladders*.) These board games provide multiple cues to numbers' magnitudes. The greater the number in a square, the greater: (a) the distance that the child has moved the token; (b) the number of discrete moves of the token the child has made; (c) the number of number names the child has spoken; (d) the number of number names the child has heard; and (e) the amount of time since the game began. Thus, children playing the game have the opportunity to relate the number

(A)   Number Board Game

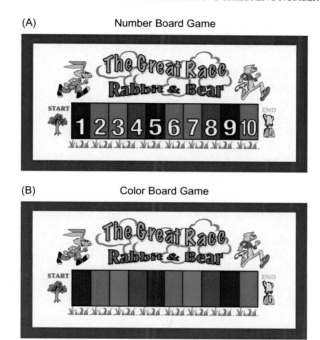

(B)   Color Board Game

FIGURE 21.3   The number and color boards [45].

in each square to the time, distance, and number of manual and vocal actions required to reach that number. Stated differently, these temporal, visual–spatial, kinesthetic, and vocal cues provide a broadly based, multi-modal foundation for a linear representation of numerical magnitudes. This theoretical analysis, together with the data on developmental and individual differences in estimation, suggested that providing children with numerical board game experience might improve their number sense and their performance on a wide range of numerical tasks. For example, given the linear relation between numbers and the spatial dimension of the board game, experience playing the game should make it possible for children to generate linearly increasing estimates on the number line task.

DOES PLAYING NUMERICAL BOARD GAMES IMPROVE CHILDREN'S NUMBER SENSE?

To test whether playing number board games promotes number sense, we randomly assigned 36 four-year-olds to play either a number board game or a color board game (Fig. 21.3) [27]. A little more than half of the children were African Americans attending Head Start or childcare centers that served impoverished populations.

At the beginning of each session, children in the number board condition were told that on each turn, they would spin a spinner that would point to "1" or "2", that they should move their token that number of spaces, and that the first player to reach the end would win. Children in the color board condition were told that on each turn, they would spin a spinner that could point to different colors, that they should move their token to the nearest square with the same color as the one to which the spinner pointed, and that the first player to reach the end would win. The experimenter also told children to say the numbers (colors) on the spaces through which they moved. Thus, children in the number board group who were on a 3 and spun a 2 would say, "4, 5" as they moved their token. Children in the color board group who were on green and spun a "blue" would say "purple, blue." If a child erred or could not name the numbers or colors, the experimenter correctly named them and then had the child repeat the names while moving the token.

The preschoolers played the number game or the color game about 20 times over four 15- to 20-min sessions within a two-week period; each game lasted about 3 min. At the beginning of Session 1 and at the end of Session 4, children were presented the 0–10 number line estimation task as a pretest and post-test.

Playing the number board game led to dramatic improvements in the low-income preschoolers' number line estimates. On the pretest, the best-fitting linear function accounted for 15% of the variance in individual children's estimates; on the post-test, it accounted for 61%. In contrast, for children in the color board game condition, the best fitting linear function accounted for 18% of the variance on both pretest and post-test. Thus, playing the number board game for four 15- to 20-min sessions over a two-week period produced substantial improvements in low-income children's number line estimation.

GENERALITY OF LEARNING ACROSS TASKS AND TIME

We [28] tested the generality of the benefits of playing the number board game, both in terms of the range of numerical knowledge that children acquire and in terms of the stability of learning over time. Effects of playing the number and color board games on understanding of the numbers one to 10 were compared on four tasks: number line estimation, magnitude comparison ("Which is bigger: N or M"), numeral identification ("Read the number on this card"), and counting ("Count from 1 to 10"). Playing the number board game was expected to produce gains on the magnitude comparison task for the same reason as on the number line task—improved understanding of numerical magnitudes. Playing this game also was expected to improve counting and numeral identification, because it provides practice and feedback on those skills too. Performance on the four tasks was assessed not only on a pretest and immediate post-test but also on a follow-up nine weeks after the final game playing session. The participants were four- and five-year-olds from Head Start centers, slightly more than half of them African American.

As in the previous study, accuracy of number line estimation increased from pretest to post-test among children who played the number board game. Gains remained present on the nine-week follow-up. In contrast, there was no change in the accuracy of estimates of children who played the color board game. The same pattern was evident on all four numerical tasks (Fig. 21.4). In all cases, preschoolers who played the number board game showed improvements that persisted over time, whereas peers who played the color board game showed neither immediate nor delayed improvements.

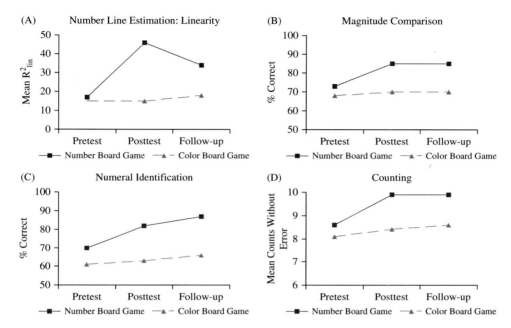

FIGURE 21.4   Performance of preschoolers from low-income backgrounds on (A) number line estimation: linearity, (B) magnitude comparison, (C) numerical identification, and (D) counting [28]. The graphs show performance on the four numerical tasks before playing the number or color board game (pretest), immediately after the fourth and final session of playing the game (post-test), and nine weeks after the final game playing session (follow-up).

The linear numerical board game is not the only focused intervention aimed at improving the numerical magnitude understanding of preschoolers from low-income backgrounds that has yielded encouraging results. A software program known as "The Number Race" [29–31] has also yielded promising findings, in this case with French preschoolers from low-income backgrounds. The focus of this program is on improving number sense access, defined as linking nonverbal number sense to symbolic representations of numbers. The construct of number sense access is similar to the present construct of translations between alternative quantitative representations. The Number Race involved adaptive computer software designed to help children compare numerical magnitudes, link symbolic and non-symbolic representations of number, and increase understanding of and skill in arithmetic. The Number Race produced gains in numerical magnitude comparison performance and a cross-format matching task that measured understanding of numerical magnitudes, though not arithmetic skill.

GAME PLAYING IN THE EVERYDAY ENVIRONMENT

The results with numerical board games raised the question of what role in numerical development, if any, board games occupy in the everyday environment. To address this issue, we obtained self-reports about preschoolers' experiences with board games, card games, and video games [28]. The self-reports were obtained from the preschoolers from low-income backgrounds who participated in the experiment described in the last section, and from age peers from middle-income backgrounds. We hypothesized that children from middle-income backgrounds would have greater experience with board games and that a child's amount of experience playing board games would correlate positively with that child's numerical knowledge.

The data were consistent with both hypotheses. Children from middle-income backgrounds reported twice as much experience with board games as children from low-income backgrounds. Interestingly, children from middle-income backgrounds reported less video game experience than their peers from low-income backgrounds. Within the low-income sample (the only group for which we had numerical proficiency data), the amount of board game experience correlated positively with all four measures of numerical knowledge. Whether preschoolers reported having played Chutes and Ladders, the commercial game that seems closest to the present board game, also correlated positively with their performance on three of the four numerical tasks. In contrast, the amount of experience with video games and with card games correlated with proficiency on only one of the four numerical tasks. Thus, both correlational and causal evidence point to a connection between playing numerical board games and acquiring numerical knowledge.

WHICH FEATURES OF BOARD GAMES INFLUENCE LEARNING?

Experiments designed to identify the critical features of the number board game have allowed tests of the theory that stimulated design of the game and have provided valuable data for future applications. Both physical features of the games and features of game-playing activity have proved important.

The linearity of the game board has proven to be one vital feature. The linear board was predicted to produce greater learning than a circular board, because the mapping between the linear physical board and the desired mental number line is simpler. The greater learning could arise either from a propensity to form a nonverbal mental number line being innate, and providing a framework to which numerical information could be linked, or from a mental number line having already started to form, due to experiences seeing people counting objects in a 1:1 number word:object fashion from left to right.

The prediction that playing the game with a linear board would produce greater learning than playing it with a circular board proved to be correct [32]. The same study demonstrated that playing the linear game, but not the circular one, leads to a higher percentage of correct answers to addition problems and to a higher percentage of errors that are close in magnitude to the correct answer. This finding was anticipated because brain areas activated in addition have been shown to be highly similar to areas activated on tasks that measure analog magnitude representations [33]. The greater impact of playing the game with the linear board on the number line, magnitude comparison, and addition tasks supports the view that playing the linear board game improves children's number sense.

A feature of game-playing activity that has proven important is counting-on from the number where the token starts the turn (as opposed to counting from one). Because children do not automatically encode written numerals before third grade [34], requiring counting-on was hypothesized to be crucial for the children to encode the numbers in the squares, which was believed crucial for them to learn the magnitudes of those numbers. The reason was that if children did not encode the symbolically expressed number (e.g., identifying the square with "8" as the "8"-square and the square with "4" as the "4"-square), they would have nothing with which to correlate the spatial, temporal, kinesthetic, and verbal cues. To the extent that identifying the number within each square was crucial to learning, and to the extent that children would not encode the number if they did not have to state the number as part of the counting-on procedure, learning would be reduced.

We tested this hypothesis by presenting kindergarten children with a 10×10 game board displaying the numbers 1–100. As predicted, kindergartners who were required to count-on by saying the numbers in the squares (e.g., "36, 37") learned much more about numerical magnitudes than children required to count "1, 2" in the same situation [35]. Both their number line estimation and their magnitude comparison improved. In addition, they were able to more accurately estimate the locations of numbers on the game board, thus demonstrating that the counting-on procedure led to better encoding of the numbers' positions on the board, which was hypothesized to be essential for learning about numerical magnitudes through playing the board game.

EFFECTS OF OTHER PRESCHOOL MATHEMATICS INTERVENTIONS

Over the years, many large-scale interventions designed to improve the mathematical skills of low-income preschoolers have been implemented. Like the board game interventions emphasized in this chapter, these multifaceted interventions show that with proper support, children from low-income backgrounds can improve their mathematical knowledge considerably. Below we review three of the interventions that have received the most convincing empirical support: Number Worlds (e.g., [36]), Building Blocks (e.g., [8]), and Pre-K Mathematics (e.g., [3]).

Number Worlds (formerly known as Rightstart) focuses on teaching children the underlying concept of number before moving on to formal addition and subtraction. As such, the program ensures that children have a good conceptualization of addition, subtraction, and numerical magnitudes using real objects (e.g., four pegs) before introducing more symbolic representations (e.g., the numeral 4). The curriculum includes a wide range of numerical activities: songs about numbers, counting games, games involving money, board games somewhat similar to the one that we have used, and so on. Within the curriculum, children spend approximately 20 min per day involved in mathematical activities.

Number Worlds has proven very successful in increasing children's numerical knowledge; after 40 sessions, 87% of low-income kindergarteners passed a test of basic numerical skills that was passed by only 25% of peers who did not receive the curriculum [37,38]. The children remained more advanced at the end of first grade (despite only receiving the intervention during kindergarten) and their first grade teachers rated them as having better number sense than other children from similar backgrounds.

The second curriculum, Building Blocks, features small- and whole-group activities, computer games and family activities designed for home use [8,39]. The curriculum focuses on varied aspects of mathematics including number, patterns, and geometry. Children spend at least 1 h focused on math each week for 26 weeks.

In a large randomized trial, 35 lower- and middle-class preschool classrooms were chosen to present the Building Blocks curriculum, another math-focused curriculum, or the curriculum used the previous year. Children who received the Building Blocks curriculum improved their math skills more than children who received the previous year's curriculum or the comparison curriculum.

A third broad preschool mathematics curriculum, Pre-K Mathematics, also combines school-based and home-based activities [3,40]. Children participate in small-group activities for 20 min twice a week throughout the school year. Parents are provided with home activities that link to the small-group activities in the school and include hands-on manipulatives along with instructions on how to perform each activity. Children from impoverished backgrounds who participated in the Pre-K Mathematics intervention showed equivalent mathematical knowledge on the post-test to middle-income children who did not participate [3].

While they are effective, these interventions are very costly, in terms of both time and resources. In addition to the money that preschools have to spend to purchase the curriculum, there is also substantial cost in terms of teacher training. For Number Worlds, teachers who implemented the curriculum received assistance from the researchers twice a week throughout the school year. For Building Blocks, teachers received 34 h of group training and 16 h of in-class coaching. For Pre-K Mathematics, teachers participated in eight days of workshops over the course of the school year, along with on-site training at least once per month. There is good reason for this extensive teacher training: without substantial and prolonged guidance, teachers often modify the curricula in ways that make it less effective [41,42].

CONCLUSIONS

The high costs of large-scale curricula were part of what motivated us to apply theoretical understanding of cognitive development, in particular findings regarding the centrality of the mental number line to mathematical understanding, to devise a focused intervention. In addition to providing information about the effectiveness of the particular intervention, this approach yielded two other types of valuable information: knowledge useful for deepening theoretical understanding of numerical magnitude representations, and knowledge useful for improving large scale interventions aimed at helping preschoolers gain numerical understanding.

Consider some of the lessons regarding acquisition of numerical magnitude representations. Some of the main conclusions are that one source of acquisition of linear representations of numerical magnitudes is playing linear numerical board games, that improved numerical magnitude representations also lead to improved ability to learn answers to arithmetic problems, and that playing linear number board games produce greater learning of both numerical magnitudes and arithmetic than playing circular ones. The results also support the view that experience that allows children to correlate symbolically expressed numbers with redundant nonverbal cues to the magnitudes associated with those symbols is crucial to the process of learning mathematics.

The lessons learned from the focused interventions also can, and we believe should, be incorporated into large-scale curricula that are aimed at improving the mathematical understanding of preschoolers from low-income backgrounds. Including games like the present ones might improve the effectiveness of the large-scale curricula; including them might also make it possible for the large-scale curricula to produce gains more quickly.

The success of focused interventions such as the one emphasized in this chapter raises the question of why such brief interventions can produce such great improvements in the mathematical knowledge of preschoolers from low-income families. One likely reason is that many of these children have had few explicitly mathematical experiences prior to the interventions. Systematic observations of home and preschool environments of young children from low-income backgrounds indicate that neither environment typically provides many experiences where the children's attention is directed to numbers [10,43]. For many children, the experience with numerical magnitudes that they receive even in the relatively brief interventions may constitute a substantial percentage of their experience connecting symbolically expressed numbers to their non-symbolic equivalents and relating symbolically expressed numbers to each other. Because of these children's limited numerical experience, because early differences in mathematical understanding tend to persist throughout schooling, and because of the large, broad, and rapid effects of early interventions that are grounded in cognitive and developmental theories and data, increasing the number of preschoolers who receive such interventions seems a goal worth pursuing.

References

[1] Organization for Economic Cooperation and Development (OECD) and Statistics Canada, Literacy, Economy, and Society: Results of the first International Adult Literacy Survey, OECD, Paris, 1995. (Ottawa: Ministry of Industry Canada).
[2] N.C. Jordan, D. Kaplan, L.N. Olah, M.N. Locuniak, Number sense growth in kindergarten: A longitudinal investigation of children at risk for mathematics difficulties, Child Dev. 77 (2006) 153–175.
[3] P. Starkey, A. Klein, A. Wakeley, Enhancing young children's mathematical knowledge through a pre-kindergarten mathematics intervention, Early Child. Res. Q. 19 (2004) 99–120.
[4] G.J. Duncan, et al., School readiness and later achievement, Dev. Psychol. 43 (2007) 1428–1446.
[5] G.J. Duncan, K. Magnusen, The nature and impact of early achievement skills, attention and behavior problems: Paper Presented at the Conference, in Rethinking the Role of Neighborhoods and Families on Schools and School Outcomes for American Children, Brookings Project On Social Inequality And Educational Disadvantage, Washington, DC, 2009, November.
[6] H.W. Stevenson, R.S. Newman, Long-term prediction of achievement and attitudes in mathematics and reading, Child Dev. 57 (1986) 646–659.
[7] E.A. Hanushek, S.G. Rivkin, School Quality and the Black–White Achievement Gap, National Bureau of Economic Research, Inc. (NBER Working Papers, 12651)
[8] D.H. Clements, J. Sarama, Effects of a preschool mathematics curriculum: summative research on the Building Blocks project, J. Res. Math. Educ. 38 (2007) 136–163.
[9] B. Blevins-Knabe, L. Musun-Miller, Number use at home by children and their parents and its relationship to early mathematical performance, Early Dev. Parenting 5 (1996) 35–45.
[10] J. Tudge, F. Doucet, Early mathematical experiences: observing young Black and White children's everyday activities, Early Child. Res. Q. 19 (2004) 21–39.
[11] S. Dehaene, The Number Sense: How the Mind Creates Mathematics., Oxford University Press, NY, 1997.
[12] National Council of Teachers of Mathematics (NCTM), Curriculum Focal Points for Prekindergarten Through Grade 8 Mathematics, National Council of Teachers of Mathematics, Washington, DC, 2006. (Pdf available at http://www.nctm.org/focalpoints/down-loads.asp).
[13] National Mathematics Advisory Panel (NMAP), Foundations for Success: The Final Report of the National Mathematics Advisory Panel, U.S. Department of Education, Washington, DC, 2008.
[14] R.S. Siegler, J.L. Booth, Development of numerical estimation: a review, in: J.I.D. Campbell (Ed.), Handbook of Mathematical Cognition, CRC Press, Boca Ratan, FL, 2005, pp. 197–212.
[15] M.D. de Havia, E.S. Spelke, Number–space mapping in human infants, Psychol. Sci. 21 (2010) 653–660.
[16] S.F. Lourenco, M.R. Longo, General magnitude represenation in human infants, Psychol. Sci. 21 (6) (2010) 873–881.

[17] S. Dehaene, S. Bossini, P. Giraux, The mental representation of parity and number magnitude, J. Exp. Psychol. Gen. 122 (1993) 371–396.

[18] M. Zorzi, K. Priftis, C. Umiltà, Neglect disrupts the mental number line, Nature 417 (2002) 138.

[19] D. Ansari, Effects of development and enculturation on number representation in the brain, Nat. Rev. Neurosci. 9 (2008) 278–291.

[20] E.M. Hubbard, et al., Interactions between number and space in parietal cortex, Nat. Rev. Neurosci. 6 (2005) 435–448.

[21] J.L. Booth, R.S. Siegler, Developmental and individual differences in pure numerical estimation, Dev. Psychol. 42 (1) (2006) 189–201.

[22] J.L. Booth, R.S. Siegler, Numerical magnitude representations influence arithmetic learning, Child Dev. 79 (4) (2008) 1016–1031.

[23] M. Le Corre, S. Carey, One, two, three, four, nothing more: an investigation of the conceptual sources of the verbal counting principles, Cognition 105 (2007) 395–438.

[24] C.A. Thompson, J.E. Opfer, Costs and benefits of representational change: effects of context on age and sex differences in symbolic magnitude estimation, J. Exp. Child Psychol. 101 (1) (2008) 20–51.

[25] M. Schneider, et al., A validation of eye movements as a measure of elementary school children's developing number sense, Cogn. Dev. 23 (3) (2008) 409–422.

[26] E.V. Laski, R.S. Siegler, Is 27 a big number? Correlational and causal connections among numerical categorization, number line estimation, and numerical magnitude comparison, Child Dev. 78 (6) (2007) 1723–1743.

[27] R.S. Siegler, G.B. Ramani, Playing linear numerical board games promotes low-income children's numerical development, Dev. Sci. 11 (5) (2008) 655–661.

[28] G.B. Ramani, R.S. Siegler, Promoting broad and stable improvements in low-income children's numerical knowledge through playing number board games, Child Dev. 79 (2) (2008) 375–394.

[29] A.J. Wilson, et al., Effects of an adaptive game intervention on accessing number sense in low-socioeconomic-status kindergarten children, Mind Brain Educ. 3 (4) (2009) 224–234.

[30] A.J. Wilson, et al., Principles underlying the design of "The Number Race", an adaptive computer game for remediation of dyscalculia, Behav. Brain Funct. 2 (1) (2006) 19.

[31] A.J. Wilson, et al., An open trial assessment of "The Number Race", an adaptive computer game for remediation of dyscalculia, Behav. Brain Funct. 2 (1) (2006) 20.

[32] R.S. Siegler, G.B. Ramani, Playing linear number board games—but not circular ones—improves low-income preschoolers' numerical understanding, J. Educ. Psychol. 101 (3) (2009) 545–560.

[33] L. Cohen, et al., Language and calculation within the parietal lobe: a combined cognitive, anatomical and fMRI study, Neuropsychologia 38 (2000) 1426–1440.

[34] D.B. Berch, et al., Extracting parity and magnitude from Arabic numerals: developmental changes in number processing and mental representation, J. Exp. Child Psychol. 74 (1999) 286–308.

[35] E.V. Laski, R.S. Siegler, Making board games even better, J. Educ. Psychol. (in press).

[36] S. Griffin, Number worlds: a research-based mathematics program for young children, in: D.H. Clements, J. Sarama, (Eds.), Engaging Young Children in Mathematics: Standards for Early Mathematics Education, Erlbaum, Mahwah, NJ, 2004, pp. 325–342.

[37] S. Griffin, R. Case, R.S. Siegler, Rightstart: providing the central conceptual prerequisites for first formal learning of arithmetic to students at risk for school failure, in: K. McGilly, (Ed.), Classroom Lessons: Integrating Cognitive Theory and Classroom Practice, MIT Press, Cambridge, MA, 1994, pp. 25–49.

[38] S. Griffin, R. Case, Evaluating the breadth and depth of training effects when central conceptual structures are taught, Monogr. Soc. Res. Child Dev. 59 (1996) 90–113.

[39] D.H. Clements, J. Sarama, Experimental evaluation of the effects of a research-based preschool mathematics curriculum, Am. Educ. Res. J. 45 (2008) 443–494.

[40] P. Starkey, A. Klein, Fostering parental support for children's mathematical development: an intervention with Head Start families, Early Educ. Dev. 11 (2000) 659–680.

[41] S. Griffin, Number Worlds: A Mathematics Intervention Program From Grade Prek-6, SRA/McGraw–Hill, Columbus, OH, 2007.

[42] S. Griffin, R. Case, Rethinking the primary school math curriculum: an approach based on cognitive science, Issues Educ. 3 (1999) 1–49.

[43] I. Plewis, A. Mooney, R. Creeser, Time on educational activities at home and education progress in infant school, Brit. J. Educ. Psychol. 60 (1990) 330–337.

[44] R.S. Siegler, J.L. Booth, Development of numerical estimation in young children, Child Dev. 75 (2) (2004) 428–444.

[45] R.S. Siegler, Improving the numerical understanding of children from low-income families, Child Dev. Perspect. 3 (2) (2009) 118–124.

Index

Printed in the United States
By Bookmasters